BRAIN DAMAGE – BRIDGING BETWEEN BASIC RESEARCH AND CLINICS

Edited by **Alina González-Quevedo**

Brain Damage – Bridging Between Basic Research and Clinics
Edited by Alina González-Quevedo

Published by InTech
Janeza Trdine 9, 51000 Rijeka, Croatia

Publishing Process Manager Marina Jozipovic

Technical Editor Teodora Smiljanic

Cover Designer InTech Design Team

Additional hard copies can be obtained from orders@intechopen.com

Brain Damage – Bridging Between Basic Research and Clinics,
Edited by Alina González-Quevedo
p. cm.
ISBN 978-953-51-0375-2

Meet the editor

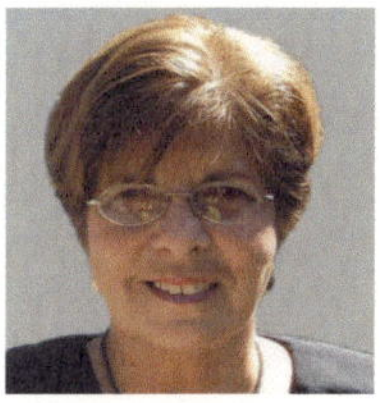

Dr Alina González-Quevedo, MD, PhD graduated from Medical School at the University of Havana in 1972 and has had specialization in Clinical Biochemistry since 1977. She worked as a Full Professor of Biochemistry at the Medical University of Havana and Senior Researcher at the Institute of Neurology and Neurosurgery, where she occupied the posts of Head of the Department of Neurochemistry (1977-2009) and Assistant Director for Research (1995-2010). Her doctoral thesis was in the pathophysiological mechanisms of Cuban Epidemic Optic Neuropathy in collaboration with the Venezuelan Institute for Scientific Research. She has also worked in other research areas such as brain barrier systems, demyelinating diseases, blood and CSF protein markers in essential hypertension and stroke, and has published more than 100 scientific papers in peer reviewed journals.

Contents

Preface

Brain damage or brain injury are very ample terms which include the destruction or degeneration of brain cells as a consequence of a wide range of internal and external factors, resulting from acute events (stroke, epilepsy or head injury) or by chronic degeneration as in Alzheimer's and Parkinson's Disease. Nevertheless, although the primary insult leading to brain damage can be distinctly different, the mechanisms underlying the death of neurons and glial cells in the brain have many common interrelated pathways (hypoxia, oxidative damage, excitotoxicity, and inflammation, among others). It should also be taken into account that when brain tissue is damaged, cells often continue to die after the initial stimulus has stopped. Thus, understanding the pathophysiological mechanisms of brain damage in different pathological settings is crucial not only to mitigate the effect of the primary insult on the brain, but also to find a way of stopping this cascade of cell death.

"Brain damage- bridging between basic research and clinics" is a book that provides an insight into this very broad area of research, focusing on topics that deal with some of the main problems confronted by modern neurosciences, spanning through neurodevelopmental and neurodegenerative disorders, changes observed in drug addictions and sleep deprivation, as well as early assessment of brain injury for preventive strategies employing sensitive biomarkers.

The first chapter deals with the etiology and evolution of fetal brain damage, reviewing the main and varied causes leading to it: genetic anomalies, nutritional deficiencies, environmental factors (alcohol, addictive drugs, and nicotine among others), prematurity, maternal illness during pregnancy, fetal inflammatory response syndrome and hypoxia. Hypoxia is central to the genesis of a significant proportion of brain injury occurring in the fetus, which gives way to a spectrum of long term brain morbidity ranging from mild motor and cognitive defects to cerebral palsy and severe cognitive disabilities. Prevention and management of fetal brain injury are topics also considered in some detail.

Cerebral palsy (CP), one of the most devastating consequences of fetal or perinatal brain injury - with a high cost to the child, the family and society -is considered in Chapter 2. Despite the technological advances that have decreased mortality in term and preterm infants, the worldwide prevalence of CP is 1.5 to 2.0 cases per 1000 births, a rate that has remained constant for nearly 40 years.

Chapter 3 deals with the toll of inborn errors of metabolism on the brain, through the experience accumulated in South India. Many body systems are affected in these disorders, but the predominant damage will be to the central nervous system (CNS). Conducting metabolic screening to diagnose and treat them early in life is of utmost importance in order to avoid irreversible damage to the brain.

As the average life span has been extended by the fast growing medical technologies, the elderly population is increasing rapidly, and with it the prevalence of age-related neurodegenerative diseases. In the following 5 chapters, mechanisms through which brain damage occurs in different neurological conditions are evaluated.

First of all, the importance of detecting subclinical target organ damage to the brain in essential hypertension is highlighted in chapter 4, as it is known to be the most important risk factor for developing stroke and vascular dementia.

Chapter 5 reviews the current understanding of the etiology and pathogenesis of Alzheimer´s Disease (AD) and Parkinson´s Disease (PD), with an emphasis on protein abnormalities and particular vulnerability of the nigral dopaminergic neurons, and the efforts that are being made for the development of disease-modifying therapies.

In chapter 6 the way in which nitrooxidative stress can contribute to major neurodegenerative diseases – such as AD, PD and glaucoma – is considered, as well as the rationales and precautions that should be evaluated when designing antioxidant therapies.

Another aspect of neurodegeneration is evaluated in chapter 7, where acute injury to the CNS – including stroke and traumatic brain and spinal cord injury – is shown to activate a neurodegenerative process whose effects are time-dependent and related to the initial severity of the primary insult.

Accumulating evidence implicates protein misfolding and aggregation as a likely common underlying cause for protein conformational disorders which include AD, PD, Huntington's disease, polyglutamine disorders, amyotrophic lateral sclerosis, and the transmissible spongiform encephalopathies or prion diseases. Chapter 8 focuses on human prion disorders, their history, etiology, symptoms, and the therapeutic strategies tried so far. The unusual properties of prion propagation have presented challenges to researchers seeking to understandthe pathogenic mechanisms of these diseases.

Chapter 9 is aimed to provide evidence on the impact of abusing drugs on cognitive functions. The author shows that most drugs of abuse can induce adverse effects which seem to impact brain circuits linked to important aspects of cognition, such as memory and learning, attention, risk taking, motivation, mood and wanting. Possible approaches to deal with this drug-induced damage from the pharmacological point of view are also discussed.

In the line of neuroprotection, it has been suggested that sleep preserves the brain in optimal conditions to support the damage occurred in different situations throughout the day (Chapter 10), possibly improving antioxidant systems, maintaining cellular integrity through the synthesis of molecules involved in cellular structures or in cellular cycle regulation, as well as improving synaptic efficiency. In this chapter the main studies that demonstrate the role of sleep on brain restoration are summarized.

Chapter 11 presents an updated view of dynamic-brain-monitoring in the intensive care unit and the author´s personal experience in this field. Very interesting results are presented in relation to the importance of quantifying brain damage in order to give more objective information for decision making and evaluating the outcome of patients.

Finally the last chapter is dedicated to carotid endarterectomy, a surgical procedure conducted in patients with pronounced carotid stenosis to prevent brain damage due to total occlusion.

Dr. Alina González-Quevedo
Institute of Neurology and Neurosurgery
La Habana
Cuba

1

The Etiology and Evolution of Fetal Brain Injury

Andrew Macnab[1,2]
[1]*Faculty of Medicine, University of British Columbia, Vancouver,*
[2]*Stellenbosch Institute for Advanced Study (STIAS), Wallenberg Research Centre at Stellenbosch University, Stellenbosch,*
[1]*Canada*
[2]*South Africa*

1. Introduction

The nine months of intrauterine life are a continuum during which a series of situations and events can occur that result in abnormalities of normal brain growth or injury to the developing brain of the fetus. Genetic mutations and hereditary syndromes can predispose the fetus to intrauterine death, mortality in early life, and various degrees and combinations of brain injury and neurological deficits. Structural brain injury occurs due to a number of well defined and some relatively obscure causes. Premature delivery puts the fetus at risk of complications during birth and in the early days of life that can compromise the brain. Such infants have systems that are physiologically too immature to function normally, making them dependent on a range of care entities many of which are known to have risks associated with their use. The end result especially when prematurity is of extreme degree, is a significant incidence of cognitive and motor deficits. Maternal infection is increasingly recognized to precipitate premature labour and produce inflammatory by-products that cross the placenta and increase the vulnerability of the fetus to brain injury. (Gotsch et al, 2007; Kendall & Peebles 2005; Mercer 2004) Various pathologies related to the placenta also compromise the well being of the fetus. Impaired fetal growth secondary to placental insufficiency is associated with a reduction in the number of brain cells formed by the time the infant is born; growth retarded infants are at increased risk of hypoxic stress and hypoxic ischemic brain injury due to failure of placental blood flow, gas exchange and fetal oxygen delivery. Suboptimal nutrition also poses the risk of hypoglycaemic brain injury immediately after birth. Post mature infants are at risk from placental failure, hypoxic ischaemic injury and birth trauma. Infants conceived with in-vitro fertilization are at increased risk of neurological disability, especially cerebral palsy. (Stromberg et al 2002) Stroke is a significant cause of neurodevelopmental morbidity in newborn infants that can result in permanent sequelae and may be underreported. (Ozduman et al 2004) The overall incidence of cerebral palsy has not been reduced significantly in spite of advances in obstetric care, and CP remains a significant cause for motor deficits and cognitive disability that become evident in early life and result in permanent disability.

Hypoxia is central to the genesis of a significant proportion of the brain injury that occurs in the fetus. Compromised oxygen delivery is a particular risk factor during labour and delivery, but the fetus is at risk of brain injury whenever cerebral ischemia occurs as a consequence of impaired cerebral blood flow. After hypoxic ischaemic injury, reperfusion of the brain and any situations that further compromise normal perfusion, oxygen and carbon dioxide transport, or the supply of metabolites required for normal brain function have the potential to complicate recovery, and can also contribute to additional brain injury. (Fellman & Raivio 1997, von Bell et al 1993) Major mechanisms linked to perinatal brain injury are hypoxic ischemic insults and haemorrhagic brain injury in term infants (those born beyond 37 weeks of gestation) and periventricular haemorrhage and white matter injury (leukomalacia) in preterm infants (those born before 37 weeks of gestation).

Hypoxic ischemic brain injury is estimated to occur in 0.5 – 0.75 per thousand deliveries. The pattern and consequences of injury depend on the severity and duration of the insult, the neurovascular and anatomical maturity of the brain which is primarily a factor related to the gestational age of the fetus, and co-related factors such as the presence or absence of infection, problems with fetal nutrition, or pre-existing abnormalities in brain growth and development. Ferriero (Ferriero 2004) has reviewed the gestation specific vulnerability of different regions of the fetal brain and individual cell lines to damage, and the central role of oxidative stress and excitotoxicity in fetal brain injury.

Infants born very prematurely are at particularly high risk for brain injury as brain development in such infants is so immature that they are vulnerable to fluctuations in brain blood flow and oxygen delivery that are insufficient to generate injury in a more mature fetus. Such fluctuations include variations in cerebral venous pressure, the degree of cerebral vasodilatation and constriction, and the distribution of cerebral blood flow, and also systemic alterations in circulating blood volume, or oxygen and carbon dioxide tension. The periventricular area of the immature preterm brain is particularly prone to injury in such ways. Haemorrhage in this area is a major cause of acute brain injury in premature infants, and the cystic changes that develop in consequence (periventricular leukomalacia – PVL) frequently result in permanent scarring. This form of periventricular haemorrhage can also be sufficiently extensive that it extends into the ventricles, where the presence of blood within the cerebrospinal fluid is irritant, and as a result often generates ventricular dilatation or causes obstructive hydrocephalus. (Volpe 2001a)

In larger premature infants and those born at term brain injury involving the cortex or basal ganglia predominates; (Okereafor et al 2008) watershed damage in the parasagital areas of the brain results from moderate hypoxic ischaemic insults, and brain stem injury when injury is more profound. (Roland et al 1988) The regionalization of injury is dictated by the selective vulnerability of different areas of the brain which depends largely on differences in metabolic demand, compensatory mechanisms that occur in response to hypoxia, the maintenance of normal levels of substrate delivery (particularly oxygen and glucose), and the maturity and type of brain cells undergoing development at the time of injury.

The immediate clinical effects of hypoxia and ischemia result in an infant who is neurologically depressed at birth, requires resuscitation to initiate breathing and sometimes cardiovascular support to stimulate heart function and ensure adequate blood pressure and circulation. Tone and behaviour are abnormal and an encephalopathy develops in the hours or days after birth where neurological abnormalities include problems with level of consciousness, tone, respiratory drive, and coordination of sucking and swallowing, and seizure activity usually occurs. In the longer term the consequences of hypoxic ischemic brain injury vary between death and complete recovery (Perlman & Shah 2001), with the spectrum of long term brain morbidity ranging from mild motor and cognitive defects to cerebral palsy and severe cognitive disabilities.

Importantly many of the causes of fetal brain injury are avoidable and some are amenable to treatment. The evolution of hypoxic ischaemic brain injury for example has two phases over time. Following the initial insult a 'latent' phase follows that is associated with a transient recovery of cerebral energy metabolism, then hours or sometimes days later a second phase occurs where cerebral energy failure and oedema within the brain cells initially injured compounds the degree of injury. (Gunn 2000) The interval between this biphasic response offers a therapeutic window during which interventions aimed at ameliorating the effects of hypoxia and ischemia are being explored.

2. Causal mechanisms for structural defects

Structural development: The structure of the fetal brain evolves throughout intra uterine life. Comprehensive reviews describe the initial proliferation of cells, generation of neurons in the cortical germinal zone, and process of normal brain growth and maturation. (Hatten 2002; Marin & Rubenstein 2003; Larroche et al 1997; Razic 2002) Normal growth involves a continuum that must be appreciated in order to fully understand the causes, evolution, and consequences of brain deficits associated with abnormalities in fetal brain development. Key influences that determine normal structure include genetic, embryonic, nutritional and environmental factors.

Genetic anomalies are the principal cause of fetal loss. (Heffner 2004) In such circumstances brain abnormalities at a macroscopic and microscopic level are commonly evident. Francis et al (Francis et al 2006) have reviewed the history and molecular genetic advances in cortical development disorders, and use microcephaly to explain the complex mechanisms underlying correct development of the human brain. Where a fetus with a genetic anomaly is born alive there may or may not be structural brain involvement. While many genetic mutations are random most are inherited, although some have variable expression. Environmental factors such as radiation or chemical exposure are uncommon but preventable causes, and parental age plays an important part. (Heffner 2004) Conception is less likely as females and males age, with the proportion of sub-optimal ova and unhealthy structurally abnormal sperm increasing exponentially with age, and there is the well recognized association between age and a number of genetic syndromes such as Trisomy 21 (Down syndrome). Infants conceived with the use of assisted reproductive technology are more likely than naturally conceived infants to have multiple major defects including chromosomal and musculoskeletal defects. (Hansen et al 2002) Some racial groups have a predisposition to specific genetic anomalies associated with structural brain abnormalities e.g. the Irish and Welsh to neural tube defects and hydrocephalus respectively.

Genetic counselling is central to diagnosis and prevention in situations where there is a family history of genetic abnormality with brain injury, birth of a prior infant with an anomaly, or predisposition to a genetic problem due to racial or age related factors. Information from autopsy is important after fetal loss, coupled with placental pathology after unexplained stillbirth. An infant born with evidence of brain injury potentially due to a genetic cause requires chromosome studies, placental pathology, and family evaluation in addition to radiological and general and often specific laboratory studies. Prognosis varies; some genetic syndromes are invariably fatal while the spectrum for brain involvement, ability and life expectancy is broad in the remainder, hence the need for identifying the chromosomal anomaly or specific syndrome and making a definite diagnosis wherever possible.

Embryonic development progresses at a rapid pace from the moment first cell division occurs, and a large proportion of the brain's structure is already formed by the time many women become aware that they are pregnant. By the end of the first trimester (3 months of gestation) all the main structures of the central nervous system are formed and it is brain growth that follows between this time and fetal maturity (40 weeks). There is always the potential for a variety of factors to negatively impact normal embryonic development, and in-vitro fertilization (IVF) has known associations with multiple pregnancy, infants of low birth weight, and a spectrum of anomalies. (Berg et al 1999, Stromberg et al 2002)

Nutritional deficiencies can negatively impact brain growth, as exemplified by the key role of periconceptual administration of folic acid in the prevention of defective neuropore closure. (Hagberg & Mallard 2000) This central role in reproductive health, normal neurological system structure, and brain function is underscored by the evolutionary adaptation of skin colour in humans to facilitate folate synthesis. When humankind's African ancestors migrated to less sunny climes, a progressive reduction in skin pigmentation became essential in order for effective folate (and vitamin D) metabolism to occur, as exposure to sunlight and transmission of ultraviolet light through the skin is required for the effective production of both folate and vitamin D. (Jablonski 2006). Dietary intake is also relevant but optimal folate levels for normal fetal neural development are difficult to achieve, especially for sub-populations at particular risk of structural anomalies. Hence, for prevention, the majority of pregnant mothers can benefit from folic acid supplementation, as evidenced by the fall in neural tube defects in populations where food items are now supplemented. Rodent models also provide convincing evidence that iron deficiency alters metabolism and neurotransmission in major brain structures, such as the basal ganglia and hippocampus, and disrupts myelination brain wide. (Lotzoff & Georgieff 2006) While evidence for the same issues affecting the human fetus is less clear, even the possibility combined with the high worldwide incidence of iron deficiency in pregnancy makes iron supplementation logical to reduce the impact of this wholly preventable form of brain pathology.

Environmental factors relevant as a mechanism for brain damage range in severity due to the high toxicity of some agents, e.g. cocaine, the effect of dosage and cumulative exposure in others such as alcohol, and the frequency of fetal exposure to agents such as nicotine in mothers who smoke. Gestational age plays a role principally in that the fetal brain is most vulnerable during the early stages of structural development. The impact of environmental factors can be multi-factorial with exposure to multiple agents increasing the risk of brain damage, and in some situations a genetic predisposition to the toxic effect of individual agents is evident e.g. related to alcohol.

Perhaps the best known association is between fetal exposure to alcohol and the Fetal Abnormality Spectrum Disorder (FASD). Heavy prenatal alcohol exposure can have serious and long-lasting effects on the developing fetal brain, that severely affect the physical and neurobehavioral development of a child. Autopsy and brain imaging studies indicate reductions and abnormalities in overall brain size and shape, specifically in structures such as the cerebellum, basal ganglia, and corpus callosum. A wide range of neuropsychological deficits have been found in children prenatally exposed to alcohol, including deficits in visulospatial functioning, verbal and nonverbal learning, attention, and executive functioning. These children also exhibit a variety of behavioural problems that can further affect their daily functioning. (Riley & McGee 2005).

The potential for adverse effects on the fetal brain from maternal drug use is exemplified by the effect of cocaine; use of the drug during pregnancy causes structural brain defects; increases the incidence of low birth weight with its attendant risks; and multiple functional deficits manifest once the child is born, some of which persist as learning difficulty into adult life. Sometimes infants exposed to cocaine in utero have ultrasound evidence of cyst formation in the frontal lobes of the brain, basal ganglia, posterior fossa, germinal matrix and septum pellucidum. These are particularly likely following drug use in the first trimester, and probably represent focal necrosis caused by complex vasoconstrictive effects of the cocaine. (Dow-Edwards 1991) This vulnerability of the fetal brain to damage in the first trimester is not unique to cocaine; many drugs and chemical agents cause structural anomalies as this is the time when key structures are being formed.

Maternal smoking increases the risk of an infant being of low birth weight (LBW) two fold; is responsible for 20% to 30% of all LBW infants; and causes such infants to weigh 150-250 g less on average than those born to non-smoking mothers. The adverse fetal effects of smoking are generated through several pathways. Placental function is impaired by vasoconstrictive cigarette smoke metabolites; these can reduce uterine blood flow by up to 38% depriving the fetus of both oxygen and nutrients. The episodic hypoxia and malnutrition that results underlie the intrauterine growth retardation that occurs in many infants born to smoking mothers. Nicotine is also a fetal neuroteratogen that targets nicotinic acetylcholine receptors in the fetal brain. Changes in cell proliferation and differentiation occur, synaptic activity develops abnormally, and cell loss and neuronal damage occurs. Even in mothers who do not smoke enough for their infants to be of low birth weight, the nicotine levels to which their fetus is exposed are high enough to produce deficits in fetal brain development (Law et al 2003)

Evaluation of structural brain damage: This is a process that combines relevant elements of the infant and maternal medical and family history, physical examination findings, and laboratory and radiological investigations, including: the infant's condition at birth (requirements for resuscitation, APGAR score, and neurological status); general appearance (appropriateness of growth for gestational age, weight, head circumference, and length, and presence of associated defects): neurological status (especially tone, cry, ability to feed, and seizure activity); fetal sonography and MRI; post-natal ultrasound and neuroradiological studies (CT scan MRI); electroencephalogram; chromosome studies; and consultation with medical specialists such as a neonatologist, geneticist and neurologist.

3. Predisposing factors for fetal brain injury

Prematurity: Brain injury in the premature infant is an extremely important problem, in part because of the large absolute number of infants affected yearly. (Volpe 1997) Considerable research documents that children born very prematurely (<32 weeks gestation) and or/extremely low birth weight (<1000 g) are at increased risk for neurobehavioral impairments (cerebral palsy, blindness, deafness), lower general intelligence, specific cognitive defects, learning disabilities, and behavioural and emotional problems. Also that the survival rate for extremely preterm infants (<26 weeks gestation or with a birth weight of <750 g) is approximately 50% but that 40% of survivors do not escape significant deficits. (Anderson & Doyle 2008) Modern neonatal care entities now enable 75-90% of preterm infants weighing < 1500g at birth to survive in Europe and the USA; however 5-10% of survivors exhibit cerebral palsy and many have cognitive, behavioural, attention-related or socialization deficits. (Halopainen & Lauren 2011)

The two principal brain lesions that underlie the neurological manifestations observed in premature infants are periventricular hemorrhagic infarction and periventricular leukomalacia. (Volpe 2001a) In the animal model relatively brief periods of hypoxaemic compromise appear to be more profound in the less mature brain in mid rather than late gestation, when they have significant effects on the fetal brain causing death of susceptible neuronal populations (cerebellum, hippocampus, and cortex) and cerebral white matter damage. (Rees & Inder 2005) Cerebellar injury is also increasingly recognized (Limperopoulos et al 2009)

Very premature infants are prone to these lesions because the structural anatomy and neurovascular immaturity of their brains predisposes them to injury from hypoxia (inadequate oxygenation) and ischemia (inadequate blood flow) which predispose them to cerebral haemorrhage. The immature brain lacks the duplication of blood supply that develops as a fetus matures and the ability to auto-regulate cerebral blood flow in response to changes in systemic blood pressure. Areas of the brain such as the germinal matrix have vascular complexes that are vulnerable to bleeding when blood pressure fluctuates. Such haemorrhage is common related to asphyxial stress and results in a pattern of injury unique to the preterm infant. In this context, prematurity is certainly the major causal factor of cerebral palsy. However, the literature also indicates that the odds of brain injury become much greater in the fetus in the presence of maternal fever, and from the effects of inflammation, or proven infection, than when the only risk factor is prematurity. (Rees & Inder 2005)

Premature and low birth weight infants are known to be at increased risk of brain injury as a consequence of intrauterine infection when microglial activation triggers excitotoxic, inflammatory and oxidative damage, (Malaeb & Dammann 2009) and of developing infections during the newborn period. Their postnatal vulnerability is because they are compromised in terms of how quickly and how effectively they can mount an immune response. This is in large part because bacterial colonization of the gut after birth is essential for digestive function, and for production of vitamin K, an essential component of the clotting mechanism without which haemorrhagic disease of the newborn can develop. This bleeding tendency can involve intracranial bleeds of sufficient severity to cause brain damage and even death. As an additional precaution, newborns are routinely given this vitamin prophylacticaly after birth. Risk factors for neonatal sepsis include prolonged rupture of membranes (beyond 18 hours the risk of infection increases 10 fold, and the occurrence of perinatal asphyxia adds additional risk); and maternal colonization with group B Streptococcus and urinary tract infection (Gerdes 2004). Prophylactic antibiotics are used in anticipation of sepsis as by the time confirmatory tests (bacterial cultures) are positive the risks of increased morbidity or mortality rises. This is due in large part to the risk of dissemination of infection e.g. to the brain and meninges causing meningitis, or because of the greater levels of toxic metabolites released when the higher counts of bacteria present as a consequence of treatment being delayed are killed by therapy.

Brain injury in premature infants as a consequence of periventricular haemorrhagic infarction and periventricular leukomalacia may be preventable. Logical approaches would include measures to prevent germinal matrix-intraventricular hemorrhage, prevent or manage impairments of cerebrovascular autoregulation and cerebral blood flow, and the use of agents such as free radical scavengers to interrupt the cascade to oligodendroglial cell death. (Volpe 2001b). Importantly, the consequences of being born prematurely also predispose infants born following fetal brain injury to additional compounding stresses and insults in the newborn period; such events also pose a threat of increased morbidity and long term neurological compromise to those who have intact brains at birth. Hence the high overall risk of motor, cognitive, and educational defects in those that survive being born prematurely. (Rees & Inder 2005, Anderson & Doyle 2008)

Low birth weight (LBW) infants are those born weighing <2500 g. LBW infants comprise both those born prematurely but appropriately grown for gestational age and those who are small because of intrauterine growth retardation. LBW infants accounts for 7.6% of all live born infants and 65% of deaths in the United States occur among LBW infants due to multiple risk factors related to the underlying cause of their small size. In most instances intrapartum morbidity is higher amongst this group, and many are also at risk during the newborn period. Brain injury in a fetus of LBW is potentially caused by many factors; where placental dysfunction is the underlying cause, acute problems may compromise placental gas exchange and precipitate fetal hypoxic ischemic stress.

Small for gestational age (SGA) infants are those with intrauterine growth retardation who when born are below the 10th centile for weight; where length and head circumference are also similarly compromised, such infants are known as symmetrically growth retarded and brain size and function are usually adversely affected. Long term deficits in neural connectivity are described (Rees & Inder 2005) and cognitive problems are common in surviving infants. SGA infants have no glycogen stores in their liver at birth and are hence prone to hypoglycaemia that can compound pre-existing fetal brain injury. In utero maternal blood glucose levels determine fetal levels, and, in addition, the fetal brain is able to metabolize lactate as an alternative energy source. However, this pathway is down regulated after birth once oral feeding begins. As a group, surviving SGA infants are at particular risk in adult life of developing cardiovascular disease, hypertension and stroke.

Maternal Illness during pregnancy poses a risk for fetal brain injury. Many are specific to pregnancy such a pre-eclamptic toxaemia, but others pre-exist prior to pregnancy and of themselves, or because of treatment they require, have the potential to cause damage, or predispose the fetus to situations such as prematurity or low birth weight that carry independent risks for neurological morbidity. Examples that pose clear risks for the fetal brain and neurological system are anticonvulsant medications and cancer therapies (Halopainen & Lauren 2011). But, while there is general recognition that any medication should be considered carefully in the context of pregnancy and wherever possible be discontinued, in some instances the wellbeing of the mother has to be weighed against the potential for risk to the fetus. However, not infrequently drugs in common use that are initially identified as problematic sometimes only come to be recognized in their true context after some years of use and appropriately rigorous research and review.

A case in point relates to selective serotonin reuptake inhibitor (SSRI) use during pregnancy and the effects of these agents on the fetus and newborn infant. Serotonin is a neurotransmitter that appears very early in fetal life and has a broad role in brain morphogenesis. Studies to evaluate the neurotoxicity of SSRI's identified a number of age-specific and site-specific effects in the fetal rat brain, especially related to the limbic system (Lattimore et al 2005). Subsequently a number of adverse effects were identified to occur in human newborns, and there was a clear association with low birth weight (Oberlander et al 2006), the need for special care in the newborn period, and an apparent increase in the incidence of prematurity (Lattimore et al 2005). This led to calls for SSRI use to be reconsidered in pregnancy, although there was debate as to whether the effects observed in the newborn were attributable to acute cessation of exposure (withdrawal) or a direct prenatal effect. However, this class of medications is widely prescribed to treat a number of psychiatric disorders, and is of particular value in severely depressed patients in pregnancy (Austin 2006). Hence, following studies of neonatal outcome and meta-analysis of existing research, the recommendation now is that the decision whether or not to discontinue SSRI use in pregnancy has to be made on a case by case basis. (Oberlander et al 2006; Lattimore et al 2005; Austin 2006)

Another challenge for care givers and concern for pregnant mothers is that the literature indicates that something as common as maternal fever during intercurrent illness can pose problems. A maternal temperature of 38 ^{0}C or higher is an independent risk factor for significantly increased fetal morbidity, and the specific risk of brain damage resulting in Cerebral Palsy is increased many fold by maternal fever. (Gotsch et al 2007; Kendall & Peebles 2005; Barks & Silverstein 2002; Grether & Nelson 1997)

Some infections are well known to cause brain injury. Those known collectively as the TORCH group (toxoplasmosis, cytomegalovirus and herpes simplex) are examples. (Hagberg & Mallard 2000) Some viral infections are associated with stillbirth, and when infants are born alive many have systemic effects due to the infectious process. Parvovirus B19 infection is an example of an illness that has been associated with severe fetal complications; fetal involvement can result in vasculitis that causes pathological changes in the central nervous system which can include stroke. (De Haan et al 2006) Fetal outcome may be normal but anaemia, hydrops fetalis and stillbirth also occur. Approximately 30–50% of pregnant women are nonimmune. Fetal infection in the first trimester poses the greatest risk. Factor V Leiden mutation can lead to activated protein C resistance which increases the risk of thromboembolism, particularly in the presence of dehydration, asphyxia and infection. Maternal infections as varied as malaria and syphilis adversely affect the fetal brain, and rubella (German measles), varicella (chickenpox) and cytomegalovirus, and labour and delivery complicated by chorioamnionitis and FIRS (Garite 2001; Wu et al; 2003; Bashiri et al 2006) are associated with an increased risk of cerebral palsy and a range of illness specific central nervous system effects. However, upper respiratory tract infections and gastroenteritis, which are common and often a concern to pregnant women, are not. (O'Callaghan et al 2011).

3.1 Fetal inflammatory response syndrome (FIRS)

Inflammatory mediators are known to precipitate premature rupture of the membranes and preterm labour, inflame and cross the placenta, and increase the risk of fetal brain injury and cerebral palsy (O'Callaghan et al 2011). Recent literature uses the term Fetal Inflammatory Response Syndrome (FIRS). (Khwaja & Volpe 2008; Back & Rivkees 2004; Gotsch et al 2007; Bashiri et al 2006; Kendall & Peebles 2005) FIRS is characterized by systemic inflammation, activation of the innate fetal immune system, and elevation of fetal plasma cytokines. Cytokines are small, peptides or glycoproteins secreted de novo in response to inflammation/infection or other immune stimulus. Usually cytokine production is responsible for the generation of a normal immune response, but in the immature fetus or premature infant born after exposure to FIRS the complex effects of cytokine activity significantly increase infant morbidity and mortality, (Gotsch et al 2007; Bashiri et al 2006; Barks & Siverstein 2002) because the balance of these agents is imperfectly controlled.

Cytokines such as Interleukin -1, -3, and -6, and Tumour Necrosis Factor mediate and regulate immunity, inflammation, and haematopoiesis (blood cell production), and are central to the mechanism for elevation of temperature and stimulation of the bone marrow to produce white blood cells in response to infection. (Bashiri et al 2006; Kendall & Peebles 2005; Barks & Silverstein 2002) Importantly, many cytokines are also vasoactive products that increase the vulnerability of the premature fetal brain to hypoxic ischemic injury, and substantial evidence indicates that when a fetus is exposed to intramniotic inflammation there is an increased risk for direct brain injury that can cause short term morbidity and cerebral palsy. (Lee et al 2007)

In the presence of inflammatory cytokines, focal variations in fetal brain perfusion occur that result in local ischemia followed by reperfusion; these perturbations cause cumulative injury to the white matter due to the primitive neuro-vascular architecture, immature auto-regulatory control mechanism, and sensitivity of maturational dependent cells to free radical damage in the immature brain (Volpe 2001b) The germinal matrix is particularly vulnerable to variations in brain blood flow and blood pressure; consequently, periventricular hemorrhage is all the more likely to occur in the preterm fetus exposed to FIRS; such haemorrhage may extend into the ventricular system to cause intraventricular hemorrhage. The literature emphasizes "the synergistic role of inflammation and hypoxia and ischemia when they occur together", and the higher incidence of hypoxic ischemic brain damage that results in a fetus exposed to maternal inflammation/infection.

The literature also supports a role for inflammatory mediators in the mechanisms of preterm premature rupture of membranes (PPROM), premature labour and delivery, and links "maternal infection and pro-inflammatory mediators in the neonatal systemic circulation with an increased risk of PVL and/or spastic diplegia." (Back 2004; Bashiri et al 2006; Barks & Silverstein 2002, Lee et al 2007; Grether 1997; Mercer 2004; Asrat 2001) Maternal cytokines are able to cross the placenta, enter the fetal circulation, cross the brain blood-brain barrier, and produce an inflammatory response in the white matter of the fetal brain which leads to brain damage. (Malaeb & Dammann 2009) Also, the incidence of fetal distress (Kilbride & Thibeault 2001) and hypoxic insults (Garite 2001) is higher following PPROM than in pregnancies with preterm labor and intact membranes. This is largely because of the increased risk of cord compression (Garite 2001; Mercer 2004; Kilbride & Thibeault 2001;

Ehrenberg & Mercer 2001) due to low amniotic fluid (oligohydramnios) as a consequence of membrane rupture, although chorioamnionitis and placental dysfunction may also be contributory. FIRS has been observed in fetuses with preterm labour with intact membranes, preterm prelabour rupture of the membranes, where there is proven fetal viral infection, and also where no microbial invasion is proven. In addition, cytokine release occurs in the fetus following contamination in the birth canal after membrane rupture. Inflammatory products entering the fetal lung then pass into the blood stream and generate an inflammatory response and systemic cytokine release in the fetus.

FIRS has been proved in a series of research studies to be a risk factor for short term perinatal morbidity after adjustment for gestational age at delivery, and also for development of long term sequelae, including brain damage (Gotsch et al 2007) "Intrauterine infection/inflammation is one of the most common causes of neonatal complications including preterm delivery, and considered to be the leading identifiable risk factor for cerebral palsy." (Bashiri et al 2006) Epidemiological evidence suggests that exposure to a combination of infection and hypoxic-ischaemic insult dramatically increases the risk of developing cerebral palsy compared with either insult alone. (Kendall & Peebles 2005) Cytokine mediated brain damage is known to occur as a direct result of an inflammatory process.

In addition to direct cytokine mediated brain damage circulating cytokines also compound the effects of any hypoxic ischemic stress experienced by the fetus. Consequently the severity of any resultant hypoxic ischemic brain damage is increased, particularly in the premature brain. (Gotsch et al 2006; Kendall & Peebles 2005) Thus causal mechanisms for the higher incidence of periventricular leukomalacia in a preterm fetus with FIRS include:

- maturation-dependent factors that render the premature infant's brain exquisitely sensitive to the occurrence of white matter injury;
- fetal distress being more common following PPROM (intrapartum fetal heart decelerations are seen in over 75% of patients);
- the higher incidence of hypoxic ischemic brain damage occurring in affected fetuses;
- reduction by cytokines of the threshold at which hypoxia becomes neurotoxic;
- the synergistic effect of inflammation with hypoxia and ischemia when they occur together;

In the context of limiting brain injury, management of cases of FIRS requires consideration of the maturity of the fetus and a balance of the risks of treating the mother and expediting delivery. "Fetal microbial invasion that results in a systemic fetal inflammatory response can, in the absence of timely delivery, progress to cause organ dysfunction, shock and perhaps death." (Gotsch et al 2007) However, the risks of brain injury associated with being born prematurely have to be weighed against those that exist from remaining in utero. In practice specialists in obstetric and newborn care must together evaluate the relative risks and act accordingly. The incidence of infection seems greatest in the first 72 hours following PPROM. (Kilbride & Thibeault 2001) Immediate induction of labor, compared with expectant management, results in lower rates of chorioamnionitis, fewer babies requiring admission to neonatal ICU, and fewer requiring treatment with antibiotics for suspected sepsis with this approach. The literature states: "For the premature fetus, once clinical chorioamnionitis occurs, rates of sepsis, pneumonia, respiratory distress syndrome and death are all increased by 2-4 fold and long-term neurologic injury is substantially more likely to occur."(Asrat 2001) There appears to be no role of expectant management in any patient with PPROM beyond 34 weeks gestation; (Canavan et al 2004) and: At 34-36 weeks gestation, the risk of severe neonatal morbidity and mortality with expeditious delivery is low. Conversely, conservative management is associated with an 8 fold risk of amnionitis; hence these women are best served by expeditious delivery with labour induction. (Mercer 2004) Even at 32 weeks of gestation, premature infants can be expected to have a 92% intact survival; it is when pregnancy is less advanced that the pros and cons of initiating delivery discussed in the literature have to be considered. The literature also indicates strategies that can be used to down-regulate the inflammatory response and treat mothers who have the signs and symptoms suggestive of infection. Some antibiotic therapies will reduce cytokine production; (Gotsch et al 2007; Kilbride & Thibeault 2001) also, because of the independent association of elevated maternal temperature with worse fetal outcome, appropriate management and control of fever is also cited as a treatment of potential benefit. (Gotsch et al 2007; Kendall & Peebles 2005)

3.2 Hypoxia

As the physiologist Haldane said: "Hypoxia not only stops the machine it wrecks the machinery." (Haldane 1922) A healthy fetus can respond to, and tolerate, the early effects of hypoxia and the degree of acidosis that occurs initially in response to the associated retention of carbon dioxide. In addition, once significantly stressed, the fetus has the physiologic ability to preferentially perfuse the deep structures of the brain with the highest metabolic rate when systemic acidosis becomes more severe. However, this compensation ultimately fails if the ongoing hypoxia remains unrecognized and unrelieved over the course of an hour or more, and the end result is extensive grey matter damage. In addition to this partial and prolonged pattern of hypoxic ischaemic injury, situations occur where the event is more acute and profound in nature. With such insults, acidosis develops relatively abruptly, little or no compensatory redistribution of blood to the deep structures of the brain occurs, and brain injury happens over a much shorter time frame.

Distinction between these two patterns is important from a preventive, diagnostic and prognostic standpoint and over issues of causation in a medico-legal context. Modern neuroimaging (CT and MRI) is the definitive way to distinguish between them based on the selective patterns of brain damage caused. Following partial and prolonged hypoxia/ischemia, the compensatory redistribution of blood results in the brain's cortical areas being less well perfused and hence the predominant regions damaged, and there is also associated hypoxic ischemic injury of multiple organs other than the brain. Where the insult is acute, near total (or profound) in nature, the deep structures of brain (thalami and basal ganglia) are predominantly damaged because there is no time for effective redistribution of cerebral blood flow to maintain their perfusion. (Roland et al 1998; Cowan et al 2003) Basal ganglia injury often predominates (Logitharajah et al 2009) and is most common in infants with acidemia and HIE. (Ruis et al 2009) Brainstem injury can be associated with severe basal ganglia, white matter and cortical injury, (Logitharajah et al 2009) and non survival. (Roland et al 1988) Secondary multi-organ injury may still occur to some degree but is usually mild or absent.

A recent review identified 5 sub-patterns of acute near total injury. (Okereafor et al 2008) In pattern 1, basal ganglia and thalami lesions were associated with severe white matter damage; pattern 2 had basal ganglia and thalami lesions with mild or moderate white matter changes; pattern 3 had isolated thalamic injury; pattern 4 moderate white matter damage only; and pattern 5 mild white matter lesions or normal findings. In 93% of infants with patterns 1 and 2 the internal capsule was abnormal - 86% of them died or developed cerebral palsy. Infants with patterns 3 and 4 developed developmental delay and diplegic cerebral palsy respectively. Those with pattern 5 had normal outcomes. Case infants were significantly more likely of African descent, born to pluriparous or hypertensive mothers, or involve uterine rupture following previous caesarean section or undiagnosed breech presentation accompanied by prolapse of the umbilical cord.

The time line of acute near-total hypoxic ischemic events can be extrapolated from data obtained in animal studies. In these studies, monkeys exposed to complete, i.e. total hypoxia and ischemia (generated experimentally by ligating the umbilical cord and preventing any respiration), could tolerate 10 minutes of hypoxic ischemic insult without permanent effects if they were delivered/resuscitated immediately after this time. Where the hypoxic ischemic event was allowed to continue beyond this period for an additional 10 minutes a cumulative increase in the level of neurological damage was then evident. Where the event extended beyond 20 minute, the fetal monkeys died, in spite of delivery/resuscitation.

In applying this data to the human fetus, it is recognized that what occurs most often is a near total (profound) interruption of brain blood flow and oxygen delivery, rather than an event where hypoxia and ischemia are absolutely total in nature. Hence the time-line for tolerance of such events, and the period over which brain damage evolves, are accepted as being longer than in the landmark animal studies conducted by Meyers. (Meyers 1973; Meyers 1975a; Meyers 1975b; Ginsberg & Meyers 1974) For this reason, it is generally agreed that approximately 15 minutes, and possibly up to 20 minutes, of sudden profound asphyxia can be tolerated by the human fetus prior to brain damage beginning (in contrast to the ten minutes seen in the animal model). Then, after this 'grace' period, damage to the brain begins to occur and over a further period of 15 to 20 minutes the extent and severity of injury becomes progressively more profound over time. And beyond this period, a human fetus is usually born dead. It is also important to recognize that the principal mechanism that causes asphyxial brain injury in the fetus is cerebral ischemia caused by the severe reduction in cerebral blood flow that occurs as a result of hypoxic myocardial depression significantly reducing cardiac output. The fetal heart has a fixed stroke volume, which means that cardiac output and the amount of blood supplied to the brain is determined by the rate of heart contraction. With hypoxia and acidosis, myocardial depression leads to a reduction in heart rate; and significant slowing of the fetal heart (bradycardia) equates with a proportional reduction in cardiac output and reduction in cerebral blood flow.

The relationships between the pattern and time course of an asphyxial insult with the site of brain injury and type of disability that results have been summarized by Robertson and Perlman (Robertson and Perlman 2006). Acute, near-total insults of moderate degree with injury to the basal ganglia and thalami result predominantly in athetoid or dystonic cerebral palsy with intact or mildly impaired cognitive development. When severe and prolonged acute insults damage the cerebral cortex in addition to deep brain structures severe spastic quadriplegia results, with associated cortical visual impairment, microcephaly and significant cognitive deficits. Prolonged partial insults of moderate degree with injury to watershed regions result in moderate spastic quadriplegia with variable cognitive deficit, but when severe, with extensive cortical brain involvement, result in spastic quadriplegia, severe cognitive impairment, cortical visual impairment, and microcephaly.

Periventricular leukomalacia (PVL) Is predominately, but not exclusively, a condition affecting the preterm infant. PVL can develop during fetal life and in the newborn period. The primary mechanism is hypoxic ischemic injury, and the ischemic component (period of inadequate blood flow) is generally regarded as the major mechanism of injury. Neurobiologic research has shown that maturational dependent oligodendroglial precursor cells are a major target in PVL, and exquisitely vulnerable to damage by free radicals generated during ischemia/reperfusion. (Volpe 2001b) The premature infant has an immature pattern of brain blood supply and a reduced ability to control brain blood flow. (Khwaja & Volpe 2008; Back & Rivkees 2004) PVL develops after periods of abnormally low blood flow in the cerebral white matter in areas where there are arterial end zones and border zones present, due to the immaturity of a preterm infant's neurovascular development. Autoregulation of cerebral blood flow is also often impaired in such infants; and where systemic hypotension occurs or there are episodes of fluctuant or inadequate cerebral blood flow for any reason, hypoxic ischemic brain damage can occur involving the vulnerable periventricular areas. (Volpe 2001a). Where a mother has prolonged premature rupture of the membranes (PPROM), her fetus is recognized to have an increased risk for a number of complications that can cause brain damage. Although not every fetus is affected directly or indirectly by the inflammatory cytokines generated under such circumstances, where such brain damage does occur this often manifests as PVL (Back & Rivkees 2004; Gotsch et al 2007)

PVL is associated with Intraventricular haemorrhage (IVH) in approximately 25% of cases; the pathogenesis of IVH is usually multifactorial. See Table 1.

- Fluctuating cerebral blood flow
- Increased cerebral blood flow
- Increased cerebral venous pressure
- Decreased cerebral blood flow followed by reperfusion
- Disorders of coagulation, platelet function and capillary integrity
- Vulnerability to hypoxic ischaemic injury

Table 1. The major pathogenic factors for IVH (Modified from Volpe 2001a)

Infants with PVL secondary to significant intrapartum hypoxic ischaemic injury will usually be abnormal on neurological exam at birth; PVL acquired intrapartum may manifest as lower limb weakness evident in the first weeks of life. (Volpe 2001a) PVL can be aggravated by or generated due to postnatal events. The commonest clinical situation in which the most important pathogenic factors combine to generate sufficient ischemia to cause PVL is when a sick preterm infant requires mechanical ventilation; i.e. vascular anatomic factors, physiologic factors, the pressure passive nature of the immature cerebral circulation, systemic variations in blood pressure, and the effects of hypocarbia (Khwaja & Volpe 2008; Volpe 2001a). If infection is the cause for assisted ventilation being required or if morbidity from a prior infection is superimposed, the probability of ischemia and/or haemorrhage compromising the periventricular vasculature is much greater.

Many infants born with PVL have a normal neurologic outcome. Those who have brain injury sufficient to generate permanent sequelae exhibit a range of problems that manifest with varying degrees of severity; including intellectual and visual deficits that are usually superimposed on spastic paresis involving the extremities where the lower limbs are predominantly affected.

Hypoxic ischaemic encephalopathy (HIE) is "an acute non-static encephalopathy caused by intrapartum or late antepartum brain hypoxia and ischemia"; (Robertson & Perlman 2006) this clinical state evolves during the first days of life following significant hypoxic ischaemic insult, and is a major predictor of neurodevelopmental disability.(Ferriero 2004) Prospective studies incorporating MRI suggest that the majority of cases of encephalopathy occur as a result of brain injury that occurs at or near the time of birth. (Cowan et al 2003) After a severe insult depression of consciousness is common in the first hours, hypotonia and reduced movement occur, particularly with cortical injury, and the onset of seizure activity is common.

The probability that hypoxic ischaemic brain injury will result in permanent neurological consequences is recognized to increase with the severity and duration of HIE. The distinguishing features of three clinical stages of HIE (mild, moderate and severe) were classified by Sarnat and Sarnat (Sarnat and Sarnat 1976) based on observations in 26 full term newborn infants exposed to perinatal asphyxia. See Table 2.

Infants who develop HIE exhibit a range of alterations in conscious level and behaviour from a hyper-alert state through irritability to lethargy and obtundation. Disorders of tone are also evident that again range from an increase through to a marked decrease. And a variety of abnormal movements occur from tremors and jitteriness through to frank seizures. Other clinical manifestations include apnoea (temporary cessation of breathing) with bradycardia and impaired oxygen saturation, shrill cry, feeding difficulty (mainly due to poor coordination of suck, but occasionally due to brain stem damage), exaggeration of the Moro and deep tendon reflexes, and decerebrate or decorticate posturing. The severity of HIE symptoms depends on the timing and duration of the causal insult. (Rees & Inder 2005) Each infant's clinical state evolves following the hypoxic episode, often with marked changes evident initially over the course of hours, and then later over days or weeks, necessitating serial examination and evaluation with EEG and neuroimaging.

An encephalopathic state develops after 1-6 per 1000 live births. Mortality is high (15-20% in some series) with most deaths occurring within a month of injury due to associated multiple organ failure or termination of care. In about 25% of cases permanent neurologic deficits remain. Not all cases of neonatal encephalopathy are due to anoxia or hypoxic ischaemic injury; (Ferriero 2004; Volpe 2001a) but epidemiological studies confirm the association of HIE with pregnancy related risks (maternal pre-eclamptic toxaemia, hypertension, FIRS, and infertility treatment) and a range of intrapartum risk factors that predispose the fetus to hypoxic ischaemic brain injury. Postnatal aggravation of intrapartum acquired injury occurs relatively rarely (10%), but is a preventable component in many instances. Prevention centres on anticipating and limiting the adverse effects on the brain of fluctuations in cerebral perfusion, respiratory distress, sepsis, metabolic instability, and any situation that increases oxygen and energy demands (e.g. as occur with protracted seizures).

STAGE	CLINICAL FEATURES	EEG	DURATION AND OUTCOME
1 - Mild	• State - Hyper-alert, irritable, jittery • Tone - normal • Suck – weak • Seizure - none	• normal (awake)	• lasts < 24-48 hours • < 1% have poor outcome
2 - Moderate	• State - Lethargic, obtunded • Tone - mild hypotonia • Suck – weak or absent • Seizures - common: variable (focal or multifocal)	• Early – low voltage • Later - periodic discharges, focal spike and wave	• lasts days • 20 - 40% poor outcome
3 - Severe	• State - Stuporous/Comatose • Tone - flaccid • Suck - absent • Seizures – decerebrate posturing	• Early – periodic pattern • Later - isopotential	• lasts days to weeks • 100% poor outcome

Table 2. The Sarnat Score (modified from Sarnat and Sarnat (Sarnat & Sarnat 1976))

Seizures: major causes of seizures include brain malformation, structural injury, or reversible metabolic disorders. The clinical signs vary from subtle movement disorders to focal or generalized brief or sustained convulsive activity. Abnormal movement often involves the eyes (blink, staring, horizontal tonic deviation), mouth (lip smacking or sucking, tongue thrusting), extremities (bicycling/rowing or jerking), or respiratory muscles (apnoea). Variations in heart rate occur (tachycardia and bradycardia), often with colour change due to a degree of oxygen desaturation. Focal clonic seizures may imply brain damage due to arterial or venous infarction. The suspicion that clinical signs represent seizures should be confirmed by electroencephalogram (EEG). MRI can help distinguish between seizures due to hypoxic–ischemic events and those caused by other forms of metabolic or genetic disease, (Huang & Castillo 2008; Alkalay 2005; Alkalay et al 2005a; Alkalay et al 2005b; Barkovich et al 1998; Efron et al 2003) and provides information on the extent of traumatic and infectious causes. Preventable/reversible causes of seizures include hypoglycemia, hypocalcemia, hyponatraemia, hypoxemia, and acidosis. However delayed treatment probably increases the risk of residual consequences; and considerable stresses are placed on the brain by the high oxygen and substrate requirements implicit when seizures are prolonged. (Tasker 2001) However, seizures do not always imply poor neurodevelopmental outcome for affected newborns.

The number of term infants who survive HIE is lower than those who are extremely premature, but the proportion who survive with long term sequelae is higher; such infants require follow up and management of their handicaps: regimens to do this have been described. (Robertson & Perlman 2006) Outcome prediction for infants with HIE has been proposed using defined periods (0-6 hours after birth, 6-72 hours after birth, and before discharge) and clinical, imaging and electrophysiological predictors, and neurological examination criteria. The purpose is to rationalize hypothermia and other intervention therapies, including the withdrawal of support, and improve knowledge related to the continuum that HIE and the evolution of the brain injury that underlies its pathology represents. (Perlman & Shah 2011).

Entities aimed at minimizing the effects of HIE are evolving. Controlled reoxygenation to avoid hyperoxia is one. Drugs with potential as therapies include novel anti-oxidative agents such as N-acetylcysteine, neuroprotective agents targeted at glutamate receptors and others such as magnesium sulphate, endocannabinoids; (Halopainen & Lauren 2011; Todd et al 2011) and controlled hypothermia shows promise. (Vannucci & Perlman 1997; Gunn & Gluckman 2007; Ferriero 2004; Schulzke et al 2007; Higgins et al 2006). The concept for cooling being beneficial during recovery from encephalopathy stems from animal studies and the neuroprotective effect of hypothermia in cases of near-drowning in children and during cardiac surgery involving periods of cardiac arrest. Early studies using short periods of cooling in encephalopathic newborns had limited and contradictory results; recent experimental studies are more promising having shown that moderate cerebral hypothermia initiated as soon as possible after the initial insult, before the onset of secondary energy failure, and continued for 48 hours or more is associated with neuroprotection (Gunn & Gluckman 2007) Randomized clinical trials that used either systemic cooling or selective head cooling in encephalopathic neonates also suggest moderate hypothermia is safe, (Gunn & Gluckman 2007; Feigin et al 2004) and that newborns with moderate encephalopathy are better from a neurodevelopmental perspective than normothermic controls at the same age in early infancy. (Gunn & Gluckman 2007) However, a 2005 working group (Higgins et al 2006) while seeing this as a "potentially promising therapy", identified significant unresolved issues; central to these is how to identify which babies are most likely to benefit (Gunn & Gluckman 2007) and the relative safety and benefit of different techniques of cooling. (Gunn & Gluckman 2007; Schulzke et al 2007). Hence studies are ongoing, as with any experimental therapy, the potential for good results must be balanced against any adverse systemic effects and long term follow up data obtained.

One element that would aid in this process and documenting the severity and evolution of brain injury is novel monitoring techniques that allow oxygen supply and demand and cerebral haemodynamics to be evaluated. An example of a technology that has been tried in this regard and continues to show potential is near infrared (NIR) spectroscopy (NIRS). NIRS is an established non-invasive optical technology using energy from the NIR spectrum to monitor changes in local blood flow and hemodynamics non-invasively within the microcirculation, and detect differences in tissue oxygen delivery, consumption and utilization. NIRS has been used to study healthy and injured brain (Wyatt 1993; Chen et al 2002; Sakatani et al 1998; Lin et al 2009), and is a promising tool for determining optimal cerebral perfusion pressure for patients with acute brain injury (Brady et al 2007). Comprehensive reviews describe the basic principles, limitations and parameters that can be quantified. (Ferrari et al 1992; Wolf et al 2007; Ferrari et al 2004; Rolfe 2002; Macnab 2009). NIR spectroscopy uses energy from the NIR spectrum to follow variations in the concentration of oxygenated (O_2Hb) and deoxygenated (HHB) haemoglobin, and employs many of the fundamental principles of physics relating to the transmission of light through tissue. However, it is the unique combination of the transparency of tissue to NIR wavelengths and the specific absorption spectra of oxygenated and deoxygenated haemoglobin that form the basis of biomedical applications of NIR spectroscopy. Reviews describe the development of instrumentation, the technical specifications of individual units and recent advances in the technology. (Ferrari et al 1992; Wolf et al 2007; Ferrari et al 2004; Rolfe 2002; Macnab 2009; Yodh & Boas 2003; Hoshi 2007) Because the initial concentration of O_2Hb and HHb in the tissue being monitored is unknown, only absolute changes in concentration relative to the initial baseline concentration can be derived using conventional NIR spectroscopy. However, with real time sampling and graphic conversion of data, the patterns and magnitude of change derived provide valuable information, as they can be used to infer physiologic change occurring within the tissue interrogated. (Hamaoka et al 2007; Ferrari et al 2011; Wolf et al 2007) Examples of such changes include:

- an increase or decrease in O_2Hb (an indirect measure of oxygen content);
- an increase or decrease in the total haemoglobin - tHb [O_2Hb + HHb] (change in blood volume);
- an abrupt decrease in O_2Hb with simultaneous increase in HHb (ischemia); and
- a gradual decrease in O_2Hb and increase in HHb (hypoxia).

The absolute ratio of O_2Hb to tHb can be determined using spatially resolved spectroscopy (SRS), (Murkin & Arango 2009; Suzuki et al 1999) which requires an instrument to have either a multiple segment photodiode chip or an array that has multiple emitter-detector distances. Such pathlength geometry allows light detection at two or more different distances from the emitter, which enables the absolute ratio of O_2Hb to tHb to be determined, and a calculation of tissue oxygen saturation to be made. On instruments with SRS capability this parameter is variously referred to as the 'tissue oxygenation index' (TOI), 'tissue saturation index' (TSI %), or 'mean tissue Hb saturation' (rSO2). (Shadgan et al 2009; Owen-Reece et al 1999; Tobias 2006)

NIR spectroscopy is an attractive technology for clinical monitoring because it is non-invasive, uses a non-toxic energy source, and can monitor physiologic change continuously with high temporal resolution. (Ferrari et al 2004; Rolfe 2000) Investigators value the ability to make comparison between sites of measurement using multichannel instruments, and conduct studies in real time. Monitoring in real time in situations where being able to identify the onset of adverse events allows potentially remediable intervention is attractive clinically, particularly where the brain or spinal cord are affected (e.g. by the onset of ischemia). (Murkin & Arango 2009; Macnab et al 2002, Macnab et al 2003) In brain studies NIRS has yielded "much credible and some important clinical research data," (Simonson & Piantadosi 1996) and a threshold for cerebral ischemia has been defined using SRS. (Al-Rawi 2005)

Early studies in newborn infants showed that changes in cerebral blood flow and blood volume occurred in the hours following hypoxic ischemic brain injury. (Wyatt 1993; von Bel 1993; Fellman & Raivio 1997) Stresses that most sick premature newborn infants experience, including painful stimuli and loud noise, also affect cerebral haemodynamics, (Gagnon et al 1999) and over time such disturbances have been suggested as a mechanism that might explain the neurological morbidity evident in many infants who do not have specific illness or adverse events to which to attribute their motor or cognitive problems. Auditory evoked changes in cerebral oxygenation are evident after hypoxic ischemic injury (Chen et al 2002). Animal studies have quantified the effects of graded hypotension on cerebral blood flow, blood volume and transit time; (Ferrari et al 1992) and with continuous time domain analysis cerebral oximetry have allowed assessment of autoregulation, which could be used as a means of optimizing cerebral perfusion pressure in patients with acute brain injury (Brady et al 2007). Most recently mapping of cortical blood flow using grids of NIRS sensors has identified cortical areas responsible for speech and language development.

Future advances in hardware and software related to MRI, spectroscopy and diffusion tensor imaging will likely allow such technologies to contribute more by delineating the site(s) and extent of neuronal injury, (Perlman 2011) and aid in evaluation and management strategies able to mitigate the long term effects of perinatal brain injury.

Multisystem involvement: The consequences of fetal hypoxic ischemic stress extend beyond the brain. The lungs of asphyxiated infants can be injured directly by hypoxia, as a consequence of inhaled meconium, secondary to left ventricular failure, or compromised from pulmonary hypertension. (Lapointe & Barrington 2011) The end result is impaired gas exchange and the need for assisted ventilation to maintain adequate oxygenation and carbon dioxide exchange. The risks of brain injury increase where such effects are superimposed on the poorly compliant lungs of a preterm infant; pneumothorax (air leak into the pleural space causing lung compression) is less common with modern ventilation techniques, but when it occurs, major disturbances in cerebral perfusion pressure result that increase the risk of serious brain haemorrhage.

Direct damage is caused to the myocardium of the heart; this and the consequences of compensatory mechanisms to preserve cerebral perfusion that divert blood flow away from other organs result in a recognizable clinical and laboratory picture; as summarized in the Table by Phelan in a recent study with definitions based on Hankins et al. (Phelan et al 2011; Hankins et al 2002) The cardiac effects of myocardial ischemia compromise conduction and mechanical (contractile) efficiency, and often require heart function to be supported with inotropic agents such as dopamine to maintain adequate circulation. Functional and conduction abnormalities are evident on cardiac echo and electrocardiogram, and elevated cardiac enzymes reflect heart muscle damage. The other multisystem effects are principally on renal, hepatic, and bone marrow function. Renal injury is the best systemic marker of potential brain injury; especially when reduced urine output (oliguria = urine output <1ml/kg/h) is associated with an abnormal neurological examination. (Perlman 2011) Absent or significantly reduced urine output in the 24 hours following hypoxic ischaemic injury is common, is often accompanied by haematuria, and reflects renal tubular damage. Blood urea and serum creatinine concentrations rise progressively and peak in the days following injury. Inappropriate secretion of antidiuretc hormone occurs, which causes fluid retention, which causes serum sodium levels to fall (hyponatraemia). The effect on the bone marrow and haemopoesis is reflected by an increase in the release of nucleated red blood cells which peaks at 6-8 hours after brain injury and falls to normal by 36-72 hours. Platelet numbers fall (thrombocytopaenia), sometimes by 12 hours, the nadir occurring at 2-3 days. (Beyene et al 2009) Thrombocytopaenia can be severe enough to cause or potentiate bleeding including within the brain. Serum calcium levels often fall; liver enzymes reflecting hepatic cellular damage increase, and blood glucose concentration can fluctuate, with low levels (hypoglycaemia) being most common.

Hypoglycaemia has recognized neurologic consequences, (Alkalay et al 2005a; Burns et al 2008; Karimzadeh et al 2011) especially when low glucose concentrations cause or accompany seizures. E.g. motor and/or psychodevelopmental delay, microcephaly (Alkalay et al 2005b), spastic quadriplegia and hemiplegia, seizures and visual impairment (Burns et al 2008). Imaging studies document the presence of oedema and hyperechogenic areas in the acute phase (Alkalay et al 2005b), and later, a high incidence of white matter injury, including a proportion with global damage (Burns et al 2008). Focal damage evident unilaterally or bilaterally has also been seen in a range of locations, including in the parietal and occipital lobes, and cortex, and in one case in the brain stem (Alkalay et al 2005a; Burns et al 2008; Barkovich et al 1998). Hyperglycaemia also has the potential to cause or aggravate brain damage, principally because of the hyperosmolar state that ensues (Efron et al 2003; Volpe 2001a).

Organ Involved	Clinical / Laboratory Features
Heart	Cardiac dysfunction requiring dopamine to support circulation Elevated creatine phosphokinase (CPK) Echocardiogram/electrocardiogram abnormalities
Kidneys	Absent or reduced urine output Elevated creatinine
Liver	Global hepatic dysfunction with elevated enzymes • serum glutamic-oxaloacetic transaminase (SGOT) • serum glutamic-pyruvic transaminase (SGPT) • lactate dehydrogenase (LDH)
Lung	Abnormal respiratory drive and lung compliance requiring assisted ventilation
Intestines	Feeding intolerance Abnormal peristalsis
Bone Marrow	Release of primitive cell lines (nucleated red blood cells) Depression of total platelet numbers

Table 3. Multisystem Involvement in the first days of life following fetal hypoxic ischaemic injury (Modified from Phelan et al 2011)

Prevention of hypoxic ischaemic brain injury centres on labour and delivery but relies on attention to multiple factors during many phases of pregnancy. Good antenatal care is fundamental to optimal maternal and fetal health. Prior medical history, particularly pregnancy outcome, needs to be considered; then regular maternal examination and investigation follow to confirm gestational age, ensure appropriate fetal growth, and plan for appropriate timing and means of delivery; supervision during labour provides the means for anticipation, monitoring and intervention that underlie good obstetric care and underpin optimal fetal outcome including the lowest chance of brain injury occurring for any reason.

In the context of intrapartum situations that put the fetus at risk of neurological sequelae, guidelines exist for most situations to anticipate, prevent, or minimize morbidity. In many situations, and with fetal hypoxia in particular, the physiological effects on the fetus generate detectable changes in the fetal heart rate. The fetal myocardium and brain are sensitive to reduction in oxygen tension, and become all the more so as elevation of carbon dioxide occurs and significant acidosis develops. Importantly, the changes in heart rate and cardiac function that result occur prior to brain metabolism being affected sufficiently for damage to begin. A non-reassuring pattern or individual changes in fetal heart rate reflecting alteration in cardiac function occur, most often in relation to uterine contractions which even during uncomplicated labour place an element of stress of the fetus. This is because the haemodynamics of placental blood flow alter as the tone of the uterus increases; blood flow through the umbilical cord on which the fetus depends is also vulnerable during contractions. During the later stages of labour, when the fetus is moving down the birth canal, cord compression, entrapment or prolapse through the cervix can occur. These situations compromise blood flow to varying degrees; in addition to oxygen delivery to the fetus being affected, perfusion and removal of carbon dioxide and acids from the fetus can become impaired. Sometimes a 'sentinel event' is detected with an abrupt and sustained drop in fetal heart rate. Such events occur in association with events such as uterine rupture, placental abruption, cord occlusion/prolapse, maternal collapse, or intra-partum haemorrhage. It is the association of such events with brain injury (Okereafor et al 2008) and the physiologic perturbations in fetal oxygenation and haemodynamics that they reflect that provide the rationale for fetal heart rate measurement and electronic fetal monitoring (EFM) (Macones et al 2008; Liston et al 2007; Am Col Obs Gyn 2005; Royal College Obs Gyn 2005). The purpose of EFM is to provide recognition of 'non-reassuring' patterns or frank abnormalities in heart rate that leads to prompt obstetric assessment, intervention(s) required to relieve compromise to the fetal circulation, or expedited instrumental delivery or emergency caesarean section.

Guidelines for electronic fetal monitoring have been generated in most jurisdictions (Macones et al 2008; Liston et al 2007; Am Col Obs Gyn 2005; Royal College Obs Gyn 2005). However, EFM became part of clinical practice following retrospective studies comparing its use to historical controls where auscultation was performed. And while case-control studies have shown correlation of EFM abnormalities with umbilical artery base excess; only 1 of 13 randomized controlled trials showed a significant decrease in perinatal mortality comparing EFM with auscultation; and meta-analysis found an increased incidence of caesarean delivery and decreased neonatal seizures but no effect on the incidence of cerebral palsy or perinatal death. (Graham et al 2008)

Placental pathology: the placenta is one of the least well understood organs in the human body, yet it is integral to fetal perfusion, gas exchange (oxygenation and carbon dioxide excretion), and nutrition, and protection of the fetus from infection. Many common maternal conditions interfere with placental function and fetal oxygenation, including hypertension, diabetes, and sickle cell anaemia. The fetus is at particular risk of brain injury in conditions where the disturbance of placental gas exchange and fetal perfusion becomes acute and severe; examples include pre-eclamptic toxaemia (which, if unchecked, also requires delivery of the fetus, regardless of the gestation achieved, in order to restore maternal blood pressure and coagulation status), and haemorrhage from placenta praevia or abruption where bleeding occurs between the placenta and the uterine wall. In one study aimed at establishing the antecedent factors and patterns of brain injury in preterm infants with HIE, placental abruption was the commonest identifiable event (Logitharajah et al 2009). Acute maternal infection and transplacental passage of inflammatory cytokines expose the fetal brain to direct and indirect damage, and the associated risks of preterm delivery where premature rupture of membranes and preterm labour occurs. Less acute situations predominantly stem from progressive failure of the placenta to function and provide nutrition and gas exchange. Growth retardation occurs with progressive slowing of fetal somatic and brain growth (intrauterine growth retardation) and increasing risk of acute placental insufficiency leading to fetal distress, again with the likelihood of hypoxia and ischemia as the predominant mechanism of brain injury. The umbilical cord, which is the conduit for blood flow and gas exchange between the placenta and fetus, is also vulnerable; compression, prolapse, occlusion, entrapment and tearing occur, each of which has recognized adverse consequences for fetal oxygenation and cerebral blood flow. Partial and prolonged and acute near total episodes of hypoxic ischaemic stress occur in consequence. Overall the incidence of interruption of adequate placental blood flow during labour is approximately 3 of every 1000 term deliveries (Perlman 2011)

Instrumental delivery: A number of situations require delivery assisted by forceps or vacuum extraction. In many instances concern over a non-reassuring pattern in the fetal heart rate or other evidence suggests fetal distress has developed, or delivery has been delayed sufficiently for the mother or fetus to be deemed at risk. The principal of forceps delivery is to place the blades of the instrument on either side of the fetal head so as to contain it within the forceps. Gentle traction is then applied to the handles of the forceps in order to dilate the cervix and allow the fetal head to progress down the birth canal. Forceps are not intended to pull the fetus through the cervix. With mis-application or undue traction applied head trauma can occur - this can result in facial injury including facial palsy, skull fracture and intracranial bleeding. Vacuum extraction involves attaching a suction cup to the baby's head and then gently applying traction to help ease the baby down the birth canal. Although permanent sequelae can result with either motor or cognitive damage, generally instrumental delivery does not result in permanent brain injury except under more extreme circumstances. This is because there are strict guidelines related to both the application of forceps and the use of vacuum extraction, all of which are intended to optimize delivery and avoid the risk of head trauma and associated brain injury. The principal risks with forceps are application when the fetal head is high in the birth canal, attempts to rotate the fetal head, or use of excessive force; and with use of the vacuum extractor application when the fetus is not sufficiently advanced down the birth canal, or for periods that are overly long or repetitive.

Infants adversely affected often show a degree of neurological depression at birth, and some have evidence of skull fractures; there can be associated underlying cortical damage (Ferriero 2004), and/or subdural or intracranial bleeding. Cerebellar injury is also described (Limperopoulos et al 2009) A small proportion of these brain injured infants then go on to develop signs of encephalopathy in the newborn period, but most recover. Occasionally the mechanical problems related to the volume of intracranial bleeding require surgical drainage. In the premature infant if bleeding occurs that extends into the intraventricular compartment this can result in post-haemorrhagic hydrocephalus.

Breech delivery. The key issues to avoid brain injury in infants presenting by the breech (bottom first - or with the part normally covered by the britches presenting) are assistance during delivery to protect the after coming head and the attendance of staff to effectively resuscitate the infant, who in many instances is born prematurely and after a degree of hypoxic stress. The central problem that predisposes the infant presenting by the breech to brain injury is that in the fetus the dimensions of the bottom are smaller than those of the head. Hence, after the body of the fetus has passed through the cervix the degree of dilatation is insufficient for the after coming head to avoid entrapment. As a result delivery is delayed and there is a risk that hypoxic ischemic brain damage will occur.

The related problem is that when the head is released by the partially dilated cervix an abrupt and significant change in intracranial pressure occurs that is associated with a comparably large and sudden alteration in cerebral blood volume. In infants who are premature in particular this change in pressure and blood volume results in fluctuations in cerebral blood flow that are sufficiently extreme for brain ischemia to be followed by hyper-perfusion that often results in brain haemorrhage. Superimposed on the period of hypoxia and ischemia caused during head entrapment this fluctuation in blood volume is often sufficient to cause bleeding into the brain and/or significant brain injury.

Preventive measures include recognition of breech presentation, and appropriate planning to ensure optimal delivery and resuscitation. This may involve operative delivery by caesarean section or protection of the after coming head with forceps during delivery, and the availability of trained staff to optimally resuscitate a potentially asphyxiated and possibly premature infant. In addition, planning is required to ensure safe transport of the mother to an appropriate level of care prior to delivery whenever possible, or the availability of local staff and/or transport team personnel to resuscitate, care for, and where necessary relocate the newborn infant to a facility capable of providing the care he/she requires after birth.

Large for gestational age infants are those weighing more than the 90th centile for their age. Such infants are often born to mothers who develop gestational diabetes. Because they are large these infants may experience difficult or delayed delivery with the inherent associated risks of hypoxic stress. Generally pregnancies compromised by gestational diabetes and accelerated fetal growth are electively ended by induction of labour prior to term. This reduces the risk of still birth and fetal morbidity from a number of causes. However, the principal risk that large gestational age infants face relates to their disordered glucose homeostasis that puts them at risk of hypoglycemia in the newborn period. This requires careful monitoring of blood glucose and provision of adequate substrate (usually in the form of frequent oral or nasogastric tube feeds, or a constant infusion of intravenous glucose) sufficient to maintain normoglycaemia. Where seizures occur due to hypoglycemia there is a recognized associated morbidity with the brain being vulnerable to injury and the risk of abnormal neurodevelopmental outcome. In addition seriously affected infants may also have a problems related to cardiac function and the maintenance of an adequate circulation due to a pericardial effusion that compromises cardiac output, and hence potentially results in impaired cerebral blood flow capable of resulting in brain injury.

Post mature infants (those born after 42 weeks of gestation) have a number of risks of brain injury related to their post maturity; these are mainly still birth or fetal distress due to placental failure or obstetric complications during delivery. Rare associations of post maturity with of brain anomaly include anencephaly, and bird-headed dwarfism.

Multiple pregnancy. The incidence of twins is 11-13 per 1000 pregnancies with a predisposition amongst African Americans. Triplet and higher-order multiple births are increasing due to IVF. Risks of brain damage exist because of a higher incidence of premature delivery and low birth weight, the risks associated with being born second (or later) and experiencing hypoxia in consequence, and a higher incidence of cord accidents than in singleton births. Congenital brain anomalies occur including anencephaly and holoprosencephaly. Vascular shunts between twins and the death of one twin can cause a variety of problems; resulting in polycythemia, stroke from emboli, and haemorrhage that can cause brain damage.

Haemorrhage. Major causes of bleeding include placental abruption (separation from the uterine wall), placenta praevia, maternal trauma, damage to the umbilical cord, and intraventricular haemorrhage. Where haemorrhage involves a significant volume of blood loss the fetus loses the ability to maintain adequate levels of oxygen delivery and tissue perfusion. While acidosis and hypoxia result brain damage occurs principally because mean blood pressure can no longer be maintained, cerebral blood flow falls and hypoxic ischemic injury follows. In the preterm infant fluctuations in cerebral perfusion during the evolution and management of haemorrhage are often damaging in their own right. Where a maternal cause exists, interventions to resuscitate the mother and intervene to address the underlying cause of the haemorrhage benefit the infant, provided they are instituted promptly and either restore fetal oxygen delivery and perfusion, or deliver the infant allowing extra-uterine resuscitation. Infants born following a haemorrhagic event need immediate assessment at birth of the adequacy of their circulation as part of their resuscitation. Such infants not infrequently require prompt intravenous fluid replacement to restore their blood volume to adequate levels for normal perfusion and oxygen delivery to occur. Delay in delivery of this component of resuscitation can compound the degree of existing hypoxic ischemic brain injury. Any pale and neurologically depressed infant needs an assessment of the adequacy of blood pressure and circulation in addition to support of respiration, oxygenation and cardiac function.

Hydrops fetalis is a condition where fluid accumulates in the fetus to an extensive degree. The majority of cases used to relate to Rhesus disease. Human parvovirus B19 infection should be considered in any case of nonimmune hydrops; (De Haan et al 2006) diagnosis is mainly through serology and polymerase chain reaction. Surveillance requires sequential ultrasound and Doppler screening for signs of fetal anaemia, heart failure and hydrops. Intrauterine transfusion in selected cases can be life saving. Cardiac arrhythmia due to supra ventricular tachycardia (SVT) can be severe enough in a fetus to cause hydrops, and is associated with significant morbidity and mortality. Several reports link SVT with neurological morbidity, including periventricular leukomalacia (PVL) and spastic diplegia (Oudijk et al 2004). SVT severe enough to compromise cardiac function and cause hydrops reduces brain blood flow sufficiently over time for ischemia and hypoxia to cause brain damage. SVT is the most common cause of non-immune hydrops, but it is also the most amenable to treatment (Porat et al 2003). Fetal heart rate monitoring is used to diagnose and follow fetal arrhythmias. Diagnosis of hydrops is made by ultrasound when generalized skin thickening of greater than 5 mm is present associated with two of the following criteria: ascites (fluid in the abdominal cavity), pleural effusion, pericardial effusion or placental enlargement (Oudijk et al 2004).

If the fetus is mature enough, delivery and post natal treatment is then possible. But if the risk from complications of prematurity is too high for safe delivery, therapeutic intervention with medication can preserve fetal well-being, as treatment with anti-arrhythmic agents ablates the arrhythmia and improves cardiac function. There is evidence that the adverse affects of SVT can be tolerated by a fetus for a period of time which makes it probable that adequate blood flow to the fetal brain continues initially. But unrecognised and untreated, worsening cardiac dysfunction leads to hydrops and compromise of brain blood flow. For this reason early diagnosis and interventional management to relieve the adverse effects of SVT on the brain are central to ensuring good neurological outcome, particularly in a premature infant with an immature brain (Oudijk et al 2004; Porat et al 2003).

In-vitro fertilization (IVF): Population based studies in Australia, Sweden and the USA document that while most children born after IVF are healthy, there are increased rates of multiple pregnancy, low birth weight, genetic anomalies, and disability (Hansen et al 2002; Schieve et al 2002; Stromberg et al 2002). Infants conceived using IVF are more likely than controls to develop neurological disability, impairment or handicap, and especially cerebral palsy; this effect is attributed largely but not solely to the high frequency of twins born, and to low birth weight and low gestational age, but an effect due to the IVF procedure per se cannot be excluded (Stromberg et al 2002). The risk of major birth defects may be as much as twice as high as for naturally conceived infants (Hansen et al 2002) and the incidence of low birth weight is higher for singletons as well as twins. (Schieve et al 2002)

Stroke: Strokes can occur in a fetus between 14 weeks of gestation and delivery, and result in cerebral palsy, mental retardation and epilepsy. In a review (Ozduman et al 2004) 78% of cases of fetal stroke with a reported outcome resulted in either death or adverse neurodevelopmental outcome. The principal causes are ischaemic, thrombotic or haemorrhagic injuries occurring in utero. Most fetal strokes are of unclear origin, but associated maternal conditions recognized to underlie some cases include platelet abnormalities, placental pathologies, medication (warfarin and antiepileptic medication associated with a decrease in vitamin K dependent coagulation factors), trauma, twin to twin transfusion, and Parvovirus B19 infection; fetal factors include cytomegalovirus infection and protein C deficiency (Ozduman et al 2004; De Haan et al 2006). Diagnosis in utero may be made on routine ultrasound. MRI is the optimal imaging modality.

4. Cerebral Palsy

Cerebral Palsy (CP) is the term used for a group of non-progressive disorders of movement and posture caused by abnormal development of, or damage to, motor control centers of the brain. CP is defined as a static neuromuscular disorder characterized by an abnormal control of movement or posture appearing early in life that is not the result of a recognizable progressive disease. (Nelson & Ellenberg 1981) CP has a prevalence of approximately 2 per 1,000 live births and is caused by a variety of congenital and acquired events before, during, or after birth. (Phelan et al 2011) CP has been investigated extensively for epidemiologic risk factors with research dating back to the 1970s. (O'Callaghan) A number of key factors have been well established to be associated with CP from population-wide databases, and with near complete ascertainment and a low likelihood of bias. These include preterm birth, low birth weight, infection in pregnancy, and twin births. (O'Callaghan et al 2011) However, a large proportion of cases have no identifiable cause, while approximately 10% are estimated to be attributable to asphyxia. (Yudkin et al 1995) Phelan identified the association of a sudden and sustained deterioration in fetal heart rate with the criteria developed by the task force on neonatal encephalopathy and cerebral palsy for intrapartum asphyxial injury in cases where a diagnosis of CP was subsequently made. In a cohort of 7242 children who developed CP, 31.3% had had one or more of six defined adverse intrapartum events (placental abruption, uterine rupture during labour, fetal distress, birth trauma, umbilical cord prolapse, and mild-severe birth asphyxia). (Gilbert et al 2011) Prematurity has the greatest impact on the future development of CP, hence the higher incidence of CP in such infants. (Gilbert et al 2011) However, birth asphyxia, birth defects and adverse labour events contribute significantly as well, suggesting that in preterm infants CP is most likely multifactorial (Sukhov et al 2011). There is also data supporting an association between CP and maternal infection late in gestation, intrauterine growth restriction, early gestational age, multiple birth, family members with cerebral palsy, breech position, smoking and drug use, low Apgar scores, male sex, caesarean delivery, and previous miscarriages. (O'Callaghan et al 2011)

By some, "intrauterine infection/inflammation is considered to be the leading identifiable risk factor for cerebral palsy" (Bashiri et al 2006) as it so commonly causes neonatal complications, including preterm delivery. And while prematurity is a major causal factor in CP, the odds of brain injury occurring become much greater in the presence of maternal fever, the effects of inflammation, or proven infection than when the only risk factor is prematurity. (Gotsch et al 2007; Bashiri et al 2006; Grether & Nelson 1997)

Criteria (with qualifying definitions) have been developed to define an acute intrapartum hypoxic event sufficient to cause cerebral palsy by the Task Force on Neonatal Encephalopathy and Cerebral Palsy (American College of Obstetricians and Gynecologists 2003). The key criteria are summarized in Table 4.

Essential criteria (must meet all four)	• Metabolic acidosis (fetal umbilical cord arterial blood) • Encephalopathic state evident in newborn period. • Evidence of cerebral palsy at follow up (spastic quadriplegia / dyskinesia) • Exclusion of other causal mechanisms for CP
Criteria that together suggest intrapartum timing, but support rather than confirm an asphyxial cause	• Sentinel event (immediately before or during labour) • Bradycardia (sudden or prolonged), or absent fetal heart rate (with persistent, late, or variable decelerations) • Apgar score at 5 minutes or beyond of 0–3 • Multiorgan involvement in the newborn period • Early brain imaging showing nonfocal abnormalities

Table 4. Criteria used to link an acute intrapartum hypoxic event with cerebral palsy

The abnormalities of muscle control that define CP are often accompanied by other neurological and physical abnormalities, and the movement impairments that occur reflect the area of brain damaged. Muscle function is variously compromised: they may be contracted and tight (spastic); exhibit involuntary writhing movements (athetosis); have difficulty with voluntary movement (dyskinesia); and/or exhibit lack of balance and coordination with unsteady movements (ataxia). Monoplegia describes involvement of muscles in one limb; diplegia involvement of both arms or both legs; hemiplegia involvement of both limbs on one side of the body; and quadriplegia involvement of all four limbs. CP is categorized first by the type of movement/postural disturbance present, then by a description of which limbs are affected, and finally by the severity of motor impairment. These three-part descriptions are helpful in providing a general picture, but cannot give a complete description of any one person with CP. The four major classifications used to describe CP are:

- Spastic
- Athetoid/Dyskinetic
- Ataxic
- Mixed

5. Investigations relevant to causation of brain injury

Assessment at birth allows the immediate needs of the newborn infant to be provided in terms of the resuscitation required to ensure transition from intrauterine to extra uterine life. This is a key element in mitigating any residual effects of intrapartum events that have damaged the brain or compromised function. It is recognized that the immediate availability of skilled personnel able to do this is an important factor in reducing morbidity, especially amongst sick and premature newborns, and one of the central responsibilities of those providing for their care. In this regard the priorities for resuscitation include establishing effective respiration and gas exchange and cardiac output and perfusion, ensuring temperature stability to avoid hypothermia, which increases oxygen requirements, and addressing any metabolic abnormalities or potential instability. Risks related to any other intrapartum causes or aggravating factors in the context of brain function or existing injury can also be addressed; examples include the presence or potential for infection to require investigation and treatment with prophylactic antibiotics.

Once the infant is adequately resuscitated, assessment also allows the gestational age of the newborn to be assessed, physical growth parameters (height, weight and head circumference) to be measured and plotted against standard values, general physical examination to be performed to identify any systemic problems, dysmorphic features, or congenital anomalies, and full examination of general status of the infant to occur. From the standpoint of actual or potentially evolving brain injury, the neurological system is examined in detail and the status of the infant documented as a baseline, and as a means of planning the next phase of care and appropriate investigations and consultation, and beginning the process of considering the ultimate prognosis. Generally an infant born with signs of neurological depression, associated with acidosis and low Apgar scores, is considered likely to have experienced hypoxia and ischemia during labour; this becomes more and more probable where signs of neurological depression and brain dysfunction (encephalopathy) evolve in the hours or days that follow birth.

Umbilical cord blood gas analysis: Levels of fetal oxygenation and acid base status at birth can be assessed from cord blood gas measurements taken at birth. Values differ between samples taken from the vein which delivers oxygenated blood to the fetus from the placenta and one of the two cord arterial vessels that return blood from the fetus to the placenta. Recent significant hypoxic ischemic stress manifests with low oxygen levels and elevated

PCO_2, and low pH, low bicarbonate and high base deficit levels (elevated acidity). Low pH values and high base deficit values in the umbilical arterial sample correlate with an increased probability of permanent neurological sequelae following fetal exposure to hypoxia and ischemia. The criteria to define an acute intrapartum event as sufficient to cause cerebral palsy include a pH <7.00 and base deficit of >12 mmol/L. (Phelan et al 2011) The threshold for moderate or severe newborn complications associated with metabolic acidosis is an umbilical artery base deficit of >12 mmol/L. (Low et al 1997) Comparison of results from reported studies demonstrates a progression of newborn complications with increasing severity of metabolic acidosis. The mean value for arterial pH is 7.26 +/- 007 (Helwig et al 1996), and a pH of <6.8 equates with the probability of neonatal death or major neurologic dysfunction (Goodwin et al 1992)

The range of normal for cord blood gas values in term infants have been reported by Liston (Liston et al 2007). The values (mean +/- SD) for umbilical artery samples are: pH = 7.27 +/- 0.069; PCO_2 = 50.3 +/- 11.1 mmHg; HCO_3 = 22.0 +/- 3.6 mEq/L; and Base deficit = -2.7 +/- 2.8 mEq/L. For umbilical vein samples, values are: pH = 7.34 +/- 0.063; PCO_2 = 40.7 +/- 7.9 mmHg; HCO_3 = 21.4 +/- 2.5 mEq/L; and Base deficit = -2.4 +/- 2.3 mEq/L.

Acidosis occurs as a consequence of cellular hypoxia (inadequate oxygenation) and tissue ischemia (inadequate blood flow). Metabolic and respiratory forms are recognized. The test used to measure tissue acidity is a blood gas where pH is the principal unit of measurement - pH values are on a logarithmic scale so that small differences represent a major change in the level of acidosis. Normal cell function only occurs within a narrow range of pH, beyond which the ability of cells to maintain normal oxygen and carbon dioxide exchange and metabolic and mechanical function is progressively compromised as the degree of acidosis increases. The association between acidosis and development of permanent brain injury from hypoxic ischemic injury usually occurs in infants who are acidotic and also neurologically abnormal at birth, and then develop clear signs of brain dysfunction (HIE) in the newborn period.

Apgar score. Named for Virginia Apgar, this is an objective index used to evaluate the condition of a newborn infant based on a rating of 0, 1 or 2 for each of the five components: colour, heart rate, response to stimulation of the sole of the foot, muscle tone, and respiration. Scores are determined by observing/examining the newborn infant at 1, 5 and 10 minutes of age. 10 is the maximum (perfect) score. Babies that have low Apgar scores are at increased risk for CP, particularly when low scores persist in spite of resuscitation being implemented. Care with interpretation is required where an infant is premature due to an associated degree of physical immaturity, and also when scores are estimated after the fact as often occurs when active resuscitation is required.

Ultrasound (US) studies and neuroradiological scans (Computerized Tomography (CT) and/or Magnetic resonance imaging (MRI): Ultrasound provided the initial method for imaging brain structure and is still clinically attractive because of the ability to study sick infants in the nursery environment. The development of CT and advent of broadly available computer generated images of the brain greatly advanced clinical diagnosis and knowledge related to brain development and injury. The outstanding contrast resolution of MRI, superimposed on the ability to image in any plane, now allows the identification of even subtle brain malformations. (Francis et al 2006) US, CT, and MRI scans are today usually done at defined intervals after birth in order to evaluate the timing and evolution of brain injury. Pathology that can be identified includes structural developmental abnormalities, oedema (brain swelling), haemorrhage, early ischemic damage, localization of injury to cortical tissue or deep brain structures (basal ganglia and thalami), onset and evolution of scarring, onset and progression of hydrocephalus or microcephaly. Cerebral oedema following hypoxic ischaemic brain injury usually subsides in 48-72 hours, allowing recovery of brain stem function; (Perlman & Shah 2011) and intrapartum or late antepartum hypoxic ischaemic changes can be distinguished from structural brain damage due to congenital or acquired causes that occurred well prior to birth.

Advanced methods of neuroimaging are the subject of recent reviews; (Glenn & Barkovich 2006; Mathur et al 2010; Counsell et al 2010; Huang & Castillo 2008) MRI, magnetic resonance spectroscopy (MRS), and diffusion-weighted MRI have shown the patterns of brain injury that evolve after hypoxic ischaemic insults, that such patterns depend on the severity of the insult and the age at which it occurs, and that brain injury evolves over days, if not weeks. (Ferriero 2004) The anatomical regions of the brain affected by hypoxic ischemic injury define whether the insult occurred acutely and was near total in nature or occurred over a more prolonged period and was partial in degree. Deep brain structures have a high metabolic rate and hence are injured in acute profound hypoxia as significant ischemia develops before compensatory changes in cerebral perfusion can occur. In contrast, in partial and prolonged hypoxia, acidosis evolves that leads to preferential perfusion of deep brain structures; but ultimately, perfusion of the cerebral cortex is compromised and this area of the brain suffers hypoxic ischemic damage.

Fetal and post-natal MR imaging have redefined the diagnosis of congenital and acquired brain injury developing in utero and during the intra-partum period (Glenn & Barkovich 2006). Fetal MR imaging is a technique that complements prenatal sonography as it has higher contrast resolution and allows direct visualization of the fetal brain, and hence more readily identifies both cerebral malformations and destructive lesions; including agenesis of the corpus callosum, cerebellar dysplasia, germinal matrix haemorrhage, intraventricular haemorrhage, multicystic encephalomalacia, periventricular leukomalacia, periventricular nodular heterotopias, poroncephaly, and sulcation anomalies (Filey et al 1991; Aubry et al 2003).

The most common abnormality observed is enlargement of the ventricles (ventriculomegaly), which may result from multiple developmental, obstructive and destructive causes; in the majority of cases there are associated anomalies within or beyond the central nervous system, which significantly increase the probability of the affected infant having developmental delay. Destructive lesions are characterized by periventricular hyperintensity, focal defects in the germinal matrix, or areas of abnormal signal intensity in the developing white matter. Haemorrhage is usually associated with hypointense areas, although signal intensity does vary depending on the stage of evolution.

For post-natal studies diffusion-weighted MR imaging and proton MR spectroscopy are the most sensitive modalities for diagnosis in the early hours following injury and recent publications describe the major findings observed (Huang & Castillo 2008).

Electroencephalogram (EEG) recording monitors the electrical activity of the brain. Seizure activity occurring in the brain but not visible clinically may be detected by EEG. Patterns of brain waves are obtained that allow the location and relative severity of various brain pathologies to be identified. Patterns of depression of cortical brain activity on EEG have been defined (Table 2) associated with varying stages and severity of hypoxic ischemic encephalopathy (Sarnat and Sarnat 1976). Serial measurements are helpful to document the evolution and recovery of abnormal brain function and the effect of therapy.

Blood counts: The presence of abnormal findings in the white blood cell (WBC) count are strongly indicative (although not diagnostic) of the presence of bacterial infection due to septicaemia (bacteria multiplying in the blood stream). (Gerdes 2004) Very low counts indicate the inability of an infant to mount an effective immune response; elevated numbers of total WBC cells, a high proportion of neutrophils (granulocytes), and elevated numbers of primitive (band) cells indicate that stimulation of the bone marrow by inflammatory cytokines has occurred, and hence such changes evolve over time. Elevation of the band cell count is the earliest change seen in the peripheral blood count in response to an inflammatory stimulus, which is the most common cause of increased release of primitive (band) cells, although hypoxia can also result in an increase in band cell number.

Measures of haemoglobin concentration or the volume of red blood cells in the circulation are used to identify anaemia and polycythemia where too few or too many red cells are circulating respectively. Both circumstances compromise oxygen delivery; anaemia by limiting the amount of oxygen that can be transported, and polycythemia by reducing the ease with which blood flows, which also increases the risk of blood vessel occlusion (thrombosis) and is one of the mechanisms underlying stroke. Also, by following serial measurements from birth, situations can be identified where bleeding occurred while the fetus was in utero. After significant blood loss, the volume of the blood in the circulation is reduced, but the haemoglobin concentration remains the same. As physiological compensation following haemorrhage occurs, fluid is drawn into the circulation to restore blood volume and, as a consequence, haemoglobin concentration and the number of red cells per unit of volume (hematocrit) fall.

Blood chemistry: The full range of biochemical abnormalities associated with brain injury is beyond the scope of this chapter. Congenital metabolic abnormalities constitute a small but complex group of conditions that require expert assessment, investigation and management. Blood glucose, and serum calcium, and electrolyte measurements, in parallel with blood gas analysis of pH, oxygen and carbon dioxide tension, bicarbonate and base deficit, are the mainstays of clinical monitoring in brain injured infants, particularly when multisystem involvement complicates the course of neonatal encephalopathy. Fetal measurement of some parameters is feasible; scalp blood sampling in particular has relevance in assessing the evolution of hypoxia and acidosis during the later stages of labour via blood gas measurement or lactate analysis, once the membranes have ruptured and the fetal head has descended into the birth canal. Lactate is a metabolite in aerobic metabolism and reflects tissue hypoxia. (Wiberg-Itzel et al 2008)

6. Prevention of fetal brain injury

Prevention of fetal brain damage requires knowledge of the aetiologies underlying injury, awareness of the availability of preventive measures, and the opportunity to employ them to address the underlying cause. In addition, situations that may aggravate existing or evolving brain injury need to be recognized and care provided that is capable of improving outcome. Treatment of the effects of fetal brain injury often begins during the newborn period and some entities contribute to better outcome. However, the many therapies that have to continue during childhood to support infants born with brain damage and those that are entailed in providing for their care in adult life are beyond the scope of this chapter.

Maternal health and diet, parental age, and mode of conception are all relevant. (Hagberg & Mallard 2000) The risk of fetal brain injury is decreased where mothers maintain a good diet, add appropriate folic acid and iron supplements, and avoid smoking, the detrimental effects of alcohol, and exposure to TORCH infections. There are benefits to becoming a mother earlier rather than later in life and from lifestyles that promote physical health and mental wellness. In vitro-fertilization is associated with an increased risk of multiple pregnancy, preterm delivery and some specific structural defects. Good antenatal care is central to optimizing the fetal environment, detection of entities that require intervention or forward planning, and allowing pregnancy to progress to term. The fetal brain probably benefits most from prevention of avoidable preterm delivery, and therapy such as antenatal steroid use to mature the fetal lung (Hagberg & Mallard 2000) when prematurity is inevitable. Post maturity with the inherent risks of placental failure and increased fetal morbidity must be avoided, especially where at risk situations exist such as gestational diabetes. Mothers who have had previous caesarean section require special planning and supervision to avoid uterine complications that can jeopardize fetal wellbeing.

Monitoring during pregnancy should screen for and detect major genetic anomalies, as termination of pregnancy is a care option for limiting the incidence of brain injury when a fetus is known to have a major anomaly. Confirmation of gestational age by monitoring fundal height and using confirmatory ultrasound also reduces the risk of prematurity. And allows monitoring of fetal growth parameters to anticipate and manage intrauterine growth retardation, and identify placental anomalies that carry a risk of increased morbidity. Surveillance for a broad range of maternal illnesses is also possible with preventive entities available to optimize fetal growth and health, and select appropriate timing, mode and location of labour and delivery.

Surveillance and monitoring of maternal and fetal wellbeing in labour requires entities that provide for anticipation, detection and management of fetal distress. Guidelines exist in most jurisdictions based on the evidence base for best practice in obstetric management where maternal wellbeing is compromised or the fetus becomes at risk. Where necessary, advance consultation with centres specializing in obstetric and newborn care should occur for advice regarding ongoing care of the mother and plans for labour and delivery. This may require transport of the mother with the fetus still in utero if care at a higher level is necessary to optimise the chances of healthy delivery and normal fetal outcome. (Jaimovitch & Vidyasagar 1993; Macnab 1994) An important consideration in this regard is that staff are available with the required skills to comprehensively resuscitate any sick newborn infant and promptly address residual morbidity from premature or complicated delivery; this is known to reduce the risks of brain injury following premature delivery, and in situations where hypoxia and ischemia or any other form of brain injury is considered a potential risk. It also follows that after birth and appropriate resuscitation newborn care entities must be available to minimize the risks of any fetal brain injury being compounded or new injury occurring in the newborn period. Measures to do this include support of respiration and circulation, provision of a neutral thermal environment, hydration and nutrition, use of prophylactic antibiotics and management of proven infections, haematological and biochemical monitoring and neuroradiological studies, and appropriate discharge planning and follow up.

7. References

[1] Alkalay A.L., H.B. Sarnat, L. Flores-Sarnat, & C. F Simmons, "Neurologic aspects of hypoglycemia', *IMAJ*, 7, 188-192 (2005a)

[2] Alkalay A.L., L. Flores-Sarnat, H.B. Sarnat, F.G. Moser & C. F Simmons, "Brain Imaging Findings in Neonatal Hypoglycemia: Case Report and Review of 23 Cases", *Clinical Pediatrics*, 44(9), 783-790 (2005b)

[3] Al-Rawi P.G., "Near infrared spectroscopy in brain injury: today's perspective", *Acta Neurochir Suppl*, 95, 453-457, (2005)

[4] American College of Obstetricians and Gynecologists, "ACOG practice bulletin. Clinical management guidelines for obstetrician-gynecologists. Number 70. Intrapartum fetal heart rate monitoring", *Obstetrics and Gynecology*, 106, 1453-1460 (2005)

[5] American College of Obstetricians and Gynecologists, American Academy of Pediatrics. Neonatal encephalopathy and cerebral palsy: defining the pathogenesis and pathophysiology. Washington, DC: American College of Obstetricians and Gynecologists; 2003

[6] Anderson P.J. & L.W. Doyle, "Cognitive and educational deficits in children born extremely preterm", *Seminars in Perinatology*, 32(1), 51-58 (2008)

[7] Asrat T., "Intra-amniotic infection in patients with preterm prelabor rupture of membranes. Pathophysiology, detection, and management", *Clin Perinatol*, 28(4), 735-751 (2001)

[8] Aubry M.C., J.P. Aubry & M. Dommergues, "Sonographic prenatal diagnosis of central nervous system abnormalities", *Childs Nerv Syst*, 19, 391-402 (2003)

[9] Austin M., "To treat or not to treat: maternal depression, SSRI use in pregnancy and adverse neonatal effects", *Psychological Medicine*, 36, 1663–1670 (2006)

[10] Back S.A. & S.A Rivkees, "Emerging concepts in periventricular white matter injury" *Semin Perinatol*, 28(6), 405-14 (2004)

[11] Barkovich A.J., F.S. Ali, H.A. Rowley & N. Bass, "Imaging patterns of neonatal hypoglycemia", AJNR Am *J Neuroradiol*, 19, 523-528 (1998)

[12] Barks J.D.E. & F.S. Silverstein, "Inflammation and neonatal brain injury" (Edo) S.M. Donn, S.K. Sinha & M.L. Chiswick, *Birth asphyxia and the brain: Basic science and clinical implications*, Futura Publishing Company, Armonk NY, 71-88 (2002)

[13] Bashiri A., E. Burstein & M. Mazor, "Cerebral palsy and fetal inflammatory response syndrome: a review", *J Perinat Med*, 34, 5-12 (2006)

[14] Bergh T, A Ericson, T Hillensjö, KG Nygren & UB Wennerholm, "Deliveries and children born after in-vitro fertilization in Sweden 1982–95 a retrospective cohort study", *Lancet*, 354, 1579–1585 (1999)

[15] Beyene S.V., P, Shah & M. Perlman, "Association between hematologic findings and brain injury due to neonatal hypoxic-ischemic encephalopathy", *Am J Perinatol*, 26(4), 285-302 (2009)

[16] Brady K.M., J.K. Lee, K.K. Kibler. P.S. Smielewski, M. Czosnyka, R.B. Easley, R.C. Koehler & D.H. Shafner, "Continuous time-domain analysis of cerebrovascular autoregulation using near-infrared spectroscopy", *Stroke,* 38, 2818-2825 (2007)

[17] Burns C.M., M.A. Rutherford, J.P. Boardman & F.M. Cowan, "Patterns of cerebral injury and neurodevelopmental outcomes after symptomatic hypoglycemia", *Pediatrics,* 122(1), 65-74 (2008)

[18] Canavan T.P., H.N. Simhan & S. Caritis, "An evidence-based approach to the evaluation and treatment of premature rupture of membranes: Part 11", *JAMA,* 59(9), 678-689 (2004)

[19] Chen S., K. Sakatani, W. Lichty, P. Ning, S. Zhao & H, Zuo, "Auditory-evoked cerebral blood oxygenation changes in hypoxic-ischemic encephalopathy of newborn infants monitored by near infrared spectroscopy", *Early Hum Dev,* 67, 113–122 (2002)

[20] Counsell S.J., Tranter S.L. & Rutherford M.A., "Magnetic resonance imaging of brain injury in the high-risk term infant", *Seminars Perinatol,* 34(1), 67-78 (2010)

[21] Cowan F., M. Rutherford, F. Groenendaal, P. Eken, E. Mercuri, G. M. Bydder, L. C. Meiners, L. M.S. Dubowitz & L.S. de Vries, "Origin and timing of brain lesions with neonatal encephalopathy", *Lancet,* 361(9359), 736-742 (2003)

[22] De Haan T.R., G.V. Wezel-Meijler, M. F. C. Beersma, J.S. von Lindern, S. G. Van Duinen & F. J. Walther, "Fetal stroke and congenital parvovirus B19 infection complicated by activated protein C resistance", *Acta Paediatrica,* 95(7), 863-867 (2006)

[23] Dow-Edwards D. L., "Cocaine effects on fetal development: A comparison of clinical and animal research findings," *Neurotoxicol Teratol,* 13(3), 347-352 (1991)

[24] Efron D., M. South, J.J. Volpe & T. Inder, "Cerebral injury in association with profound iatrogenic hyperglycemia in a neonate", *Eur J Ped Neurol,* 7, 167-171 (2003)

[25] Ehrenberg H.M. & B.M. Mercer, "Antibiotics and the management of preterm premature rupture of the fetal membranes", *Clin Perinatol,* 28(4), 807-818 (2001)

[26] Feigin V., N. Anderson, A. Gunn, A. Rogers, & C. Anderson, "The emerging role of therapeutic hypothermia in acute stroke", *Lancet Neurol,* 2, 529 (2004)

[27] Fellman V. & A.K. Raivio, "Reperfusion injury as the mechanism of brain damage after perinatal asphyxia", *Pediatr Res,* 41, 599–606 (1997)

[28] Ferrari M., D.A. Wilson, D.F. Hanley & R.J. Traystman, "Effects of graded hypotension on cerebral blood flow, blood volume, and mean transit time in dogs", *Am J Physiol,* 262(6), H1908–H1914 (1992)

[29] Ferrari M., L. Mottola & V. Quaresima, "Principles, techniques and limitations of near infrared spectroscopy", *Can J Appl Physiol,* 29(4), 463-487 (2004)

[30] Ferrari M., M. Muthalib & V Quaresima, "The use of near-infrared spectroscopy in understanding skeletal muscle physiology: recent developments", *Phil Trans R Soc A,* 369, 4577-4590 (2011)

[31] Ferriero D.M., "Neonatal brain injury", *New Engl J Med,* 351(19), 1985-95 (2004)

[32] Filly R.A., R.B. Goldstein & P.W. Callen, "Fetal ventricle: importance of routine obstetric sonography", *Radiology,* 181, 1-7 (1991)

[33] Francis F., G. Meyer, C Fallet-Bianco, S. Moreno, C. Kappeler, A. Cabrera Soccorro, F P.D. Tuy, C. Beldjord & J. Chelly, "Human disorders of cortical development: from past to present", Eur J Neurosci, 23, 877-893 (2006)

[34] Gagnon R.E., A. Leung, A.J. Macnab "Variations in regional cerebral blood volume in neonates associated with nursery care events", *Am J Perinatol,* 16(1), 7-11 (1999)
[35] Garite T.J., "Management of premature rupture of membranes" *Clin Perinatol,* 28(4), 837-847 (2001)
[36] Gerdes J.S., "Diagnosis and management of bacterial infections in the neonate', *Pediatr Clin N Am,* 51, 939-959 (2004)
[37] Gilbert W.M., B.N. Jacoby, G. Xing, B. Danielsen & L.H. Smith, "Adverse obstetric events are associated with significant risks of cerebral palsy", *Am J Obstet Gynecol,* 204(5), e15-6 (2011)
[38] Ginsberg M.D. & R.E. Meyers, "Fetal brain damage following maternal carbon monoxide intoxication: an experimental study", *Acta Obstet Gynec Scand,* 53, 309-317 (1974)
[39] Glenn G.A & Barkovich A.J., "Magnetic resonance imaging of the fetal brain and spine: an increasingly important tool in prenatal diagnosis, Part 1", *Am J Neuroradiol,* 27:1604-1611 (2006)
[40] Goodwin T.M., I. Belai, P. Hernandez, M. Durand & R.H. Paul, "Asphyxial complications in the term newborn with severe umbilical acidemia", *Am J Obstet Gynecol,* 167, 637-641 (1992)
[41] Gotsch F., R. Romero, J.P. Kusanovic, S. Mazaki-Tovi, B.L. Pineles, O. Erez, J. Espinoza & S.S. Hassan, "The fetal inflammatory response syndrome" *Clin Obstet Gynecol,* 50(3), 652-83 (2007)
[42] Graham E.M., Ruis K.A., Hartman A.L., Northington F.J. & Fox H.E., "A systematic review of the role of intrapartum hypoxia-ischemia in the causation of neonatal encephalopathy", *Am J Obstet Gynecol.* 199(6):587-952 (2008)
[43] Grether J.K. & K. B. Nelson, "Maternal infection and cerebral palsy in infants of normal birth weight", *JAMA,* 278(3), 207-211 (1997)
[44] Guay J. & J Lachapelle, "No evidence for superiority of air or oxygen for neonatal resuscitation: a meta- analysis", Can J Anesth, doi 10.1007/s12630-011-9589-0 (2011)
[45] Gunn A.J., Cerebral hypothermia for prevention of brain injury following perinatal asphyxia", *Current Opinion in Pediatrics,* 12(2), 111-115 (2000)
[46] Gunn A.J., & P.D. Gluckman, "Head cooling for neonatal encephalopathy: The state of the art", *Clinical Obstetrics and Gynecology,* 50(3), 636-651 (2007)
[47] Hagberg H. & C. Mallard, "Antenatal brain injury: aetiology and possibilities of prevention", *Seminars in Neonatology,* 5(1), 41-51 (2000)
[48] Haldane J.S., "Respiration", Yale University Press, New Haven (1922).
[49] Halopainen I.E. & H.B. Lauren, "Glutamate signaling in the pathophysiology and therapy of prenatal insults", Pharmacol Biochem Behav, (2011), doi:10.1016/j.pbb.2011.03.016
[50] Hamaoka T., K.K. McCully, V. Quaresima, Y. Yamamoto & B Chance. "Near-infrared spectroscopy/imaging for monitoring muscle oxygenation and oxidative metabolism in healthy and diseased humans", *J Biomed Optics,* 12(6), 062105 (2007)
[51] Hankins G.D. V., Koen S., Gei A.F., Lopez S. M., Van Hoek J. W., Anderson G.D., "Neonatal organ system injury in acute birth asphyxia sufficient to result in neonatal encephalopathy. *Obstet Gynecol,* 99, 688-91 (2002)

[52] Hansen M., J. J. Kurinczuk, C. Bower & Sandra Webb, "The Risk of Major Birth Defects after Intracytoplasmic Sperm Injection and in Vitro Fertilization", *N Engl J Med,* (346), 725-730 (2002)

[53] Hatten M.E., "New directions in neuronal migration", *Science,* 297, 1660-1663 (2002)

[54] Heffner L.J., "Advanced maternal age- How old is too old?" *N Engl J Med,* 351, 1927-1929 (2004)

[55] Helwig J.T., J.T. Parer, S.J. Kilpatrick & R.K. Laros, "Umbilical cord acid-base state: What is normal?" *Am J Obstet Gynecol,* 174(6), 1807-1814 (1996)

[56] Higgins R., T.N.K. Rau, J. Perlman, D.V. Azzopardi, L.R. Blackmon, R.H. Clark, A.D. Edwards, D.M. Ferriero, P.D. Gluckman, A.J. Gunn, S.E. Jacobs, D Jenkins-Eicher, A.H. Jobe, A.R. Laptook, M.H. LeBlanc, C. Palmer, S. Shankaran, R.F. Soll, A.R. Stark, M.Thoresen, J. Wyatt, & the hypothermia workshop speakers and discussants, "Hypothermia and perinatal asphyxia: executive summary of the National Institute of Child Health and Human Development workshop", *J. Pediatr,* 148, 170-175 (2006)

[57] Hoshi Y., "Functional near-infrared spectroscopy: current status and future prospects," *J Biomed Optics,* 12(6), 062106, (2007)

[58] Huang B.J. & M. Castillo, "Hypoxic-ischemic brain injury: imaging findings from birth to adulthood", *Radiographics,* 28, 417-439 (2008)

[59] Jablonski N., "Skin. A natural history", University of California Press (2006)

[60] Jaimovich D.G. & G. Vidyasagar, "Transport medicine", *Pediatr Clin N Am,* 40(2), (1993)

[61] Karimzadeh P., S. Tabarestani & M. Ghofrani, Hypoglycemia-occipital syndrome: A specific neurologic syndrome following neonatal hypoglycemia?", *J Child Neurol,* 26, 152-159 (2011)

[62] Kendall G. & D. Peebles, "Acute fetal hypoxia: the modulating effect of infection", *Early Hum Dev,* 81, 27-34 (2005)

[63] Khwaja O. & J.J. Volpe, "Pathogenesis of cerebral white matter injury of prematurity", *Arch Dis Child Fetal Neonatal Ed,* 93, F153-F161 (2008)

[64] Kilbride H.W. & D.W. Thibeault, "Neonatal complications of preterm premature rupture of membranes. Pathophysiology and management", *Clin Perinatol,* 28(4), 761-785 (2001)

[65] Lapointe A. & K.J. Barrington, "Pulmonary hypertension and the asphyxiated newborn", *J Pediatr,* 158, e19-24 (2011)

[66] Larroche J.C., F. Encha-Razavi, & F. de Vries, "Central nervous system", Ed. E Gilbert-Barnes (ed) *Potter's pathology of the fetus and infant,* Mosby, St. Louis, 1028-1150 (1997)

[67] Lattimore K.A., S.M. Donn, N. Kaciroti, A.R. Kemper, C.R. Neal & D.M. Vazquez, "Selective serotonin reuptake inhibitor (SSRI) use during pregnancy and effects on the fetus and newborn: A meta-analysis", *J Perinatol,* 25, 595-604 (2005)

[68] Law, K.L. L.R. Stroud, L.L. LaGasse, R. Niaura, J. Liu & B.M. Lester, "Smoking during pregnancy and newborn neurobehavior", *Pediatrics,* 111, 1318-1323 (2003)

[69] Lee S.E., R. Romero, H. Jung, C.W. Park, J.S. Park JS & B.H. Yoon. "The intensity of the fetal inflammatory response in intraamniotic inflammation with and without microbial invasion of the amniotic cavity', *Am J Obstet Gynecol,* 197(3), 294.e1-294.e6 (2007)

[70] Limperopoulos C., R.L. Robertson, N.R. Sullivan, H. Bassan & A.J. du Plessis, "Cerebellar injury in term infants : clinical characteristics, magnetic resonance imaging findings and outcome", *Pediatr Neurol,* 41(1), 1-8 (2009)
[71] Lin P. Y., S.I. Lin, T. Penney & J.J. Chen, "Applications of near infrared spectroscopy and imaging for motor rehabilitation in stroke patients", *J Med Biol Eng,* 29(5), 210-221 (2009)
[72] Liston R.M., D. Sawchuck & D. Young, "Fetal health surveillance: Antepartum and intrapartum consensus guideline", *J Obs Gyn Canada,* 29(9, Suppl 4), S3-S56 (2007)
[73] Logitharajah P., M.A. Rutherford & F.M. Cowan, "Hypoxic-ischemic encephalopathy in preterm infants: antecedent factors, brain imaging, and outcome", *Pediatr Res,* 66(2), 222-229 (2009)
[74] Lotzoff B. & M.K. Georgieff, "Iron deficiency and brain development", *Seminars in Pediatric Neurology,* 13(3), 158-165 (2006)
[75] Low J.A., B.G. Lindsay & J. Derrick, "Threshold of metabolic acidosis associated with newborn complications", *Am J Obstet Gynecol,* 177, 1391-1394 (1997)
[76] Macnab A.J., "Paediatric interfacility transport: Standards of care, organization and principles", *Pediatr Anaesth,* 4, 351-357 (1994)
[77] Macnab A.J., R.E. Gagnon & F.A. Gagnon, "Near infrared spectroscopy for intraoperative monitoring of the spinal cord", *Spine,* 27(1), 17-20, (2002)
[78] Macnab A.J., R.E. Gagnon, F.A. Gagnon & J. LeBlanc, "NIRS monitoring of brain and spinal cord: Detection of adverse intraoperative events", *Spectroscopy,* 17, 483-490, (2003)
[79] Macnab A.J., "Biomedical applications of near infrared spectroscopy", Eds. A. Barth & P.I. Haris, *Biological and Biomedical Spectroscopy Volume 2 Advances in Biomedical Spectroscopy*, IOS Press, Amsterdam, 305-402 (2009)
[80] Macones G.A., G.D. Hankins, C.Y. Spong, J. Hauth & T. Moore, "The 2008 national institute of child health and human development workshop report on electronic fetal monitoring: Update on definitions, interpretation, and research guidelines", *JOGNN,* 37, 510-515 (2008)
[81] Malaeb S. & O. Dammann, "Fetal inflammatory response and brain injury in the preterm newborn", *J Child Neurol,* 24, 1119-1126 (2009)
[82] Marin O. & J.L. Rubenstein, "Cell migration in the forebrain", *Annu Rev Neurosci,* 26, 441-483 (2003)
[83] Mathur A.M., Neil J.J. & Inder T.E., "Understanding brain injury and neurodevelopmental disabilities in the preterm infant: the evolving role of advanced magnetic resonance imaging", *Seminars Perinatol,* 34(1):57-66 (2010)
[84] Mercer B.M., "Preterm premature rupture of the membranes: diagnosis and management", *Clin Perinatol,* 31, 765-782 (2004)
[85] Meyers R.E., "Two classes of dysergic brain abnormality and their conditions of occurrence", *Arch Neurol,* 29, 394-399 (1973)
[86] Meyers R.E., "Four patterns of perinatal brain damage and their conditions of occurrence in primates", (Eds) B.S. Meldrum & C.D. Marsden, *Advances in Neurology volume 10,* Raven Press, New York (1975)
[87] Meyers R.E., "Fetal asphyxia due to umbilical cord compression: metabolic and brain pathologic consequences", *Biol Neonate,* 26(1–2), 21–43 (1975)

[88] Murkin J.M. & M. Arango, "Near-infrared spectroscopy as an index of brain and tissue oxygenation", *Br J Anaesth, 103 (Suppl. 1),* i3-i13, (2009)
[89] Nelson K.B. & J.H. Ellenberg, "Apgar scores as predictors of chronic neurologic disability", *Pediatrics,* 68, 36–44 (1981)
[90] Oberlander T.F., W. Warburton, S. Misri, J. Aghajanian & C. Hertzman, "Neonatal outcomes after prenatal exposure to selective serotonin reuptake inhibitor antidepressants and maternal depression using population-based linked health data", *Arch Gen Psychiatry,*63, 898-906 (2006)
[91] O'Callaghan M.E., A.H. MacLennan, C.S. Gibson, G.L. McMichael, E.A. Haan, J.L. Broadbent, P.N. Goldwater, & G.A. Dekker, for the Australian Collaborative Cerebral Palsy Research Group, Epidemiologic associations with cerebral palsy", *Obstetrics and Gynecology,* 118(3), 576-582, (2011)
[92] Okereafor A., J. Allsop, S.J. Counsell, J. Fitzpatrick, D. Azzopardi, M.A. Rutherford & F.M. Cowan, "Patterns of brain injury in neonates exposed to perinatal sentinel events", *Pediatrics,* 121, 906-914 (2008)
[93] Oudijk M.A., R.H. Gooskens. P. Stoutenbeek, L.S. De Vries, G.H. Visser & E.J. Meijbooms, "Neurological outcome of children who were treated for fetal tachycardia complicated by hydrops", *Ultrasound Obstet Gynecol,* 24, 154-158 (2004)
[94] Owen-Reece H., M. Smith, C.E. Elwell & J.C. Goldstone, "Near infrared spectroscopy", *Br J Anaesth,* 82, 418–26, (1999)
[95] Ozduman K., B. R Pober, P. Barnes, J. A. Copel, E.A.Ogle, C.C. Duncan & L. R Ment, "Fetal Stroke", *Ped Neurol,* 30(3), 151-162 (2004)
[96] Perlman J.M., "Interruption of placental blood flow during labor: potential systemic and cerebral organ consequences", *J Pediatr,* 158, e1-4 (2011)
[97] Perlman M. & P.S. Shah, "Hypoxic ischemic encephalopathy: challenges in outcome and prediction", J Pediatr, 158, e51-54 (2011)
[98] Phelan J. P., L. M. Korst, & G. I. Martin, "Application of Criteria Developed by the Task Force on Neonatal Encephalopathy and Cerebral Palsy to Acutely Asphyxiated Neonates", *Obstet Gynecol,* 118(4), 824-830 (2011)
[99] Porat S., E.Y. Anterby, Y. Hamani & S. Yagel, "Fetal supraventricular tachycardia diagnosed and treated at 13 weeks of gestation: a case report", *Ultrasound Obstet Gynecol,* 21, 302-305 (2003)
[100] Razic P., "Evolving concepts of cortical radial and areal specification", *Progr Brain Res,* 136, 265-280 (2002)
[101] Rees S. & T. Inder, "Fetal and neonatal origins of altered brain development", *Early Human Development,* 81(9), 753-761 (2005)
[102] Riley E.P. & C.L. McGee, "Fetal alcohol spectrum disorders: An overview with emphasis on changes in brain and behavior", *Exp Biol Med,* 230(60), 357-365 (2005)
[103] Robertson C.M.T. & M. Perlman, "Follow-up of the term infant after hypoxic-ischemic encephalopathy", Paediatr Child Health, 11(5) 278-282 (2006)
[104] Roland E.H., A. Hill, M.G. Norman, O. Flodmark & A.J. Macnab, "Selective brainstem injury in an asphyxiated newborn", *Ann Neurol,* 23(1), 89-92 (1988)
[105] Roland E.H., K. Poskitt, E. Rodriguez, B.A. Lupton & A. Hill, "Perinatal hypoxic-ischemic thalamic injury: clinical features and neuroimaging", *Ann Neurol,* 44(20), 161-166 (1998)
[106] Rolfe P., "In vivo near-infrared spectroscopy", *An Rev Biomed Eng,* 2, 715-754 (2000)

[107] Royal College of Obstetricians and Gynaecologists, "The use of electronic fetal monitoring. The use and interpretation of cardiotocography in intrapartum fetal surveillance. Evidence-based clinical practice guideline number 8. Clinical effectiveness support unit. London, UK: Royal College of obstetricians and Gynaecologists Press. www.rcog.org.uk/resources/public/pdf/efm.guideline.final2may2001.pdf (2005)

[108] Ruis K.A., K.A. Ruis, C.U. Lehmann, F.J. Northington, F.J. Lin & E.M. Graham, "Neonatal brain imaging and the identification of metabolic acidemia and hypoxic-ischemic encephalopathy", *J Matern Fetal Neonatal Med,* 22(10), 823—828 (2009)

[109] Sakatani K., Y. Xie, W. Lichty, S. Li & H. Zuo, "Language-activated cerebral blood oxygenation and hemodynamic changes of the left prefrontal cortex in post stroke aphasic patients: a near infrared spectroscopy (NIRS)", *Stroke,* 29, 1299–1304(1998)

[110] Sarnat H.B. & Sarnat M.S., "Neonatal encephalopathy following fetal distress: a clinical and electroencephalographic study", *Arch Neurol,* 33(10), 696-705 (1976)

[111] Schieve L.A., S. F. Meikle, C. Ferre, H. B. Peterson, G Jeng & L. S. Wilcox, "Low and Very Low Birth Weight in Infants Conceived with Use of Assisted Reproductive Technology", *N Engl J Med,* (346), 731-737 (2002)

[112] Schulzke S.M., S. Rao & S.K. Patole, "A systematic review of cooling for neuroprotection in neonates with hypoxic ischemic encephalopathy - are we there yet?", *BMC Pediatrics,* 7, 30 (2007) doi: 10.1186/1471-2431-7-30

[113] Shadgan B., Reid W. D., Gharakhanlou R., Stothers L. & Macnab A. J., "Wireless near-infrared spectroscopy of skeletal muscle oxygenation and hemodynamics during exercise and ischaemia", *Spectroscopy,* 23 233-41 (2009)

[114] Simonson S.G. & C.A. Piantadosi, "Near-infrared spectroscopy, clinical applications", *Crit Care Clin,* 12(4), 1019-1029, (1996)

[115] Stromberg B., G. Dahlquist, A. Ericson, O. Finnstrom, M. Koster & K Stjernqvist, "Neurological sequelae in children born after in-vitro fertilization: a population based study", *Lancet,* 360(9344), 718-719 (2002)

[116] Sukhov A., Y. Wu, G. Xing, L.H. Smith & W.M. Gilbert, "Risk factors associated with cerebral palsy in preterm infants", *J Mat Fetal Neonatal Med,* doi:10.3109/14767058.2011.564689 (2011)

[117] Suzuki S., S. Takasaki, T. Ozaki & Y. Kobayashi, "A tissue oxygenation monitor using NIR spatially resolved spectroscopy", *Proc SPIE,* 3597, 582-592 (1999)

[118] Tasker R.C., "Seizures" Eds. A.J. Macnab, D.J Macrae & R. Henning. *Care of the critically ill child.* Churchill Livingstone London, Toronto, New York. (2001)

[119] Tobias J.D., "Cerebral oxygenation monitoring: near-infrared spectroscopy", *Expert Rev Med Devices,* 3(2), 235-243, (2006)

[120] Todd K.G., L.L. Jantzie & P. Cheung, "Oxidative stress in neonatal hypoxic-ischemic encephalopathy", Eds. N. Gadoth & H.H. Gobel, Oxidative stress and free radical damage in neurology. *Oxidative stress in applied basic research and clinical practice,* 47-63 doi: 10.1007/978-1-60327-514-9_4 Springer Science and Business Media LLC (2011)

[121] Vannucci R.C. & J.M. Perlman, Interventions for perinatal hypoxic-ischemic encephalopathy. *Pediatrics,* 100, 1004–1014 (1997)

[122] Volpe J.J., "Brain injury in the premature infant - from pathogenesis to prevention", *Brain and Development,* 19(8), 519-534 (1997)

[123] Volpe J.J., "Intracranial hemorrhage: Germinal matrix-intraventricular hemorrhage of the premature infant. (Ed) J.J. Volpe, *Neurology of the newborn*, Fourth Edition, Saunders, Philadelphia, Pa. 428-493 (2001a)

[124] Volpe J.J., "Neurobiology of periventricular leukomalacia in the premature infant", *Pediatr Res*, 50(5), 533-562 (2001b)

[125] von Bel F., C.A. Dorrepaal, J.N.L. Benders, P.E.M. Zeeuwe, M.V.D. Bor & H.M. Berger, "Changes in cerebral hemodynamics and oxygenation in the first 24 h after birth asphyxia", *Pediatrics*, 92, 365–371 (1993)

[126] Wiberg-Itzel E., C. Lipponer, M. Norman, A, Herbst, D. Prebensen, A. Hansson, A.L. Bryngelsson, M. Christoffersson, M. Sennstrom, U.B. Wennerholm & L. Nordstrom, "Determination of pH or lactate in fetal scalp blood in management of intrapartum fetal distress: randomized controlled multicentre trial", *BMJ*, 336(7656), 1284-1287 (2008)

[127] Wolf M., M. Ferrari & V. Quaresima, "Progress of near-infrared spectroscopy and topography for brain and muscle clinical applications", *J Biomed Optics*, 12(6), 062104 (2007)

[128] Wu Y.W., G.J. Escobar, J.K. Grether, L.A. Croen, J.D. Greene & T.B. Newman, "Chorioamnionitis and cerebral palsy in term and near-term infants", *JAMA*, 290, 2677-2372 (2003)

[129] Wyatt J.S., "Near infrared spectroscopy in asphyxial brain injury", *Clin Perinatol*, 20, 369–378 (1993)

[130] Yodh A.G. & D.A. Boas, "Functional Imaging with diffusing light", Ed. T. Vo-Dinh, *Biomedical Photonics Handbook*, CRC Press, Florida, USA, 21-1 – 21-45 (2003)

[131] Yudkin P.L., A. Johnson, L.M. Clover & K.W. Murphy. "Assessing the contribution of birth asphyxia to cerebral palsy in term singletons", *Pediatr Perinatal Epidemiol*, 9, 156 -70 (1995)

2

Brain Damage and Long-Lasting Sequels in Childhood: What Does Cerebral Palsy (CP) Mean at the Beginning of the XXI Century?

D. Truscelli
Rehab Unit, Pediatrics Department at the Universitary Hospital of Bicêtre (Paris)
France

1. Introduction

1.1 A great question: The patient and a "legal" definition of CP

In an article from DMCN[1], a question is discussed by many authors, with the aim to consider carefully, CP syndrome versus disease, that is to say a human being suffering from his birth on from a lot of sequels subsequent to brain damage.

The common CP factor consists in permanent posture and movement disorders, with or without mental difficulties, leading to the more patent functional handicap, in standing, sitting, walking, and stiff or impaired upper limb movements. Nowadays, it seems no more adequate to sum up the CP patients by their motor troubles but it is necessary to think over the other factors of limitation to integrate the normal social mainstream at any age, from perception, behaviour, cognition, communication troubles and epilepsy seizures.

CP, an umbrella term? So, might it be really necessary to extend the historical and usual definition of the CP syndrome admitted as sequels of non progressive cerebral damage, whist may occur during the development of the fœtus' brain or of the new born baby's one. From an epidemiological and scientific point of view, it does not seem relevant to include patients suffering from similar neurological sequels but after cerebral tumours or traumatisms, brain infections, epileptic attacks, genetic (such as Lesch-Nyhan syndrome, glutaric aciduria disease) and degenerative brain diseases.

In fact, in a medical practise, so called CP patients from different aetiological causes are attended to, cured, treated and followed up in same clinics or medical centres, often with similar rehab techniques, similar drugs, similar surgical decisions on musculoskeletal problems, and secondary orthopedic ones; there, the children's various learning difficulties are analysed to support them in their scholarship. Here, too, the parents may find a necessary help and support to cope with the daily life constraints and talk about their concern in the future with caregivers, social workers and other parents.

1.2 Brain damage, mental capacities and development

Physical (mechanical) limitation and mental development may be different, it depends on the aetiology of the disease, on the type and extent of the cerebral lesions. The independence between poor body state and intellectual power has been pointed out by G. Tardieu who in 1952 described the IMC, (standing for Infirmité Motrice Cérébrale =IMC) as a little part (1/3) out of the global term of CP, known at that time as infantile encephalopathies. The most mental impaired patients were not to be neglected or to be let aside. Tardieu wished to adopt a basic experimental attitude to check his hypothesis. How strong is the voluntary and conscious patient's participation during rehab sessions to recover part of his motor abilities? The subject's role by his interaction is obvious to understand: rehab techniques and relationship with a caregiver allow a better learning and memorizing.

The hypothesis was not checked, now it is known that functional improvement is not completely linked with a mental potential : a lot of CP children with poor mental means are able to walk easily enough -as they can - sometimes by odd pattern even without any rehab session! (see further innate circuitery).

Another important aim, in the nineteen fifties, was a social necessity, to underline and prove that IMC with good mental capacities were eligible to go to normal public schools. In France it was very difficult, even impossible, to go to school with a motor impairment from cerebral palsy*. It may seem stunning to emphasize that mental development is possible without a necessary sensori-motor experience, but that is so! The sole mental representation of action (as described by Piaget), the access to symbolism and abstraction do not come from manipulation but from a process of perception and cognition work. Some athetosic patients (especially kernicterus victims) without any capacity to take and seize an object or to touch it carefully, may reach a high mental level, without any perception trouble. Some of them with limited motor oral means to express themselves, can build up an inner language, learn literacy and are able to typewrite by sophisticated software and to use remote commands. Before electronics performances existed, and sometimes even to day, because it is cheap and easy to make, they are used to show photos, pictures or ideograms from a board or notebook, by visual signs, mimics or simple gesture to pass a message to their parents or friends. *Many CP adults in wheelchairs and using electronic software, best bear witness*[2] *to their scholar success or relative failure, to their effort to integrate society or to keep their difficulties in everyday life under control.*

But it is true, risk is high that cerebral damage affects the cerebral networks which participate in the mental development: some recent studies predict about 50% of global cases.

1.3 CP and somatic troubles in child and adult life

Although the cerebral damage itself is not progressive, its clinical expression is "not unchanging" over time. Parents and caregivers know and are afraid of loss of mobility performances, weight of somatic problems, as nutritional failure, feeding difficulties,

* After the 2nd world war many epidemics, all was done for the poliomyelitic children and adults, to let them come back to their previous social status.

sialorrhea, gastro-oesophageal reflux and its complications (insomnia), constipation, respiratory difficulties, sphincterian problems, skin damages. Later, one has to cope with early aging and numerous new health problems, not only psycho-medical ones but also social consequences and lifetime high cost.

One has to try and attenuate them as far as possible!

2. Prevalence

For the last 50 years, when the means of prevention of the neonatal problems and delivery conditions have been organized, the rate of 2 CP children per 1000 children born alive has not changed. In all countries, the most numerous CP are male patients and first born in the family.

The number of premature births is as high as 8%, especially with the babies born at or before 31 weeks of gestational age[3].

A lot of recent studies point out the responsibility of prenatal causes of CP. So, up to date research is carried out in the field of neuro-protection of the foetus animal (mice) brain against excito-toxic challenge: the purpose is to apply to the mother and/or new born baby the experiments that have proved beneficial.

3. Etiology

Since 1960, morbidity has been changing. Kernicterus has disappeared, thanks to efficient preventive measures; miserable delivery conditions have been improved by monitoring system, planned caesarean sections; the legal dispositions to protect pregnant women and the quality of neonatal reanimation, in specific units, has played a great role.

Nowadays, more and more patients with CP, around 50% , are ex-premature infants.

15% are term-born but under hypoxic conditions from obstetrical complications or circulatory attacks on the part of the mother or the child or both, before or during delivery.

The hemiplegic palsies represent 20% of the total cases and have often no recognised explanation; the Xray exams often discover impressive cerebral lesion(s), with a real discrepancy according to the state of the baby.

But, it is necessary to know that no radiological cause may be detectable in some infants who have abnormal mental/motor development, it requires a lot of biological complementary exams to determine the pathogenesis of the so-called CP, especially if a hereditary cause is suspected.

4. Early diagnosis of CP is advised

Putting the diagnosis as soon as possible, from 7/9 months after birth, is usual.

For which purpose? From a rehab point of view, the early diagnosis plan is to avoid that the baby has an interval of therapeutic silence, which can be considered as dangerous.

It would allow "to stimulate the brain plasticity"[4] and so develop the sensori-motor synaptic activity; all these measures would be able to lead the baby to progress and reach a personal autonomy. From a human position, it would also help the parents to deal with their questioning about an unforeseen future.

Here, we shall not explain classical and necessary exam of paediatricians but we shall focus on innovative efforts to understand how the brain damage reveals itself.

We insist that paediatricians have to be aware of not misinterpreting the transient motor abnormalities and CP permanent neurological troubles, in the first year of life.

Many expert clinicians have opened new tracks to find out the first signs of a qualitative motor deficiency, which breaks the natural pattern of the motor development from head - to - toes and allows an early diagnosis.

We cannot really go on speaking about a quantitative psycho-motor delay, because the child is a premature and would need more time to be at a normal level.

The concept of corrected age according to the degree of prematurity must be precisely discussed if applied to ex-premature babies of more than 6/9 months of civil age.

A poor Apgar score at five minutes' life is not sufficient to predict the future neurological development, it depends on other parameters surrounding prenatal and birth conditions.

The long lasting presence of the archaic reflexes (such as automatic walking) is no longer considered as abnormal. But what is quite different is to observe the presence of asymetric **neck** reflexes[†], regularly induced by passive head rotation of the patient, and stereotyped , which means a severe brain impairment!

With the young baby under 12/18 months, CP seems like being a disorganisation of the motor development more than a delay in the sequential milestones development. Parents are expecting more and more performances from their baby, who looks "strange", because he is both, stiff and flaccid, unable to adapt his posture to the mother's carrying, to shape or control his reactions and actions: to some degree such a CP baby because of his body stiffness may seem to progress better than a normal child, due to his hypertonic up-righting reactions that are considered as very good and advanced performances at such a young age!

Each medical doctor or physiotherapist involved in the diagnosis is used to some different techniques, according to his professional formation, to evaluate how the infant manages its integration between extension and flexion against gravity.

All of them are very careful, knowing a child cannot participate to the assessment because he may be tired from his birth conditions or other somatic reasons or because he is convalescing. At that time, afraid of putting a false positive or negative diagnosis, medical doctors or caregivers are obliged to make a new assessment under better clinical conditions.

† different is the asymetric and changing attitude of a normal baby, known as "fencer attitude"

Is it possible to do a very early diagnosis with a very young and frail premature, because he is at high risk of permanent cerebral damage? Many doctors claim to be cautious and ready to refer to the X ray imaging and other complementary exams to gather items of high risk or to be certain. Indeed, in addition, infant sex and preterm premature rupture of membranes or preterm labour are, also, independent predictors of CP.

Reanimation methods often play a role in restoring the baby's health!

5. The" innate motor circuitery" has modified the knowledge of the infantile motor development

This ciçrcuitery differs from the archaic reflexes, which disappear progressively when cerebral high level control becomes predominant. It represents the basis of the involuntary and automatic regulation which is not learnt at the contact with environment, it is done genetically. These pre-programmed reactions, which keep their spatial shape all life long, become more and more efficient, because the muscular bodies have been growing at the same time as baby's will to participate. Some authors speak of maturation of the cerebral system.

Since 1970 approximately, a new conception of the motor development (nativism[5]) has allowed to us to insist on the examination of the innate patterns involving structural and global motor organisation (*a celluloid doll body is designed according to the general pattern shaping a baby: the lower limb have semi-flexed knees, the feet are at right angle on the legs, upper limbs with semi-flexed elbows, hands opened; in supine position, in the hand of a girl, the doll "bears its head" aligned with trunk*!)

Briefly, the baby possesses all the natural resources to progress by himself. We know that the basic organisation is obvious in the term born infant and gives him a general motor pattern, which follows a positive evolution during the first year of life. So we can describe a lot of reactions, the head and trunk up righting ones, pull - to - sit, antigravity lateral reactions, ventral suspension, lift manoeuvre, lateral protecting reactions, if someone pushes him on one side…

If the innate circuitery - managing the spontaneous motor expression and automatic reactivity against gravity- failed or is altered at any degree, it means that a more or less important structural injury, is present in the cerebral motor network. This posturo-motor damage is permanent does not depend on intellectual development. The damage cannot deeply be modified by any exercise, passive or active : all life long, because he has lost the automatic quick control, the patient will have to keep or recover his balance under conscious control and voluntary motor command : it represents a relevant clue for care givers to think of very difficult or impossible walking. The patient must progress, while standing by or acting, in using a slow and never perfect correction; if he cannot do it or does not know how or has not a sufficient mental level , he is submitted to the gravity weigh and falls into it.

Moreover, when a baby sinks into gravity, this damage prevents him from acquiring an independence of the axis and limbs. To achieve a rotation of the head, if eye-hand coordination or spatial orientation is necessary, he cannot pursue a target with his eyes, and all his body is involved in the movement

6. Assessment

Some authors as G Cioni[6] -following H. Prechtl teaching- are more interested in the attitude patterns of the pre-term infant in the cradle, the variability of the postures, the aspect of the spontaneous movements of the extremities, in time and space. Presence of synchronized and stiff spasms is a sign of neurological disorder when the baby is awakened and does not cry.

Other practitioners are involved in a dynamic examination[7] exploring the global reactivity against gravity, if the baby general health is sufficient. We can say that during the non – functional period in the baby development, the assessment of the automatic responses opens new tracks towards an early diagnosis. The pathological responses are similar whatever the baby's neurological future will be. The patients who are likely to become hemiplegic can show differences between both sides. Knowing the dramatic developmental changes in the infant's brain, which may question about CP diagnosis, A. Grenier [8] comes up with an original idea in pointing out the clinical "signs of normality" in the young baby's motor behaviour and communication. His know-how in manipulating the baby to relax him and to lead him to perform some motor coordination, is magical.

Best prediction is achieved through a combination of multiple, complementary tools[9].

7. Scoring

The well known Gross Motor Function Measure (website: www-fhs.mcmaster.ca/canchild) is one of the method to evaluate globally CP disorder -whatever the neurological trouble is- and to follow up the patient progress; it consists in an examination of 88 items in 5 chapters concerning pro and supine decubitus/ rolling up, all fours crawling / on knees moving, sitting, standing position, walking; the assessment allows to give a score number. This number is reliable if the examiner has been taught by a special instructor, and does not hesitate to ask for a second or third exam, if the results are uncertain.

8. Specific neurological troubles

After the first year of life, as the baby is growing, the classical troubles appear:

CP child seems close to the neurological characteristics of the various cerebral syndromes; they have been classified: hemiplegic form, Little disease (syndrome of premature birth), athetosic syndromes and dyskinetic troubles etc. In the most severe cases, feeding problems, epilepsy, auditive and visual disorders, dysarthria, somatic troubles are very usual. One says generally that CP children escaped psychic disturbances in their childhood, but as teenagers are not unlikely to develop depressive syndromes or trends towards suicide.

8.1 Hemiplegic forms

This unilateral impairment seems to appear classically after a silent interval after birth, but it is not quite true.

Many signs are often pointed out by parents or nurses: they observe that the motor development is a little delayed and that one side of the body does not do what the other does spontaneously, in every day life nursing. for example, to dress the baby. If the practitioner knows how to test the basic organization he can provide items of diagnosis.

From 6 months, it is easier and easier to determine the extent of the hemiplegic palsy because the baby enters the so-called functional period.

The X ray exam confirms the lesions and its extent, usually a cerebral infarctus, inner accident hidden during pregnancy.

In a lot of cases, the motor development is not so much impaired, and lets the parents think of a not so bad general prognosis, by forgetting other factors of cerebral injury. Walking is acquired in the second year of life, but quickly everybody worries about equines posture and other troubles from foot to hip.

Treatment consists in physiotherapy associated to braces, orthesis and botox `infiltrations to reduce factors of stiffness, spasticity included.

We have to confirm presence or not, of lateral homonymous hemianopsia and gnosic troubles in the impaired hand.

Everything has to be checked up as it is important for future autonomy and access to a professional job: side of the impaired hand , remaining capacities to be a grip or a press (30% of the cases) sole use of the forearm (30%). In the last 30% of the cases, the hand is for ever unused or is an ignored tool.

Language most often is saved in right hemiplegic forms, but a following up of the mental capacities is necessary to survey the general development, often not as good as expected to try to prevent school learning difficulties.

Epilepsy is frequent, and often uneasy to be managed by usual drugs.

8.2 Little disease

It is the sequel of 15/20% of the ex -premature infants. We remind that prematurity is defined by a pregnancy of less than 35 gestational age weeks.

The best known disease is the Little diplegia or spastic diplegia, which affects the 2 lower limbs and trunk; apparently the upper limbs are saved , the communication is correct.

In the vertical suspension and lift manoeuver, whereas the normal child spreads his legs, putting his feet at right angle, the pathological pattern is well known: the CP child crosses his legs, and sets his feet in full extension. If the caregiver puts down the child on the ground, the feet remain in equines.

Walking may be acquired later, with a lot of difficulties, such as equines pattern, knee and hip flexed, and hampered by weakness of the trunk. The more difficult walking is, the more frequent orthopedic complications are; all the joint levels of the lower limb may be impaired. The hips are especially affected and need to be followed up regularly, clinically and by X rays.

The rehab management consists in physiotherapy procedures, handling to facilitate corrected positions, use of support positions for sitting, at home or at school.

Soft tissues surgery takes place to maintain a certain quality of the joint motor range and length of the muscles, before a bone surgery becomes necessary. It depends on the functional outcome and patient 's way of life.

The complications are more frequent in the severe cases, for example quadriplegia , in which the voluntary command is low or impossible and when the patient is not able to mobilize himself. The participation of mental impairment is to be considered.

Anyway, surgery can modify the local area where it is done, improving flexibility and range of movement but cannot modify the global functional level.

8.3 The associated neuropsychological troubles

The late syndrome of the premature infant has been known, since 1964[10].

It is not a synonymous with motor trouble, because it is a perceptivo-cognitive disorder, subsequent to posterior brain lesions along the visual pathways, handicapping the development of skills that require visuo-mental and planning capacities. Numerous visual troubles are obvious as such squinting, lack of visual fixation and great difficulty in visual pursuit; sometimes, gnosic visual troubles may interfere in the mental representation.

Finally, the child is largely impaired by a great clumsiness, called dyspraxia. Dyspraxia is an execution trouble disrupting a finalized and coordinated gesture, learnt many times by education, it is due to a lack of successive fittings to reach a target; so, in dressing, then using spoon and fork for eating, playing of building up a tower with cubes, making a puzzle, drawing etc.

For example, difficulties in handwriting (dysgraphy) come from a lack of eye-hand coordination and control of the shape of the letters: however, the child is not unable to draw signs provided that they do not correspond to a given shape.

He can symbolize very well about a very poor design.

It is important to highlight that dyspraxia[11] should be not diagnosed on a sole symptom but on a net of clues , according to age: parents complaints on poor developmental performances as above mentioned, the results of the psychological tests showing a great discrepancy between language subtests and spatio-temporal ones and the assessment from an advised occupational therapist.

School learnings may be impaired at different levels, except language development which generally is good. As handwriting remains poor and slow, not profitable in time, the use of an electronic keyboard may be a means to write; but if visual control does not improve enough, the device cannot resolve the top-down problem and entirely compensate the difficulties in performing the task, which still remains slow and faulty. On the other hand, the same cerebral lesions may also affect intellectual capacities in counting and later in mathematics which do not follow an appropriate development.

In case of very great prematurity, under 32 gestational age weeks, the motor disorders are not so frequent but many other neuropsychological troubles may be pointed out involving memory, executive function, attention: as time goes on, secondary and progressive difficulties, related to the strain of school learning and of the necessary high level abilities, heavily bear upon the pragmatic life.

Athetosic syndromes are rare , 7%, including dystonic syndromes.

They are related to hypoxic-ischemia brain lesions on the basal ganglia and thalamus area, in the term-born babies. Kernicterus has disappeared.

The disease looks strange because the patients have mobile spasms, especially on the extremities. All the body, even oral muscles, is often involved, leading to dysarthria, feeding problems and sialorrhea, putting them at a disadvantage.

These patients are not paralyzed but suffering from involuntary movements and spasms, which noise the voluntary gestures forcing them to use strange ones to reach the target. The involuntary movements appear around 18 months; they disappear during rest or sleep time, are enhanced by anxiety or anguish. If the motor areas brain lesions are not extended, they do not provoke neuropsychological disturbances, such as in the late premature syndrome, and allow skills in day life gestures and a challenging behaviour!

But if the lesions are extended further, various CP cases with involuntary movements are associated to many learning disabilities in the field of cognition, communication, and behaviour.

Oral dysfunction leads to many problems, of which underlying components have to be analysed. The lips and tongue adjustments for taking liquids and/or food are impaired, and hamper the stimulation of various swallowing phases. Tongue and face gnosic exam is to be done as soon as possible to complete assessment[12]; silaorrhea and feeding difficulties are responsible for long feeding sessions and cause anxiety and frustration for infant and parents. Then they may lead to a risk of a chronic lack of hydratation, malnutrition, wrong positioning of teeth, and difficult dental hygiene. On the other hand, feeding troubles can induce severe false passages by food choking and determine pulmonary complications. As the CP child does not manage coughing and blowing his nose, he can suffer from ORL chronic infections. Specific cares are to be done to inhibit hyperextension of the body, to facilitate jaw closure and thus feeding sessions and to prevent local complications, sometimes even lethal. In case of the most severe impairment out of any improvement, gastrostomy by tube feeding is discussed.

Speech is impaired or impossible and requires alternative means of communication, from the most simple support to the best sophisticated ones, depending on patient capacities and needs, in order to preserve language development as far as possible.

If the child has access to signing gesture we can consider to learn him Makaton[13] signs and pictograms to communicate with his peers. The Bliss symbolic resources is a pictographic language for international communication, used for language-related disabilities, not especially for CP impairments.

Classification may be based on topography of the sequels, and one speaks of diplegia, triplegia, quadriplegia ... The principle of classification does not provide clues to treat a complex disease: factorizing must be preferred. The goal is to point out not only obvious deficits but also to detect the remaining, and sometimes hidden, capacities that compose a human being's functioning and behaviour adaptation.

9. Overwiev

"Parental concern on significant developmental motor delay may well be appropriate while the professional response is dilatory or non-existent" wrote AL Scherzer and I Tscharnuter in 1982[14]. This still may be true. But, nowadays, the Xray exams can predict a high risk of persistent abnormalities or assert a fixed motor lesion, early in baby's life. Radiology plays a new role, MRI especially, to appreciate the pathogenesis of the CP. The sophisticated exam may help to put a precise diagnosis but in the great majority of the cases it does not provide information enough to build up a prognosis. But "abnormal" radiological aspects can be misleading: we know new born babies that have been announced to the parents as severely impaired because of abnormal basal ganglia neuro-imaging, whose motor and intellectual development is normal at 4/6 months!

So the clinical exam is not to be neglected[15] and a regular follow up is necessary. Wise and relevant medical attitude is to take time to consider, something such as infant's convalescing time, if all the clues are sufficient for the diagnosis' disclosure.

Anyway we have to remember that there is a CP human being whose progressive needs have to be recognized and taken into account. Parents have to take part in neuro rehabilitation projects: "during the past two decades, awareness of the role of the family in the child's life has increased and the term 'family-centred services' (FCS) [16] has been introduced to facilitate care for children with special needs and their families". Moreover a new strategy merits further investigation, a therapy approach focusing on changing the task and the environment rather than children's impairments![17]

Anyway, nothing may be done without parents' consent, in the respect of their availability, emotional state, religious faiths. At the end, the financial conditions of the family life must be not forgotten either.

10. Rehabilitation techniques. There is not ONE school of physiotherapy

Conductive Education, Infant Health and Development Program, Infant Behaviour Assessment and Intervention Program represent categories of global approach. Treatment according to Vojta, is envisaged stimulating patterns of active mobilization by nociceptive stimulus, applied by therapist or any voluntary worker without attention to family function.

From the work and publications of Bertha Bobath, other methods are applied, keeping a neuro-developmental action project. In France, many practitioners use the methods taught by Le Métayer[18]. He insists on a global motor approach, as in the Bobath method, to teach movements patterns and not a sequence of mosaic of activation of specific muscles.

But, following the G. Tardieu studies on muscle contracture, he advocates to analyze the musculo-skeletal state, fearing that an unsuitable "peripheral tool" interferes with care: the impact of physiotherapy might not be relevant enough.

Indeed, the muscle stiffness must be analyzed and measured: is it an active contracture such as spasticity (defined as velocity-dependant increase in tonic stretch reflex) or other factors included in the upper motor neuron syndrome? Or a passive contracture because of a shortening of the muscle, or a mixed form? We remind that the CP muscle keeps a normal structure and is able to adapt its length to a cast immobilization[19] position, and that muscular shortening means serial reduction of the sarcomeres and modification of the visco-elasticity properties[20]. If clinical measures are not sufficient, EMG exam can be used to obtain details. Now there is an hype towards a 3D gait analysis to highlight the different intricate causes, but it is reserved to walking patients !

So, according to the muscular properties, it is possible to use passive stretching[21] by serial casts or other devices to combat soft tissue tightness, (especially the sural triceps) and improve the range of movement, on condition to correct the joint and bones displacements or not to dislocate their structure, in the aim of maintaining the cast. The results are often good during the young age, but do not last, so treatment has to be repeated regularly. After adolescence, passive stretching does not work.

Treatment of the neural and biomechanical components of "increased tone" consists on passive and active movement, positioning in lying, sitting and standing, use of splinting[22]. Scientific data research on the CP muscle, submitted to strains of the pathological CP motor pattern and its evolution, according to age, is necessary to prevent the muscle from secondary local complications and the limitation of general progress.

In upper limb there are two kinds of treatment: one takes into account the muscular flexibility and the joint/bone orthopedic state, and the second involves the occupational therapist in the management of day life gestures and patient's motility. The therapists need to communicate between them to let the patient, whatever his age, in the best conditions related to his environment. More and more, the debate is between a child focused-treatment or an environment- focused treatment.

"Everything not useful is finally harmful".

The goal of botulinum toxin injection is to relax muscles' stiffness at the point of injection, in reducing local muscular overactivity such as spasticity[23]; but it is not a final goal, there must be a purpose behind it; a pragmatic approach is necessary.

So, first of all, how may the patient use or take benefit of removal of spasticity, according to his dysfunction? Spasticity is one of the three components of the upper motor neuron syndrome associated to weakness of the voluntary command and shortening of muscle. Command weakness is often neglected behind the obvious stiffness.

So, we must be sure that this expected result does not provoke too much muscular weakness and finally does not give functional benefit. It is a challenge. It would be interesting to study the other factors which play a role to carry out the rehab project, such as patient's perceptive development, mental capacities, participation, level of interaction with a multidisciplinary team.

Another point: it has been proved, after more than 15 years of practise, that local relaxation improvement thanks to BTX injections has not a long duration, and does not provide functional improvement.

11. Role of medical treatment

For many reasons, drugs are used and very often, to reduce acute or chronic health difficulties. Treatment also concerns management of behaviour troubles, or pain, or epilepsy. On other hand, a lot of oral drugs are required to reduce general hypertony, involuntary movements, as diazepam, dantrolene, baclofen etc. with or without use of BTX. Advantages and side-effects must be analyzed before any new or repeated prescription.

12. Surgery

It would be prudent to keep in mind this phrase "Just one body for one life".

When manual and instrumental physiotherapy means are overpassed, one can think of surgery operations. On soft tissues, it is a tenotomy of various kinds, which can provide flexibility in a sagittal or frontal cross-section. But the younger the patient is, the more transient the benefit is, because of the patient weight and stature growth. In childhood, we can predict a successful result in the short term, *but same causes reproducing same effects*, we can fear the recurrence at long term. The orthopaedic corrections can be discussed, on joint and bone deformities, such as the rotation deformities, hip dysplasia or luxation, fixed flexed knee etc..[24]

Concerning upper limb surgery, the results are a little disappointing. A reshaped hand and wrist action cannot provide more functional ability than the previous state. BTX injections, associated with surgery to open the palm may be dangerous by reducing fingers strength etc..

Secondary complications on muscle an/or bone are frequent and have to be taken into account and watched over previously, as early as possible.

If hypertonicity is not reduced by previous treatment, neuro- surgical treatments such as posterior radicotomy (or dorsal rhizotomy) or baclofen pump to interrupt the pathways leading factors of hypertonicity can be proposed.

Briefly, any surgical option can provide local or peripheral improvements, but cannot change the functional level; CP patients, with minor or moderate impairments, who spontaneously have acquired aided or non-aided walking and achieved a certain independence, may have a general benefit! The same remark concerns the upper limb operations.

12.1 Overview on outcome

In a remarkable review[25], the authors report that there are specific ages to achieve performances: "sitting by 24 m, walking by 72/84 m". In the CP cerebellar forms, walking with a certain instability may be possible later. The length of time is interesting and shows that a better and earlier rehab intervention cannot deeply change the motor prognosis.

13. Neuro-imaging

Brain abnormalities are present in 70 to 90% of the global cases.

In very preterm infants the standard practise is the ultra sound scanning, with interesting results. MRI[‡] is more sensitive but a difficult exam to perform.

Peri-ventricular-Leukomalacia (PVL) or White matter injury on MRI imaging is conventional.

CP is frequently linked to white matter injury in children born preterm; DTI[26] is a powerful technique providing details of White matter microstructure, and reflects disruption of thalamus connections as well as descending pathways.

Findings include decreased grey matter volumes, basal ganglia, thalamus areas, cerebellar abnormalities as well as injury in subplate neurons. With advances in neonatal care the incidence of cystic forms of PVL has fallen whereas the identification of deep white matter injury (non-cystic) has risen.

Dyskinetic[27] CP and its subtypes occur mainly in the term born babies, suffering from perinatal insults. In some selected cases, the neuropathological descriptions of status dysmyelinatus, affecting mainly the pallidum in kernicterus, and status marmoratus, refering to the marbled appearance of the striatum and thalamus after hypoxia–ischemia have been described. In great majority, MRI findings are thalamus/basal ganglia lesions, associated to cortical lesions.

14. Alternative devices: Augmentative and alternative means of communication[28]

It is difficult to give a non-speaking patient, young or not, an alternative means of communication. Parents have built up a specific mode of interaction, assert they understand their child: it is true and not true, it depends on the message. The child 's emotional state, his pleasure or distress, or basic needs may be passed on. But there is high risk not to give a correct meaning to some attitudes or behaviour, associated to a certain vocalizations or noises or handicapped movements. Generally speaking, communication is based on (consistent?) yes/no questioning by the parents who are used to looking for a response from a passive child. But the first communication mode is not sufficient and cannot be adapted to new situations such as going to school and introducing communication with a teacher or friend. To integrate a new system and to implement the communication, one has to work in a multidisciplinary team.

---

‡ MRI= magnetic resonance imaging

N Jollieff and H Mc Conachie noted in 1992, at EACD meeting, that four questions can be asked about communication aids: who, what, when, how?

Who. First, a medical exam is necessary to meet the family and let them speak about the antecedents and the diagnosis disclosure of the severe CP disease; feeding problems, often combined with the physical impairment, and their evolution must be assessed. Moreover, visual and hearing quality must be checked, sometimes by a specialist. Then, a psychologist and speech therapist have to evaluate the early infant-mother relationship, child's pre-requisite skills and attention, his verbal comprehension level , whereas the social worker deals with child's and parents' needs.

What. It concerns the type of aid and the means to handle the apparatus, or to touch a keyboard or to use a remote command. So, the occupational therapist is involved in appreciating the limits of the physical impairment, and advising some recommendations. We have noted in the classification's chapter that the devices are various, simple ones allowing the young patient to show pictures in order to communicate with words written under the picture or symbols, other ones more complicated using a grammatical system to make phrases. Some electronic devices are able to give voice to the patient's grammatical work or telegraphic comment. We have to take into account the weariness of the patient and the speed of his contribution and whether the impact on the environment is successful.

Why. The aim is to transfer current communication mode onto more technical system.

How. In many cases, the organization of funding and training has frequently failed because of a lack of an identified co-ordinator, the recommendations have not been followed up, or the patient has not obtained his device (speech synthesizer for example) as expected. The use of computers with adapted remote commands may offer a new facility to those who are able to learn reading and writing, according to their scholarship levels.

The patient's parents and teachers have to be trained to use any alternative device and facilitate the patient's practise.

It is recommended that the multidisciplinary teams keep in touch with alternative and augmentative communication (AAC) [29] organizations (ISAAC organization, for example) to carry out multicentre research in the field.

15. CP teenager[30] and adult life[31]

Cerebral palsy is often seen as a disorder involving children only. But children with CP nearly always grow up to become adults with CP, and with continuing improvements

in survival. Deaths in children with CP, never common, have in recent years become very rare, unless the child is very severely and multiple disabled.[32]

It has become increasingly important to plan appropriate service provision for such adults.

Critical questions that need answering include to review current understanding of physical processes that may contribute to loss of function and premature aging.

It is very important to try to maintain evidence-based care for adults.

Any young adult CP patient who is living in the society mainstream complains that, after years of regular following up in childhood, he cannot find out medical doctor or experienced physiotherapist, or other caregiver , to deal with his needs.

Experienced team is missing also in private or public night and day institutions which attend to CP adults.

Although the neurological injury is non-progressive, CP adults with the disorder often develop well known musculoskeletal complications, but also joint problems, hip/ knee arthrosis, ankle and toes deformities etc. which may lead to severe pain, chronic fatigue, and a premature decline in mobility and function, as they age.

This advance in research of good health and life time span, however heartening, poses new challenges to the medical community.

16. Social cost

In France, the social security entirely covers the CP infants health expenses and medical follow up, physiotherapy charges, equipment and so on. When a CP child enters a rehab and schooling centre, it is free. The most important lifetime costs[33] are the social care costs during childhood.

To inquire about up dated available family aids, in France, according of patient's age and handicap, French parents or parents living in France may refer to the magazine "Déclic" (http://www.magazine-declic.com/Magazine/).

The compensatory allowance concerns handicapped people whose disabilities rate is at least 80% and who need the help of another person for activities of daily living, from 20 to 65 years. Later, the handicapped patients receive a special aid.

In France, many associations are involved in supporting actions towards physically impaired people problems[§]. They have created multidisciplinary outpatients and inpatients centres and have organized professional and permanent courses to ensure an updating formation to the carers[34], other foundations[35] are involved in research on CP causes and quality of care.

17. Pain, distress and quality of life = QOL

The CP life is full of pain(s) and distress periods. Some seem to be related to their chronic disability and physical handicap, some other to the usual human questioning on wasting one's life.

There is a lot of specific questionnaires to help caregivers to understand (highlight) why and where a child or adult patient suffers. For the patients with severe and/or polyhandicapped [36] CP impairments, the San Salvadour scale is very useful. There are also self assessment scales to measure pain intensity. But nothing is better than an examination to discover whether pain is precisely situated or extended or long lasting. We know the risk of

§ APF = national association

misdiagnosis, such as unilateral strong back pains vs. renal colic, repeated claims of fatigue, lack of appetite and general malaise vs. severe constipation (fecaloma) etc..

Pain does not come, or seldom, from the physical impairment (except very severe forms or intense involuntary movements) but more often from an awkwardness in parents or caregivers handling, helping to dress, to feed, or to mobilize! There are pragmatic rules to follow regarding the daily life CP assistance and to check if the patient's equipment and orthoses are appropriate for him.

A part of peripheral pain may be related to the moral weight of the handicap and sometimes it is difficult to separate the respective part between physical and moral causes; the complaint may not correspond to the real neurological deficit.

Some patients expect too much from surgical operations and are deeply disappointed of the result, apparently successful, because they have imagined -or dreamt - being cured and not repaired!

However, patients with deteriorated walking function have greater pain frequency[37], pain intensity, the impact of pain on daily activities, and physical fatigue and reduced balance. Thanks to a meticulous examination of the patient (neurological, orthopaedic, and somatic exam) and a questioning in the close environment, we can try to resolve a lot of pain sources and reduce uneasiness.

Even though it is difficult, there is always something to do, by medical drugs, psychological support, changing support position, orthopaedic measures. It depends of age, motor level, and social position and patient's will.

Distress. The repeated question from the patients is, why me? And on the other hand, feeling of guilt of their difference and non-achievement in life aspirations and in social integration are factors of a depressive attitude. It is not infrequent to discover alcoholic excess, tobacco addiction or other display of personal discouragement …

Nevertheless, some adult patients, thanks to their resilience[38] property, manage to live the best life they may, by a "CP way of life"[39]!

18. References

[1] Rosenbaum P and al. DMCN feb 2007, 49, s, 2, 8-15
[2] A. Jollien "le métier d'homme " Paris Seuil 2002
[3] Ghada Beaino and al. Predictors of cp in very preterm infants: Epipage prospective study DMCN 2010, 52, 119-125
[4] JC Tabary: Plasticité synaptique et autonomie. Mot Cérébr 30, n°2, juin 2009
[5] J. Melher et E. Dupoux, Naître humain. Ed, Odile Jacob, Paris 1990
[6] Cioni G and al. Comparison between observation of spontaneous movements and neurologic examination in pre term infants. J Pediatrics 1997, 130 (5) 704-11
[7] M. Le Métayer.Contribution à l'étude des niveaux d'évolution motrice. J kinésither 1963 M Le Métayer. Evolution des stratégies rééducatives in D. Truscelli: les IMC réflexions et perspectives sur la prise en charge Masson 2008
[8] A Grenier. "la motricité libérée du nouveau-né" Médecine et enfance 2000

[9] Hadders Algra M. Neuromotor manifestation of CP during infancy DMCN 2009, 51, suppl 31-35
[10] Stambak M and al. Les dyspraxies de l'enfant, in Psychiatrie de l'enfant. 1964 7 381-496
[11] M Mazeau.L'enfant dyspraxique et les apprentissages. Masson Paris 2010
[12] Le Métayer: Evaluation des gnosies faciales et linguales. Mot cérébr 28, n°4 , déc 2007
[13] M Walker. Makaton la communication pour tous. Colloque ISAAC; Dijon 2006.
[14] Early diagnosis and therapy in CP, M Dekker NY 1982
[15] Amiel-Tison Cl, Julie Gosselin , Sheila Gahagan, Pediatrics oct 2005
[16] Tineke Dirks, M Hadders Algra.The role of the family in intervention of infants at high risk of cerebral palsy: a systematic analysis. DMCN September 2011, pages 62–67,
[17] Darrah J and al. Context therapy: a new intervention approach for children with CP. DMCN 2011, 53, 7, 615-620
[18] Le Métayer M. Rééducation cérébro-motrice. (2è ed.)Paris Masson 1999
[19] Tardieu G, and al. For how long must the soleus muscle be stretched each day to prevent contracture? DMCN 1988 30,3-10
[20] Jared RH Foran and al. Structural and mechanical alterations in spastic skeletal muscle. DMCN 2005, 47,713-717
[21] Tamis Pin and al. The effectiveness of passive stretching in children with CP. DMCN 2006 48, 855-862
[22] Physiotherapy management of established spasticity, by S Edwards in spasticity rehab 1998. ed G Sheean. Churchill com
[23] JM Gracies and al. BOTOX dilution and endplate targeting in spasticity: a double blind controlled study. Archives of physical medicine and rehab vol 90 ,1, jan 2009
[24] G Thuilleux. Problémes orthopédiques chez les IMC, p 200-290. In D Truscelli. Les infirmities cérébrales Paris Masson 2008
[25] Campos da Paz A and al. Walking prognosis in CP: a 22 year retrospective analysis DMCN 1994 36 130-134
[26] A H Hoon and al. Sensory and motor deficits with CP born preterm with diffusion tensor imaging abnormalities in thalamocortical pathways DMCN 2009 51 697-704
[27] I Krageloh Mann. Dyskinetic CP prevalence and neuroimaging [27]DMCN 2007 49 244-244
[28] E Cataix-Nègre. Communiquer, autrement. Solal 2011
[29] Mc Conachie H, Pennington L. In-service training for schools on AAC. European J of Disorders communication 32, (spec n°) 277-288, 1997
[30] Alvin P Marcelli D Médecine de l'adolescent, IMC : by D.Truscelli, A. Lespargot, F de Barbot p 279-282. Paris Masson ed. 2005
[31] P Haak CP and aging DMCN 2009 51 s4 16-23
[32] E Zucman. Auprès de la personne handicapée. Vuibert Espace Ethique 2007
[33] M Kruse and al. Lifetime costs of CP DMCN original article 2009
[34] Institut de formation en IMC et polyhandicap, www. Institutmc.org, APF and others
[35] www.lafondationmotrice.org

[36] Collignon P, Guisiano B, Combes JC. La douleur chez l'enfant polyhandicapé. *In :* Ecoffey C, Murat I. *La douleur chez l'enfant.* Flammarion Med Sci, Paris, 1999 : 174-178.
[37] L K Vogtle. Pain in adults with CP: impact and solutions. DMCN 2009, 51, s4,113-121
[38] B Cyrulnik. Un merveilleux malheur. Ed Poche 2002
[39] R Fernandez. Joie de vivre des IMC. Mot Cerebr 2002 23 165-167

3

Inborn Errors of Metabolism and Brain Involvement – 5 Years Experience from a Tertiary Care Center in South India

Kannan Vaidyanathan, M. P. Narayanan and D. M. Vasudevan
Metabolic Disorders Laboratory, Department of Biochemistry, Amrita Institute of Medical Sciences and Research Center, Kochi, Kerala, India

1. Introduction

Inborn errors of metabolism (IEM) comprise a large group of more than 500 different rare genetic disorders. They arise due to mutations in genes encoding a single enzyme in metabolic pathways. Some of these disorders are very rare, whereas certain other disorders are more common. There are considerable racial and ethnic differences in the incidence pattern of these disorders. Aminoacidurias like phenylketonuria are common in the Western population; in Asian countries including India, organic acidurias like propionic acidurias, methyl malonic acidurias and maple syrup urine disease are more common. Clinical presentation of IEM is varied and it affects multiple organ systems, including CNS. Indeed CNS involvement is one of the most common presenting symptoms. The diseases can appear immediately after birth; or sometimes it may be delayed, even appearing in adult life.

In this chapter we shall describe our experience with metabolic screening in the last 5 years. This is followed by a presentation of some important case histories along with their laboratory work-up. We then go on to discuss the current global status in diagnosis and management of these diseases. It should be emphasized at the beginning itself that our laboratory (Metabolic Disorders Laboratory, Amrita Institute of Medical Science, Kochi, Kerala, S. India) is a referral center for the state of Kerala as well as the neighboring states in South India. Hence the studied population represents children who are suspected to have IEM or are high-risk individuals, or who have been referred from other hospitals in this part of India. Hence the results described do not reflect the population incidence.

If these patients are not diagnosed and treated early in life, they go on to have irreversible damage. Many body systems are affected, and the predominant damage will be to the central nervous system. The babies may develop permanent mental retardation, growth retardation, intractable seizures, cerebral palsy etc.

2. Objectives

8361 patients were screened for different metabolic disorders during the time period from September 2006 to August 2011. The screening panel included tests for aminoacidurias, organic acidurias, disorders of carbohydrate metabolism (including galactosemia, glycosuria, fructosuria, pentosuria, mucopolysaccharidoses etc), congenital adrenal hyperplasia, pheochromocytoma, hyperhomocysteinemia, porphyrias etc.

3. Methods

Patients admitted to Amrita Institute of Medical Sciences, Kochi and other hospitals in Kerala State, South India with signs and symptoms suggestive of metabolic disorder were tested. Neurological symptoms of the patients included psychomotor delay, mental retardation, seizures, dystonia, ataxia, lethargy, coma, encephalitis, speech delay, hyperactivity etc. Non-neurological symptoms were failure to thrive, organomegaly, vomiting, skin rashes, metabolic acidosis, hyperammonemia, hypoglycemia, lactic acidosis and ketonuria.

The breakup of different tests are as follows - (1) Total number of tests - 8361 (2) Urine screened for metabolic disorders (panel including amino acids, organic acids, carbohydrates, ketone bodies etc) - 1940 (3) Amino acid screening by HPLC - 519; Organic acid screening by HPLC - 420 (4) Homocysteine estimation - 953 (5) VMA estimation - 582 (6) Porphyrias - 266 (7) 17 α hydroxy progesterone estimation (for congenital adrenal hyperplasia) - 1155 (8) Adenosine deaminase estimation - 2406 and (9) Other tests - 540 (Myoglobin, 5 HIAA, lipoprotein electrophoresis, glucose 6 phosphate dehydrogenase, homocystinuria etc). Methodologies are given under each concerned section.

4. Results

The breakup of positive cases is as follows - Aminoacidurias - 32, organic acidurias - 51 (confirmed cases), hyperhomocysteinemia - 285, pheochromocytomas and neuroblastomas - 44, elevated adenosine deaminase levels - 358 and congenital adrenal hyperplasia - 309. Further discussion is limited to aminoacidurias, organic acidurias, hyperhomocysteinemia, pheochromocytomas and neuroblastomas, since other disorders will not affect the brain.

We have divided this chapter into 3 major sections: Each of these sections will discuss the results and recent review of literature. Some rare and interesting cases are also discussed under the concerned sections. Section 1 – Aminoacidurias and organic acidurias; Section 2 – Homocysteine, Section 3 - Pheochromocytoma and neuroblastoma. Section 1 on aminoacidurias and organic acidurias is divided into 4 sub-sections: 1.1 - Maple syrup urine disease, 1.2 - Methyl malonic acidurias and propionic acidurias, 1.3 - Phenylketonuria and 1.4 - Nonketotic hyperglycinemia.

5. Section 1: Amino acidurias and organic acidurias

5.1 Materials and methods

1940 urine samples were initially screened for different aminoacidurias and organic acidurias. Simple screening tests and thin layer chromatography were used for screening. 519 samples were analyzed further for aminoacidurias and 420 samples were analyzed for organic acidurias by HPLC. 20 ml fresh urine samples and 3 mL EDTA blood samples were collected under aseptic precautions for the analysis.

5.1.1 HPLC method of amino acid analysis

Analytical Conditions were as follows - Column- LUNA C-18, Mobile phase A: 5 mM sodium phosphate buffer with pH 7.0, Mobile Phase B: 100% Acetonitrile. Gradient Elution,

Flow Rate- 1.0 ml/ min, Temperature- 40 °C, Detection- Absorption (254 nm). Samples were deproteinized and treated with phenyl isothiocyanate (PITC) and triethylamine (TEA) prior to injection (pre column derivatization).

5.1.2 HPLC method of organic acid analysis

Analytical Conditions were as follows - Column: 4.6 mm * 250 cm, Lichrocart 250-4 Lichrosorb RP -18 (Phenomenex), Mobile phase: 0.01M KH_2PO_4/H_3PO_4 (pH 3.5), Flow rate: 1 ml/min, Detection: U V 206 nm, PDA detector, Column Oven Temperature: 25 C. Urine samples were also deproteinized prior to injection.

5.1.3 Results

We detected a high incidence of aminoacidurias and organic acidurias in this population. Among organic acidurias, higher prevalence of propionic aciduria (PAA), 16 cases, and methylmalonic aciduria (MMA), 15 cases, were seen. 13 cases of maple syrup urine disease (MSUD), 1 case of isovaleric aciduria and 6 cases of alkaptonuria were detected. 5 cases of tyrosinemia, 4 cases of nonketotic hyperglycinemia (NKH) and 3 cases of phenyl ketonuria (PKU) were also confirmed. There was one case of non- PKU hyperphenylalaninemia. One patient was detected to have hypermethioninemia (484 µmol/L). Mild elevation of individual amino acids was seen in a number of cases and was not considered to be characteristic of any individual aminoaciduria. This included glycine (59 cases), alanine (44 cases), proline (17 cases), histidine (8 cases) and lysine (2 cases). This probably is a representation of increased catabolic state in these patients.

5.1.4 Review of literature

Lou et al (2011) studied 552 children at high risk by MS/MS in China and report 64 children with IEM including predominantly organic acidurias and some aminoacidurias. Niu et al (2010) did population screening on about 1.5 million Taiwanese neonates by MS/MS and found that PKU, MSUD, GA-1 and MMA were the commonest disorders. Cakmakci et al (2010) reports the use of proton MR spectroscopy and diffusion weighted MR imaging in the diagnosis of children with neurometabolic brain disorders including MSUD, Canavan disease and galactosemia. Walter et al (2009) studied cord blood in a large cohort of 24, 983 births for various IEM. Cord blood screening did not detect PKU, MSUD, argininosuccinic acidurias, MMA, glutaric aciduria type 2, MCAD deficiency etc which was diagnosed later. They conclude that cord blood screening is not recommended for IEM.

Wasant et al (2008) identified 12 cases of organic acidurias in 365 patients over 3 years from Thailand. The cases include alkaptonuria, IVA, PA, MMA, GA-I, GA-II and MCD. Shigematsu et al (2010) identified 1065 cases of IVA from 146, 000 neonates screened over three years in a Japanese population.

5.2 Section 1.1: Maple syrup urine disease

5.2.1 Case report

We report here two cases of maple syrup urine disease (MSUD). Patient 1 presented at 3 months of age with excessive irritability, abnormal posturing since birth and delayed developmental milestones. History of sibling death at Day 15 of life. The clinician reported abnormal urine odor and clinical suspicion was MSUD, isovaleric aciduria or PKU. Laboratory analysis revealed ketonuria and metabolic acidosis. HPLC analysis of amino acid confirmed MSUD (Figure 1). Child died immediately afterwards.

Patient 2 presented at Day 12 with metabolic acidosis, abnormal urine odor, ketonuria and hepatosplenomegaly. Blood and urine studies revealed the diagnosis of MSUD. Aggressive treatment was started including branched chain amino acid restricted diet and supplementation. Patient has survived until 3 years of age, without any episode of exacerbation afterwards. Patient is on follow up. Levels of leucine, isoleucine and valine came down to normal level (Table 1).

In the case of the first patient (Patient 1), diagnosis was delayed and hence treatment could not be instituted and the baby died. But in the second case (Patient 2) diagnosis and treatment was started early in life and outcome was better. These two case studies indicate the importance of early diagnosis and treatment in MSUD.

5.2.2 Biochemical abnormalities

The name originates from the characteristic smell of urine (similar to burnt sugar or maple sugar) due to excretion of branched chain keto acids. Maple syrup urine disease (MSUD) or branched chain ketoaciduria is caused by deficiency of branched chain keto acid dehydrogenase complex (BCKAD). The basic biochemical defect is deficient decarboxylation of branched chain keto acids (BCKA). It leads to accumulation of branched chain amino acids (BCAA) Leucine, Isoleucine and Valine and corresponding branched chain α keto acids (BCKA). Five distinct phenotypes are present: Classic, Intermediate, Intermittent, Thiamine-responsive and Dihydrolipoyl dehydrogenase (E3) deficient.

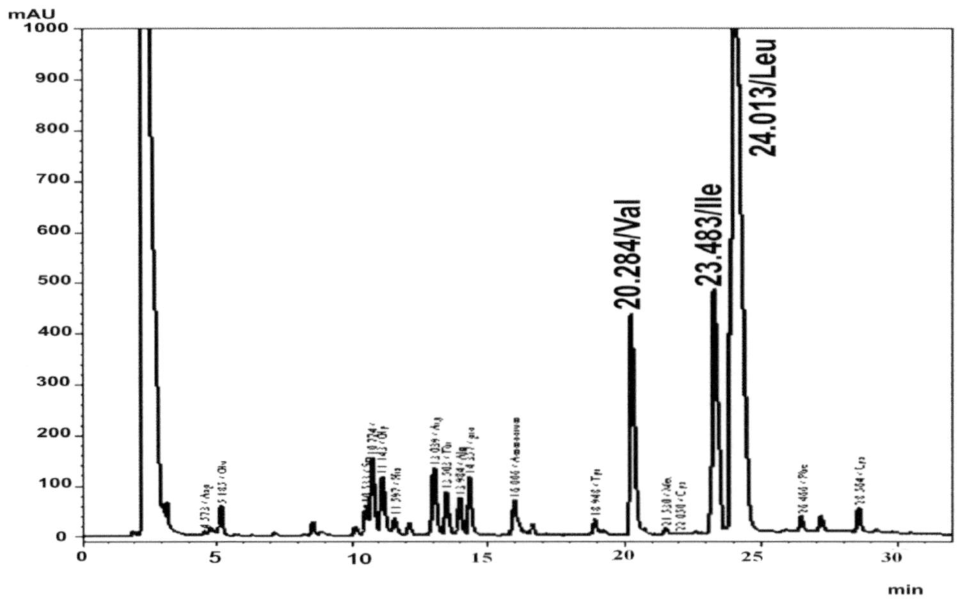

Fig. 1. Chromatogram of patient 1 (Leucine 2240 μmol/L, Valine 411 μmol/L, Isoleucine 180 μmol/L; Normal Leu <150, Val <255 and Ile <80 μmol/L)

	Valine (μmol/l)	Leucine (μmol/l)	Isoleucine (μmol/l)
11.04.2009	518	3020	437
25.07.2009	194	1708	350
15.03.2010	98	424	166
06.08.2010	135	479	69

Table 1. Serial levels of Branched chain amino acids in patient 2 diagnosed with MSUD –

Classic MSUD is the most common and is the most severe type. It has a neonatal-onset type of encephalopathy. Other types generally have onset by 2 years. BCAA, generally Leucine, is elevated in blood and urine. Presence of alloisoleucine is diagnostic. It has autosomal recessive inheritance. Worldwide frequency is 1 in 1,85,000.

BCAA comprise 35% of indispensable amino acids in muscles. Majority of untreated classic patients die within the early months of life from recurrent metabolic crises and neurologic deterioration. Treatment involves long-term dietary management and aggressive intervention during acute metabolic decompensation. Age at diagnosis and subsequent metabolic control are the most important determinants of long-term control. Patients in whom treatment is initiated after 10 days of age rarely achieve normal intellect.

Disease starts in the first week of life. It is characterized by convulsions, severe mental retardation, vomiting, acidosis, coma and death within the first year of life. Urine contains branched chain keto acids, valine, leucine and isoleucine. Rothera's test is positive, but unlike in cases of ketoacidosis, even boiled and cooled urine will give the test. Diagnosis depends on enzyme analysis in cells. Diagnosis should be done prior to 1 week after birth. Giving a diet low in branched chain amino acids. Mild variant is called intermittent branched chain ketonuria. This will respond to high doses of thiamine. This is because the decarboxylation of the BCKA requires thiamine. Liver transplantation has been successfully tried in some cases of MSUD.

5.2.3 Review of literature

Chen et al (2010) has reviewed 15 cases of MSUD from China and they suggest that early diagnosis and treatment can help prevent neurologic signs. Pangkanon et al (2008) report 13 cases of MSUD in Thai infants. All patients had neurological manifestations and psychomotor retardation. Lee et al (2008) report 47 Filipino patients with MSUD which is the commonest IEM in Philippines. They report that clinical outcome is poor in their series of patients.

Barschak et al (2009) report MSUD is associated with lipid peroxidation. They also report reduced amino acids methionine and tryptophan, which are amino acids with antioxidant activity. Mescka et al (2011) report protective effect of carnitine against oxidative stress induced by MSUD.

Ribeiro et al (2008) report that the major metabolites accumulating in MSUD disturb brain aerobic metabolism by compromising the citric acid cycle and the electron flow through the respiratory chain. They hypothesize that this might explain the neurological features in MSUD.

Brunetti-Pierri et al (2011) report successful use of phenylbutyrate in bringing down branched chain amino acid levels in MSUD. Shellmer et al (2011) studied 14 patients who received liver transplantation for MSUD and found that liver transplantation reduced further CNS damage in these patients. Strauss et al ((2010) has suggested novel therapeutic modalities in the management of MSUD based on their experience in treating 79 patients over 20 years.

Zinnanti et al (2009) report that rapid brain leucine accumulation displaces other essential amino acids resulting in neurotransmitter depletion and disruption of normal brain growth and development in mouse model. They also report that administration of norleucine reduces branched chain amino acid accumulation in brain, blood and milk. Norleucine also substantially delayed encephalopathy in intermediate type MSUD. They conclude that brain damage in MSUD might be due to two factors - (1) Neurotransmitter deficiencies and growth restriction associated with BCAA accumulation, and (2) Energy deprivation through Krebs' cycle disruption associated with BCAA accumulation.

Ibarra-Gonzalez et al (2007) report increased mortality and disabilities, especially neurological, in a cohort of 36 patients with MSUD from Mexico. Kowalik et al (2007) report deficiency of iron, zinc, copper, Vitamin B1, B2, niacin and Vitamin C in treated MSUD patients. Wajner et al (2007) report that BCAA inhibited Na-K ATPase pump in the brain and alanine prevented this inhibition. They conclude that this mechanism might contribute to neurological damage in MSUD, as Na-K ATPase pump is a critical enzyme for normal brain development and functioning. Bridi et al (2005) also report that alpha keto acids accumulating in MSUD stimulate lipid peroxidation and reduce antioxidant defense in cerebral cortex.

There are a large number of studies which report on CT and MR scans of the brain in MSUD [Cakmakci et al (2010), Tu et al (2005), Sener (2004), Schonberger et al (2004) and others]. Bindu et al (2007) have described neuroradiological findings in 3 patients with intermediate MSUD from South India.

5.3 Section 1.2: Methylmalonic aciduria and propionic aciduria

5.3.1 Results

We have detected 16 cases of propionic acidurias and 15 cases of methyl malonic acidurias in our study. Most of these patients had neurological manifestations and presented with metabolic acidosis and/or hyperammonemia. 60% of patients had neurological abnormalities including psychomotor delay, mental retardation, seizures, dystonia, ataxia, lethargy, extrapyramidal symptoms, encephalopathy, coma, visual deficiency, speech delay etc.

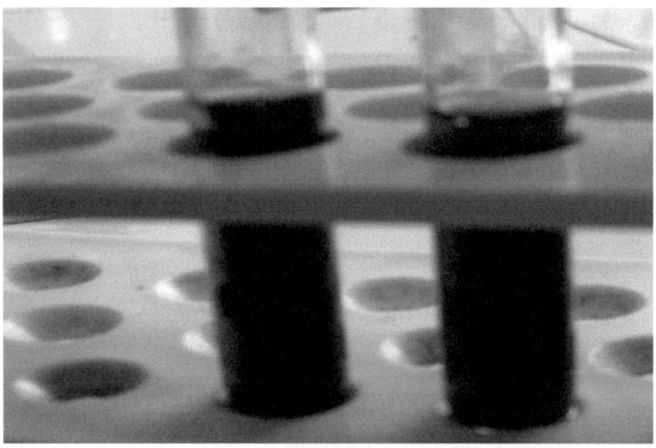

Fig. 2. Screening test for methyl malonic aciduria (Emerald green is positive test; other test tube is control urine sample)

Abnormal MRI findings were found in 11 patients including macrocephaly, cerebral atrophy and cerebral edema. Further details of this work can be seen in our paper (Narayanan et al, 2011; Vaidyanathan et al, 2011). Figure 2 gives a screening test for methyl malonic acid.

5.3.2 Biochemical abnormalities

Propionyl CoA is primarily converted to methyl malonyl CoA, which is subsequently converted to Succinyl CoA. Enzymes involved are propionyl CoA carboxylase, methyl malonyl CoA racemase and methyl malonyl CoA mutase. Biotin is needed for first and cobalamin for the third enzyme. Propionyl CoA carboxylase has two non-identical sub-units α and β, biotin binds to α sub-units, located on chromosomes 13 and 3 respectively. Methyl malonyl CoA mutase has 2 identical α sub-units, located on chromosome 6. Holocarboxylase deficiency and biotinidase deficiency are known. Other known disorder is multiple carboxylase deficiency. PCC deficiency leads to propionic acidemia, and elevated 3 hydroxy propionate, methyl citrate, tiglyl Glycine, and unusual ketone bodies in urine. Severe metabolic ketoacidosis in neonatal period is seen. Alkali therapy and protein restriction are needed.

Inherited deficiency of the mutase enzyme or abnormalities in cobalamin can result in methyl malonic aciduria. Neonatal or infantile metabolic ketoacidosis are the hallmarks. Patients with abnormal binding ability of enzyme to cobalamin, cannot be treated by cobalamin therapy. These cases may be treated with dietary protein restriction and antibiotic therapy. Other patients respond to cobalamin or hydroxycobalamin therapy. This can be used in combination with dietary protein restriction. Therapy has been found to reduce methyl malonate levels. Mutations leading to impaired adenosyl cobalamin and methyl cobalamin and deficient activity of methyl malonyl CoA mutase and N5 methyl tetrahydro folate reductase. Homocysteine methyl transferase have methyl malonic aciduria combined with homocystinuria. Features include failure to thrive, developmental retardation, megaloblastic anemia and macrocytosis. Therapy includes protein restriction, pharmacological doses of hydroxocobalamin and betaine supplementation.

Both disorders are inherited as autosomal recessive disorders. Prenatal diagnosis is possible by enzyme assays on chorionic villus biopsy or cultured amniotic cells and chemical determinations on amniotic fluid or maternal urine.

5.3.3 Review of literature

Liu et al (2010) reports 24 mutations in the MMACHC gene to be responsible for cblC type of combined methyl malonic aciduria and homocystinuria in 79 unrelated Chinese patients. 5 mutations are responsible for 80% of cases and suggest a role for mutation detection in early diagnosis. Cosson et al (2009) reports on long term outcome of 30 French patients with methyl malonic acidurias. 15 patients had neonatal onset, 13 had severe neurological involvement, 14 had chronic renal failure and 5 died during a metabolic crisis. Patients with a mut(0) phenotype had a severe phenotype and early and more severe CRF than patients with mut-/cblA phenotype.

Chandler et al (2007) reports successful use of adenoviral mediated gene therapy for methylmalonic aciduria in murine models and human patients with MUT gene mutation. Yang et al (2006) and other authors report that in China methylmalonic acidurias is more commonly associated with homocysteinemia. Filippi et al (2010) describes the use of N –

carbamyl glutamate in the emergency management of hyperammonemia in neonatal acute onset propionic aciduria and methylmalonic aciduria. Perez et al (2009) describes pseudoexon exclusion by antisense therapy in MMA. Haas et al (2009) report that Coenzyme Q (10) is significantly decreased in MMA patients.

Wajner et al (2009) identified 34 patients with MMA and 18 patients with PA from Brazil in 15 years. Zwickler et al (2008) reviews MMA patients in 14 centers in Germany and outlines the management principles. Most centers used hydroxocobalamin or cyanocobalamin for cobalamin-responsive patients while cobalamin - nonresponsive patients are supplemented with carnitine. Intestinal decontamination by antibiotic therapy, D-A-CH or Dewey recommendations for protein therapy and precursor-free amino acid supplements were used by most centers. Zhang et al (2007) studied the clinical picture of 96 patients with MMA over a 10 year period. Most of the patients had neurological abnormalities including developmental delay, seizures, psychomotor degeneration and motor disorders. A significant proportion of patients had MMA along with homocysteinemia.

Longo et al (2005) describes neurological abnormalities in MMA patients detected by MRI and 1H-MRS. Burlina et al (2003) and Rossi et al (2001) also describe neurological damage in MMA. Bodamer et al (2005) studied creatine metabolism in MMA patients and found that guanidinoacetate is elevated. They suggest that guanidinoacetate may be responsible for neurotoxicity in MMA. Vara et al (2011) discusses the importance of liver transplantation in propionic aciduria (PA) patients. Liver transplantation reduces the risk of metabolic decompensation and improves the quality of life. Romano et al (2010) report that cardiomyopathy in PA is reversible with liver transplantation.

Ah Mew et al (2010) also reports that NCG reduces ammonia and glutamine and induces ureagenesis in PA. Schwahn et al (2010) also reports of NCG in PA. Chandler et al (2011) describes the use of gene therapy using adeno associated virus (AAV8) for the treatment of PA. Ribas et al (2010) report that PA and MMA induce DNA damage and L - carnitine prevents this damage. Haberlandt et al (2009) report seizures in 9 patients with PA and hypothesize that some intermediates might be involved in the pathogenesis of epilepsy. Rigo et al (2006) suggests the involvement of NMDA receptors in the pathogenesis of neurological manifestations.

de Keyzer et al (2009) report multiple OXPHOS deficiency in liver, kidney, heart and skeletal muscle in patients with MMA and PA. Desviat et al (2009) report high frequency of large gene deletions in PA patients. This finding underscores the need for gene dosage analysis in additional to mutation testing in PA patients. Perez Cerda et al (2004) report the utility of prenatal diagnosis by molecular methods in 19 unrelated families with PA.

5.4 Section 1.3: Phenylketonuria (PKU)

5.4.1 Case report

We hereby report two patients with PKU. Patient 3 is a 21 year old woman with sub-normal intelligence and suspected to have phenylketonuria, though not confirmed previously (Phenylalanine level - 1427 μmol/L, Normal <65 μmol/L). Patient 4 is 19 years old and is the sibling of Patient 2 (Phenylalanine level 1177 μmol/L). She also had sub-normal intelligence. Both patients had pleasant social manners. At the time of presentation, Patient 3 was pregnant and had hence sought advice. Three months after presentation, Patient 4 also became pregnant. Both patients were confirmed to have phenylketonuria by urine and blood tests for phenylalanine. Phenylalanine restricted diet was advised, but compliance was not satisfactory and phenylalanine levels remained above 1000 µmol/L. Patient 3 delivered and child suffered from clinical and laboratory signs of maternal hyperphenylalaninemia. Child died in the immediate post natal period. The child of the other patient died in utero.

5.4.2 Biochemical abnormalities

Hyperphenylalaninemias are due to disorders of phenylalanine hydroxylation reaction. The minimum requirements for phenylalanine metabolism to occur are the enzyme phenyl alanine hydroxylase (PAH), molecular oxygen (O_2), L-Phenyl Alanine and tetrahydrobiopterin (BH_4). Other components include dihydrobiopterin (DHPR), reduced pyridine nucleotide, 4α carbinolamine dehydratase (for BH_4 recycling), GTP cyclohydrolase (GTP - CH) and 6 pyruvoyl tetrahydropterin synthase (6 PTS). Hyperphenylalaninemia is defined as Phenylalanine levels above 120 µM (2 mg/dl). Normal plasma level of phenyl alanine is 58±15 µM.

Phenylalanine cannot be converted to tyrosine. So phenylalanine accumulates. Phenylalanine level in blood is elevated. So alternate minor pathways are opened. Phenyl ketone (phenyl pyruvate), phenyl lactate and phenyl acetate are excreted in urine. Phenyl pyruvate inhibits pyruvate decarboxylase enzyme in brain, but not in liver. Hence myelin formation defects and mental retardation are seen. Brain effects are due to phenylalanine and its metabolites (phenyl ketones, namely Pyruvate, lactate, acetate, acetyl glutamine and ethyl amine) that accumulate via alternate pathway. Myelination and protein synthesis are affected and there is deficient neurotransmitter supply. Peculiarities of gait, stance and sitting posture are additional features. Brain calcification may be seen in DHPR deficient type.

Phenylketonuria is well known for the neurological manifestations. The classical PKU child is mentally retarded with an IQ of 50. About 20% inmates of psychiatric hospitals may have PKU. Agitation, hyperactivity, tremors and convulsions are often manifested. This may be because phenylalanine interferes with neurotransmitter synthesis. The child often has hypopigmentation, explained by the decreased level of tyrosine. Phenyl lactic acid in sweat may lead to mousy body odor.

5.4.3 Maternal hyperphenylalaninemia

Female child, on growing to adulthood may become pregnant (maternal hyper phenylalaninemia). Then again special diet is to be given, because the increased phenylalanine level will affect the brain development of the fetus. Maternal hyperphenylalaninemia (PKU embryo-fetopathy) cause embryopathy/ fetopathy comprising impaired growth, congenital cardiac malformations, microcephaly and mental retardation in the embryo/fetus. Fetal phenylalanine level is 1.5 - 2 fold higher than maternal blood level. Further fetal blood brain barrier concentrates phenylalanine to another 2-4 fold. Intraneuronal phenylalanine level of 600µmol interferes with brain development. Phenylalanine restricted diet should be started at least 3 months prior to planned pregnancy. Phe level in mother to be maintained at 60-180 µmol/L. Linoleic and linolenic acid supplements should be maintained at high level.

5.4.4 Review of literature

Oddason et al (2011) report 27 patients diagnosed with PKU in Iceland since 1947. Classical PKU is the commonest type. Macdonald et al (2011) in a study from UK report that PKU patients, especially older, are not fully compliant with treatment and hence have higher than acceptable phenylalanine levels. At the same time, van Rijn et al (2011) report that well-controlled adult PKU patients can tolerate larger dietary variations in phenylalanine levels. ten Hoedt et al (2011) report that high phenylalanine levels can directly affect mood and sustained attention in adult PKU patients (Randomized, double-blind, placebo-controlled, crossover trial).

Ribas et al (2011) suggest that oxidative stress may play a role in pathogenesis of PKU. Sanayama et al (2011) provide experimental evidence for the same and report that oxidative stress status is closely linked with phenylalanine levels. Sitta et al (2011) report that administration of L-carnitine and selenium can reduce oxidative stress in PKU patients.

Hanley (2011) in a review states that "non-PKU mild hyperphenylalaninemia" (MHP) also might have neuropsychological function deficits and therefore may need treatment with tetrahydrobiopterin and/or phenyl alanine restricted diet. Campistol et al (2011) discusses on the extent of neuro-congitive dysfunction in mild PKU (mPKU) and conclude that further studies are needed on mPKU to clearly answer this question. van Spronsen (2011) addresses the question on treatment of mPKU and reaches similar conclusion.

Vernon et al (2010), Trefz et al (2010), Harding (2010), Burton et al (2010), Somaraju & Merrin (2010) and others report that saptopterin hydrochloride, a synthetic analog of tetrahydrobiopterin, is a promising new drug in the treatment of PKU. This modality of treatment is especially important considering the report by Enns et al (2010) who state that PKU treated with diet alone has sub-optimal outcome with relation to neurocognitive, psychological and physical parameters. Lee et al (2009) and others however, report better outcome with dietary treatment alone. Blau et al (2010) reports on the management practices in PKU in 165 PKU centers in 23 European countries. They emphasize that treatment recommendations vary tremendously in different countries and hence there is an urgent need to pool long-term data in registries to generate evidence based international guidelines. Ahring et al (2009) and van Spronsen (2009) give similar reports.

Rocha and Martel (2009) report the use of large neutral amino acids in the treatment of PKU. The same carrier transports phenylalanine as well as large neutral amino acids into the brain; hence their use diminishes toxicity due to phenylalanine. Weigel et al (2008) report low free carnitine levels in PKU patients given low phenylalanine diet. They suggest that carnitine level should be monitored in PKU patients. Sitta et al (2009) reach similar conclusions. A study by Maillot et al (2008) reports on the importance of maintaining blood phenylalanine during pregnancy. They conclude that maintenance of maternal blood phenylalanine level within the target range predicts good offspring outcomes; and further suggests that variations even within that range should be avoided.

5.5 Section 1.4: Nonketotic hyperglycinemia

5.5.1 Case report

We report here one male baby (Patient 5) with intractable seizures who was 7 days old. All antiepileptic drugs were tried without any response. The parents were complaining about medical negligence. HPLC analysis of amino acid revealed nonketotic hyperglycinemia (NKH) (Figure 3). Even though the child could not be revived; this case shows the importance of workup for inborn errors of metabolism to reach a diagnosis. In this case, the diagnosis was important for the doctor to counsel the parents appropriately.

5.5.2 Biochemical abnormalities

It is due to defect in **glycine cleavage system**. Glycine level is increased in blood, urine and CSF. Severe mental retardation and seizures are seen. There is no effective management. Large quantities of Glycine accumulate in all body tissues including CNS. Diagnosis is established by CSF: plasma Glycine concentration >0.08. Patients have a neonatal phenotype and present in the first few days of life with lethargy, hypotonia and myoclonic jerks and progressing to apnea and death. Surviving infants have intractable seizures and profound mental retardation. Later-onset children have progressive spastic diplegia and optic atrophy, but mental retardation and seizures may not be seen. Transient NKH is also reported. It is inherited as an autosomal recessive disorder. In neonatal NKH CSF: plasma ratio may be 0.09-0.25 and in atypical NKH it is 0.09 - 0.10. Normal ratio is 0.012 - 0.040.

5.5.3 Review of literature

Aburahma et al (2011) report that elevated CSF/plasma glycine level is encountered in a variety of clinical conditions and hence cannot be considered to be pathognomonic of nonketotic hyperglycinemia (NKH). This report is significant because NKH is a disease with very bad prognosis. Lang et al (2008) discusses the difficulties of diagnosing transient NKH.

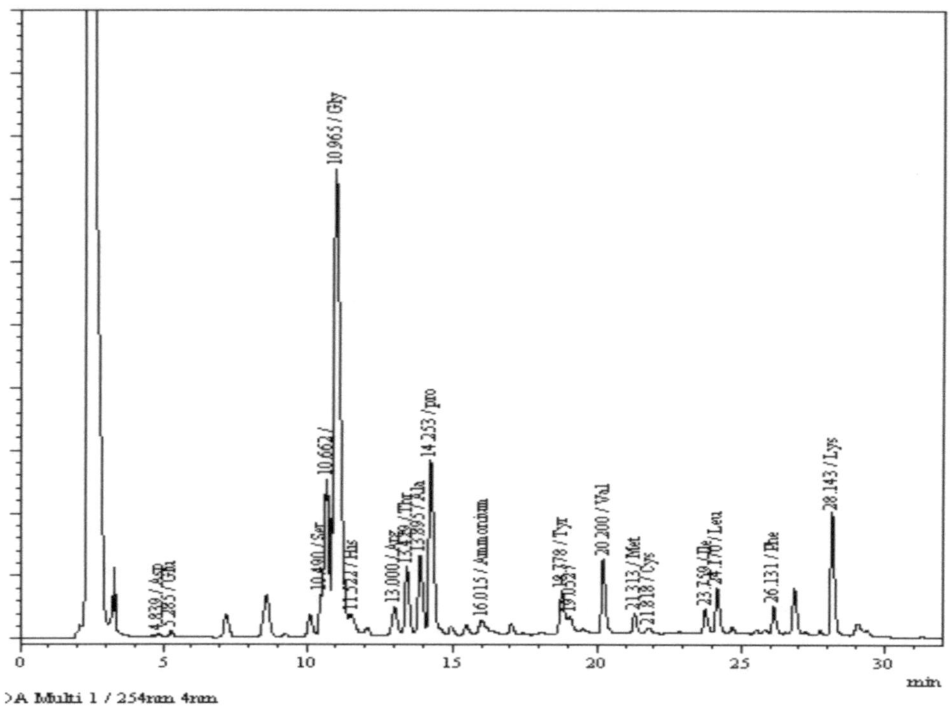

Fig. 3. Chromatogram of patient 5 showing elevated glycine levels (Glycine 1311 μmol/L, Normal Glycine < 275 μmol/L)

Leipnitz et al (2009) report lipid peroxidation and reduced antioxidant levels in NKH. Kanno et al (2007) reviews the genetic causes of NKH. NKH can be caused by genes in the glycine cleavage system, including GLDC, AMT and GCSH. They report significant number of GLDC mutations by MLPA (multiple ligation-dependent probe amplification) analysis. Conter et al (2006) and Kure et al (2006) also report significant number of mutations in these genes.

Tan et al (2007) report that currently tandem mass spectrometry employed for newborn screening does not identify NKH without significant error rate. Raghavendra et al (2007) and others report significant neurological abnormalities in patients with NKH. Generally NKH is a disease refractory to treatment. A number of authors report the use of sodium benzoate and dextromethrophan in the treatment of NKH, some of them with and others without any beneficial effect.

6. Section 2: Hyperhomocysteinemia

6.1 Materials and methods

Homocysteine estimation was done by ELISA method (BioRad Laboratories Inc.). 5 ml blood was drawn from the patients. 953 patients were analyzed during this 5 year period, 110 patients were from the Department of Cardiology, 656 from the Department of Neurology and the remaining from other departments.

6.2 Results

285 patients had elevated homocysteine levels. 226 cases had hyperhomocysteinemia from the Department of Neurology (226/656, 34.5%), 31 had hyperhomocysteinemia from the Department of Cardiology (31/110, 28.2%), and the remaining were other cases like peripheral artery disease, deep vein thrombosis etc. Neurological disorders included different types of stroke including medullary stroke, ischemic stroke, young stroke, transient ischemic attack, sagittal sinus thrombosis, lacunar thalamic stroke and recurrent stroke. All patients with hyperhomocysteinemia from the Department of Cardiology were suffering from Coronary artery disease (CAD).

6.3 Biochemical abnormalities

Normal homocysteine level in blood is 5-15 μmol/L. In diseases, it may be increased to 50 to 100 times. Moderate increase is seen in aged persons, vitamin B12 or B6 deficiency, tobacco smokers, alcoholics and in hypothyroidism. Substantial increase is noticed in congenital enzyme deficiencies. Large amounts of homocysteine are excreted in urine. In plasma, homocysteine (with -SH group) and homocysteine (disulfide, -S-S- group) exist. Both of them are absent in normal urine; but if present, it will be the homocysteine (disulfide) form. If homocysteine level in blood is increased, there is increased risk for coronary artery diseases. Homocystinuria/ hyperhomocysteinemia may be due to many causes. These include impaired activity of CBS (genetic CBS deficiency, INH therapy), methionine synthase defect, MTHFR defect, impaired metabolism of vitamin B12, renal insufficiency, pyridoxine and folate deficiency etc.

6.4 Review of literature

Hyperhomocysteinemia is associated with a number of diseases including coronary artery diseases, stroke, retinal vein thrombosis, diabetic peripheral neuropathy, schizophrenia, preeclampsia, chronic pancreatitis etc. Herrmann and Obeid (2011) have reviewed the role of hyperhomocysteinemia in neurodegenerative diseases like Alzheimer's disease, vascular dementia, cognitive impairment and stroke. Damelan et al (2010) report hyperhomocysteinemia is ischemic stroke patients from France. Valentino et al ((2010) report elevated blood and CSF levels of homocysteine in amyotropic lateral sclerosis (ALS).

Sniezawska et al (2011) report that antiepileptic drug (AED) treatment in epileptics leads to increase in homocysteine and asymmetric dimethyl arginine (ADMA) levels. Greater increase in homocysteine is observed in patients with MTHFR CT (C677T) and MTHFD1 GG (G1958A) polymorphisms. Linnebank et al (2011) report reduced serum Vitamin B12 and folate levels on treatment with AED. Zhuo et al (2010) report that normalization of homocysteine values in rat models with hyperhomocysteinemia resulted in improvement of cognitive defects and brain amyloidosis.

Paoli et al (2010) report that protein N homocysteinylation induces the formation of toxic amyloid like amyloid protofibrils. The authors hypothesize that this could be responsible for pathophysiology of hyperhomocysteinemia. da Cunha et al (2010) report increase in inflammatory markers in brain and blood of mice after acute homocysteine administration. This study suggests that inflammation may be at least partially responsible for neurological and cardiovascular response of homocysteine. Green et al (2010) report that homocysteine lowering vitamins do not lower S adenosyl homocysteine levels in older people. They suggest that S adenosyl homocysteine might be a better indicator for vascular events. They hypothesize that this might explain the lack of clinical benefit of B vitamins in some patients with hyperhomocysteinemia. Almawi et al (2009) and others have investigated the role of MTHFR C677T polymorphism and high homocysteine levels in patients with stroke. Dutta et al (2009) report mild increase in serum homocysteine levels in Indian patients with idiopathic mental retardation.

7. Section 3: Pheochromocytoma, neuroblastoma

7.1 Materials and methods

VMA estimation was done using column method (BioRad VMA by column test). 24 hr urine samples were collected following dietary restrictions for 3 days. Samples were collected in 6N HCl and stored in the refrigerator during collection time. If the pH was more than 3.5, the samples were rejected. The analysis was done following manufacturer's guidelines. 582 samples were collected during this time period.

7.2 Results

44 patients had elevated VMA levels. This included 24 cases of pheochromocytoma, 15 cases of neuroblastoma and 5 cases of paraganglioma. The analysis correlated positively with histopathology studies. All patients with pheochromocytoma and paraganglioma were above 10 years of age; whereas 60% cases of neuroblastoma cases were below 10 years of age. The sensitivity and specificity of our results were 88% and 86% respectively. All neuroblastoma cases showed elevated VMA level.

7.3 Biochemical abnormalities

Catecholamines are important biological compounds, essential to maintain the proper functioning of the body. Secretion of excessive catecholamines can produce stress, palpitation, paroxysmal hypertension, congestive heart failure, thyroid hormone deficiency and arrhythmias. Measurement of catecholamines and its metabolites is primarily used in the diagnosis of Neuroendocrine tumors; Neuroblastomas, Pheochromocytomas and paragangliomas. Most common metabolites of catecholamines are Vanillylmandelic acid (VMA), urinary free catecholamines, metanephrine, normetanephrine, homovanillic acid (HVA), plasma catecholamines, plasma metanephrines and chromogranin A. Most of the metabolites are measured by spectrophotometric assays, nowadays replaced by HPLC and mass spectrometry. Vanillylmandelic acid (VMA) is a major catecholamine metabolite formed by the actions of catechol-O-methyl transferase and MAO. VMA is excreted by kidney and represents 40%-50% urinary excretory product of norepinephrine and epinephrine. Norepinephrine is the major source of VMA.

Neuroblastomas are the most common solid extra-cranial tumors in children, and account for 7-10 % of all tumors. In about 90% of cases of neuroblastoma, elevated levels of catecholamines or its metabolites are found in the urine or blood. Pheochromocytomas are chromaffin-cell tumors; 80-85 % arises from the adrenal medulla and 15-20 % arises from extra-adrenal chromaffin tissues (paragangliomas). They are characterized by excessive production of catecholamines. If not diagnosed or if left untreated, the excessive secretion of catecholamines by these tumors can have devastating consequences. Paraganglioma is a rare neuroendocrine tumor that arises from extraadrenal sympathochromaffin tissue, usually in the abdomen. 10% of the catecholamine producing tumors are paragangliomas that develop in head, neck, thorax and abdomen. About 97% are benign and 3% metastatic.

7.4 Review of literature

Elevated urinary catecholamines have been described in 90 - 95 % of patients with neuroblastomas [Smith et al (2010)]. Studies suggest that dopamine nervous systems are involved in the pathogenesis of autistic disorder. Quantification of urine homovanillic acid (HVA) and vanillylmandelic acid (VMA) by GC/MS are very important in the study of dopamine metabolism in autistic children [Kaluzna-Czaplinska et al (2010)]. Allenbrand and Garg (2010) also report quantification of urine HVA and VMA by GC/MS. Li et al (2010) describe that the ratio of HVA/VMA ratio is useful as a disease marker in neuroblastomas and pheochromocytomas. Aydin et al (2010) report that VMA is a poor prognostic factor in patients with neuroblastoma.

Hickman et al (2009) report that in patients with pheochromocytoma, plasma free metanephrines displayed superior diagnostic sensitivity and specificity compared with other biochemical markers of catecholamine output and metabolism. Boyle et al (2007) came to a similar conclusion. Lionetto et al (2008) describe an HPLC-tandem mass spectrometric method for the simultaneous quantification of VMA, HVA and 5-HIAA in human urine.

8. Conclusions

We have detected a high incidence of metabolic disorders in our population. The commonest disorders detected were organic acidurias, congenital adrenal hyperplasia and hyperhomocysteinemia. Aminoacidurias like PKU are rare; whereas organic acidurias (PAA, MMA and MSUD) are more common. Prompt identification and treatment is important and early diagnosis helps to institute treatment measures which prevents further morbidity and reduces mortality rates.

Acknowledgements: We thank Kerala State Council for Science, Technology and Environment (KSCSTE), Indian Council of Medical Research (ICMR) for the financial support; Sumithra K, Rajesh PC and Anoop PA for the technical assistance.

9. References

Aburahma S, Khassawneh M, Griebel M, Sharp G, Gibson J. Pitfalls in measuring cerebrospinal fluid glycine levels in infants with encephalopathy. J Child Neurol. 2011 Jun;26(6):703-6. Epub 2011 Feb 18.

Ah Mew N, McCarter R, Daikhin Y, Nissim I, Yudkoff M, Tuchman M. N-carbamylglutamate augments ureagenesis and reduces ammonia and glutamine in propionic acidemia. Pediatrics. 2010 Jul;126(1):e208-14. Epub 2010 Jun 21.

Allenbrand R, Garg U. Quantitation of homovanillic acid (HVA) and vanillylmandelic acid (VMA) in urine using gas chromatography-mass spectrometry (GC/MS). Methods Mol Biol. 2010;603:261-9.

Almawi WY, Khan A, Al-Othman SS, Bakhiet M. Case-control Study of methylenetetrahydrofolate reductase mutations and hyperhomocysteinemia and risk of stroke. J Stroke Cerebrovasc Dis. 2009 Sep-Oct;18(5):407-8.

Aydin GB, Kutluk MT, Yalcin B, Varan A, Akyuz C, Buyukpamukcu M. The prognostic significance of vanillylmandellic acid in neuroblastoma. Pediatr Hematol Oncol. 2010 Sep;27(6):435-48.

Barschak AG, Sitta A, Deon M, Busanello EN, Coelho DM, Cipriani F, Dutra-Filho CS, Giugliani R, Wajner M, Vargas CR. Amino acids levels and lipid peroxidation in maple syrup urine disease patients. Clin Biochem. 2009 Apr;42(6):462-6. Epub 2008 Dec 24.

Bindu PS, Shehanaz KE, Christopher R, Pal PK, Ravishankar S. Intermediate maple syrup urine disease: neuroimaging observations in 3 patients from South India. J Child Neurol. 2007 Jul;22(7):911-3.

Blau N, Belanger-Quintana A, Demirkol M, Feillet F, Giovannini M, MacDonald A, Trefz FK, van Spronsen F; European PKU centers. Management of phenylketonuria in Europe: survey results from 19 countries. Mol Genet Metab. 2010 Feb;99(2):109-15. Epub 2009 Sep 13.

Bodamer OA, Sahoo T, Beaudet AL, O'Brien WE, Bottiglieri T, Stockler-Ipsiroglu S, Wagner C, Scaglia F. Creatine metabolism in combined methylmalonic aciduria and homocystinuria. Ann Neurol. 2005 Apr;57(4):557-60.

Boyle JG, Davidson DF, Perry CG, Connell JM. Comparison of diagnostic accuracy of urinary free metanephrines, vanillyl mandelic Acid, and catecholamines and plasma catecholamines for diagnosis of pheochromocytoma. J Clin Endocrinol Metab. 2007 Dec;92(12):4602-8. Epub 2007 Jul 17.

Bridi R, Braun CA, Zorzi GK, Wannmacher CM, Wajner M, Lissi EG, Dutra-Filho CS. alpha-keto acids accumulating in maple syrup urine disease stimulate lipid peroxidation and reduce antioxidant defences in cerebral cortex from young rats. Metab Brain Dis. 2005 Jun;20(2):155-67.

Brunetti-Pierri N, Lanpher B, Erez A, Ananieva EA, Islam M, Marini JC, Sun Q, Yu C, Hegde M, Li J, Wynn RM, Chuang DT, Hutson S, Lee B. Phenylbutyrate therapy for maple syrup urine disease. Hum Mol Genet. 2011 Feb 15;20(4):631-40. Epub 2010 Nov 23.

Burlina AP, Manara R, Calderone M, Catuogno S, Burlina AB. Diffusion-weighted imaging in the assessment of neurological damage in patients with methylmalonic aciduria. J Inherit Metab Dis. 2003;26(5):417-22.

Burton BK, Bausell H, Katz R, Laduca H, Sullivan C. Sapropterin therapy increases stability of blood phenylalanine levels in patients with BH4-responsive phenylketonuria (PKU). Mol Genet Metab. 2010 Oct-Nov;101(2-3):110-4. Epub 2010 Jun 27.

Cakmakci H, Pekcevik Y, Yis U, Unalp A, Kurul S. Diagnostic value of proton MR spectroscopy and diffusion-weighted MR imaging in childhood inherited neurometabolic brain diseases and review of the literature. Eur J Radiol. 2010 Jun;74(3):e161-71. Epub 2009 Jun 21.

Campistol J, Gassio R, Artuch R, Vilaseca MA; PKU Follow-up Unit. Neurocognitive function in mild hyperphenylalaninemia. Dev Med Child Neurol. 2011 May;53(5):405-8. Epub 2011 Mar 21.

Chandler RJ, Chandrasekaran S, Carrillo-Carrasco N, Senac JS, Hofherr SE, Barry MA, Venditti CP. Adeno-associated virus serotype 8 gene transfer rescues a neonatal lethal murine model of propionic acidemia. Hum Gene Ther. 2011 Apr;22(4):477-81. Epub 2011 Feb 16.

Chandler RJ, Tsai MS, Dorko K, Sloan J, Korson M, Freeman R, Strom S, Venditti CP. Adenoviral-mediated correction of methylmalonyl-CoA mutase deficiency in murine fibroblasts and human hepatocytes. BMC Med Genet. 2007 Apr 30;8:24.

Chen Z, Luo F, Wu XJ, Shi LP. Maple syrup urine disease of neonates: report of two cases and review of literature. Zhonghua Er Ke Za Zhi. 2010 Sep;48(9):680-4.

Conter C, Rolland MO, Cheillan D, Bonnet V, Maire I, Froissart R. Genetic heterogeneity of the GLDC gene in 28 unrelated patients with glycine encephalopathy. J Inherit Metab Dis. 2006 Feb;29(1):135-42.

Cosson MA, Benoist JF, Touati G, Dechaux M, Royer N, Grandin L, Jais JP, Boddaert N, Barbier V, Desguerre I, Campeau PM, Rabier D, Valayannopoulos V, Niaudet P, de Lonlay P. Long-term outcome in methylmalonic aciduria: a series of 30 French patients. Mol Genet Metab. 2009 Jul;97(3):172-8. Epub 2009 Mar 24.

da Cunha AA, Ferreira AG, Wyse AT. Increased inflammatory markers in brain and blood of rats subjected to acute homocysteine administration. Metab Brain Dis. 2010 Jun;25(2):199-206. Epub 2010 Apr 28.

Damelan K, Kom A, Kossivi A, Koffi BA, Emile A, Kodjo GE. Hyperhomocysteinemia among ischaemic stroke victims in the teaching hospital of Lome. Ann Biol Clin (Paris). 2010 Nov-Dec;68(6):669-73.

de Keyzer Y, Valayannopoulos V, Benoist JF, Batteux F, Lacaille F, Hubert L, Chretien D, Chadefeaux-Vekemans B, Niaudet P, Touati G, Munnich A, de Lonlay P. Multiple OXPHOS deficiency in the liver, kidney, heart, and skeletal muscle of patients with methylmalonic aciduria and propionic aciduria. Pediatr Res. 2009 Jul;66(1):91-5.

Desviat LR, Sanchez-Alcudia R, Perez B, Perez-Cerda C, Navarrete R, Vijzelaar R, Ugarte M. High frequency of large genomic deletions in the PCCA gene causing propionic acidemia. Mol Genet Metab. 2009 Apr;96(4):171-6. Epub 2009 Jan 20.

Dutta S, Chatterjee A, Sinha S, Chattopadhyay A, Mukhopadhyay K. Correlation between cystathionine beta synthase gene polymorphisms, plasma homocysteine and idiopathic mental retardation in Indian individuals from Kolkata. Neurosci Lett. 2009 Apr 10;453(3):214-8. Epub 2009 Feb 21.

Enns GM, Koch R, Brumm V, Blakely E, Suter R, Jurecki E. Suboptimal outcomes in patients with PKU treated early with diet alone: revisiting the evidence. Mol Genet Metab. 2010 Oct-Nov;101(2-3):99-109. Epub 2010 Jun 22.

Filippi L, Gozzini E, Fiorini P, Malvagia S, la Marca G, Donati MA. N-carbamylglutamate in emergency management of hyperammonemia in neonatal acute onset propionic and methylmalonic aciduria. Neonatology. 2010;97(3):286-90. Epub 2009 Nov 4.

Green TJ, Skeaff CM, McMahon JA, Venn BJ, Williams SM, Devlin AM, Innis SM. Homocysteine-lowering vitamins do not lower plasma S-adenosylhomocysteine in older people with elevated homocysteine concentrations. Br J Nutr. 2010 Jun;103(11):1629-34. Epub 2010 Jan 21.

Haas D, Niklowitz P, Horster F, Baumgartner ER, Prasad C, Rodenburg RJ, Hoffmann GF, Menke T, Okun JG. Coenzyme Q(10) is decreased in fibroblasts of patients with methylmalonic aciduria but not in mevalonic aciduria. J Inherit Metab Dis. 2009 Aug;32(4):570-5. Epub 2009 Jun 7.

Haberlandt E, Canestrini C, Brunner-Krainz M, Moslinger D, Mussner K, Plecko B, Scholl-Burgi S, Sperl W, Rostasy K, Karall D. Epilepsy in patients with propionic acidemia. Neuropediatrics. 2009 Jun;40(3):120-5. Epub 2009 Dec 17.

Hanley WB. Non-PKU mild hyperphenylalaninemia (MHP) - The dilemma. Mol Genet Metab. 2011 May 14. [Epub ahead of print]

Harding CO. New era in treatment for phenylketonuria: Pharmacologic therapy with sapropterin dihydrochloride. Biologics. 2010 Aug 9;4:231-6.

Herrmann W, Obeid R. Homocysteine: a biomarker in neurodegenerative diseases. Clin Chem Lab Med. 2011 Mar;49(3):435-41.

Hickman PE, Leong M, Chang J, Wilson SR, McWhinney B. Plasma free metanephrines are superior to urine and plasma catecholamines and urine catecholamine metabolites for the investigation of phaeochromocytoma. Pathology. 2009 Feb;41(2):173-7.

Ibarra-Gonzalez I, Fernandez-Lainez C, Belmont-Martinez L, Vela-Amieva M. Increased mortality and disability in a cohort of Mexican children with maple syrup urine disease. Gac Med Mex. 2007 May-Jun;143(3):197-201.

Kaluzna-Czaplinska J, Socha E, Rynkowski J. Determination of homovanillic acid and vanillylmandelic acid in urine of autistic children by gas chromatography/mass spectrometry. Med Sci Monit. 2010 Sep;16(9):CR445-50.

Kanno J, Hutchin T, Kamada F, Narisawa A, Aoki Y, Matsubara Y, Kure S. Genomic deletion within GLDC is a major cause of non-ketotic hyperglycinaemia. J Med Genet. 2007 Mar;44(3):e69.

Keskinen P, Siitonen A, Salo M. Hereditary urea cycle diseases in Finland. Acta Paediatr. 2008 Oct;97(10):1412-9. Epub 2008 Jul 9.

Kowalik A, Narojek L, Sykut-Cegielska J. Compliance of the diet restricted with leucine, isoleucine and valine in maple syrup urine disease (MSUD) children. Rocz Panstw Zakl Hig. 2007;58(1):95-101.

Kure S, Kato K, Dinopoulos A, Gail C, DeGrauw TJ, Christodoulou J, Bzduch V, Kalmanchey R, Fekete G, Trojovsky A, Plecko B, Breningstall G, Tohyama J, Aoki Y, Matsubara Y. Comprehensive mutation analysis of GLDC, AMT, and GCSH in nonketotic hyperglycinemia. Hum Mutat. 2006 Apr;27(4):343-52.

Lang TF, Parr JR, Matthews EE, Gray RG, Bonham JR, Kay JD. Practical difficulties in the diagnosis of transient non-ketotic hyperglycinaemia. Dev Med Child Neurol. 2008 Feb;50(2):157-9.

Lee JY, Chiong MA, Estrada SC, Cutiongco-De la Paz EM, Silao CL, Padilla CD. Maple syrup urine disease (MSUD)-Clinical profile of 47 Filipino patients. J Inherit Metab Dis. 2008 Nov 10. [Epub ahead of print]

Lee PJ, Amos A, Robertson L, Fitzgerald B, Hoskin R, Lilburn M, Weetch E, Murphy G. Adults with late diagnosed PKU and severe challenging behaviour: a randomised placebo-controlled trial of a phenylalanine-restricted diet. J Neurol Neurosurg Psychiatry. 2009 Jun;80(6):631-5. Epub 2009 Feb 9.

Leipnitz G, Solano AF, Seminotti B, Amaral AU, Fernandes CG, Beskow AP, Dutra Filho CS, Wajner M. Glycine provokes lipid oxidative damage and reduces the antioxidant defenses in brain cortex of young rats. Cell Mol Neurobiol. 2009 Mar;29(2):253-61. Epub 2008 Oct 2.

Li Q, Batchelor-McAuley C, Compton RG. Electrooxidative decarboxylation of vanillylmandelic acid: voltammetric differentiation between the structurally related compounds homovanillic acid and vanillylmandelic acid. J Phys Chem B. 2010 Jul 29;114(29):9713-9.

Linnebank M, Moskau S, Semmler A, Widman G, Stoffel-Wagner B, Weller M, Elger CE. Antiepileptic drugs interact with folate and vitamin B12 serum levels. Ann Neurol. 2011 Feb;69(2):352-9. doi: 10.1002/ana.22229. Epub 2011 Jan 19.

Lionetto L, Lostia AM, Stigliano A, Cardelli P, Simmaco M. HPLC-mass spectrometry method for quantitative detection of neuroendocrine tumor markers: vanillylmandelic acid, homovanillic acid and 5-hydroxyindoleacetic acid. Clin Chim Acta. 2008 Dec;398 (1- 2):53-6. Epub 2008 Aug 8.

Liu MY, Yang YL, Chang YC, Chiang SH, Lin SP, Han LS, Qi Y, Hsiao KJ, Liu TT. Mutation spectrum of MMACHC in Chinese patients with combined methylmalonic aciduria and homocystinuria. J Hum Genet. 2010 Sep;55(9):621-6. Epub 2010 Jul 15.

Longo D, Fariello G, Dionisi-Vici C, Cannata V, Boenzi S, Genovese E, Deodato F. MRI and 1H-MRS findings in early-onset cobalamin C/D defect. Neuropediatrics. 2005 Dec;36(6):366-72.

Lou Y, Yin N, Chen FQ, Cheng YY, Xu LJ, Dai F, Song XT. Selective screening of inborn errors of metabolism by using the tandem mass spectrometry: pilot study of 552 children at high risk. Zhongguo Dang Dai Er Ke Za Zhi. 2011 Apr; 13 (4): 296 – 9.

Macdonald A, Nanuwa K, Parkes L, Nathan M, Chauhan D. Retrospective, observational data collection of the treatment of phenylketonuria in the UK, and associated clinical and health outcomes. Curr Med Res Opin. 2011 Jun;27(6):1211-22. Epub 2011 Apr 19.

Maillot F, Lilburn M, Baudin J, Morley DW, Lee PJ. Factors influencing outcomes in the offspring of mothers with phenylketonuria during pregnancy: the importance of variation in maternal blood phenylalanine. Am J Clin Nutr. 2008 Sep;88(3):700-5.

Mescka C, Moraes T, Rosa A, Mazzola P, Piccoli B, Jacques C, Dalazen G, Coelho J, Cortes M, Terra M, Regla Vargas C, Dutra-Filho CS. In vivo neuroprotective effect of L-carnitine against oxidative stress in maple syrup urine disease. Metab Brain Dis. 2011 Mar;26(1):21-8. Epub 2011 Mar 5.

Narayanan MP, Vaidyanathan K, Vinayan KP, Vasudevan DM. Diagnosis of major organic acidurias in children: Two years experience at a tertiary care centre. Ind J Clin Biochem (Oct - Dec 2011) 26(4): 347 - 353.

Niu DM, Chien YH, Chiang CC, Ho HC, Hwu WL, Kao SM, Chiang SH, Kao CH, Liu TT, Chiang H, Hsiao KJ. Nationwide survey of extended newborn screening by tandem mass spectrometry in Taiwan. J Inherit Metab Dis. 2010 Oct;33(Suppl 2):S295-305. Epub 2010 Jun 22.

Oddason KE, Eiriksdottir L, Franzson L, Dagbjartsson A. Phenylketonuria (PKU) in Iceland. Laeknabladid. 2011 Jun;97(6):349-352.

Pangkanon S, Charoensiriwatana W, Sangtawesin V. Maple syrup urine disease in Thai infants. J Med Assoc Thai. 2008 Oct;91 Suppl 3:S41-4.

Paoli P, Sbrana F, Tiribilli B, Caselli A, Pantera B, Cirri P, De Donatis A, Formigli L, Nosi D, Manao G, Camici G, Ramponi G. Protein N-homocysteinylation induces the formation of toxic amyloid-like protofibrils. J Mol Biol. 2010 Jul 23;400(4):889-907. Epub 2010 May 25.

Perez B, Rincon A, Jorge-Finnigan A, Richard E, Merinero B, Ugarte M, Desviat LR. Pseudoexon exclusion by antisense therapy in methylmalonic aciduria (MMAuria). Hum Mutat. 2009 Dec;30(12):1676-82.

Perez-Cerda C, Perez B, Merinero B, Desviat LR, Rodriguez-Pombo P, Ugarte M. Prenatal diagnosis of propionic acidemia. Prenat Diagn. 2004 Dec 15;24(12):962-4.

Raghavendra S, Ashalatha R, Thomas SV, Kesavadas C. Focal neuronal loss, reversible subcortical focal T2 hypointensity in seizures with a nonketotic hyperglycemic hyperosmolar state. Neuroradiology. 2007 Apr;49(4):299-305. Epub 2007 Jan 3.

Ribas GS, Manfredini V, de Marco MG, Vieira RB, Wayhs CY, Vanzin CS, Biancini GB, Wajner M, Vargas CR. Prevention by L-carnitine of DNA damage induced by propionic and L-methylmalonic acids in human peripheral leukocytes in vitro. Mutat Res. 2010 Sep 30;702(1):123-8. Epub 2010 Jul 24.

Ribas GS, Sitta A, Wajner M, Vargas CR. Oxidative Stress in Phenylketonuria: What is the Evidence? Cell Mol Neurobiol. 2011 Jul;31(5):653-62. Epub 2011 Apr 23.

Ribeiro CA, Sgaravatti AM, Rosa RB, Schuck PF, Grando V, Schmidt AL, Ferreira GC, Perry ML, Dutra-Filho CS, Wajner M. Inhibition of brain energy metabolism by the branched-chain amino acids accumulating in maple syrup urine disease. Neurochem Res. 2008 Jan;33(1):114-24. Epub 2007 Aug 8.

Rigo FK, Pasquetti L, Malfatti CR, Fighera MR, Coelho RC, Petri CZ, Mello CF. Propionic acid induces convulsions and protein carbonylation in rats. Neurosci Lett. 2006 Nov 13;408(2):151-4. Epub 2006 Sep 25.

Rocha JC, Martel F. Large neutral amino acids supplementation in phenylketonuric patients. J Inherit Metab Dis. 2009 Aug;32(4):472-80. Epub 2009 May 13.

Romano S, Valayannopoulos V, Touati G, Jais JP, Rabier D, de Keyzer Y, Bonnet D, de Lonlay P. Cardiomyopathies in propionic aciduria are reversible after liver transplantation. J Pediatr. 2010 Jan;156(1):128-34.

Rossi A, Cerone R, Biancheri R, Gatti R, Schiaffino MC, Fonda C, Zammarchi E, Tortori-Donati P. Early-onset combined methylmalonic aciduria and homocystinuria: neuroradiologic findings. AJNR Am J Neuroradiol. 2001 Mar;22(3):554-63.

Sanayama Y, Nagasaka H, Takayanagi M, Ohura T, Sakamoto O, Ito T, Ishige-Wada M, Usui H, Yoshino M, Ohtake A, Yorifuji T, Tsukahara H, Hirayama S, Miida T, Fukui M, Okano Y. Experimental evidence that phenylalanine is strongly associated to oxidative stress in adolescents and adults with phenylketonuria. Mol Genet Metab. 2011 Jul;103(3):220-5. Epub 2011 Mar 29.

Schonberger S, Schweiger B, Schwahn B, Schwarz M, Wendel U. Dysmyelination in the brain of adolescents and young adults with maple syrup urine disease. Mol Genet Metab. 2004 May;82(1):69-75.

Schwahn BC, Pieterse L, Bisset WM, Galloway PG, Robinson PH. Biochemical efficacy of N-carbamylglutamate in neonatal severe hyperammonaemia due to propionic acidaemia. Eur J Pediatr. 2010 Jan;169(1):133-4. Epub 2009 Aug 14.

Sener RN. Diffusion magnetic resonance imaging patterns in metabolic and toxic brain disorders. Acta Radiol. 2004 Aug;45(5):561-70.

Shellmer DA, DeVito Dabbs A, Dew MA, Noll RB, Feldman H, Strauss KA, Morton DH, Vockley J, Mazariegos GV. Cognitive and adaptive functioning after liver transplantation for maple syrup urine disease: a case series. Pediatr Transplant. 2011 Feb;15(1):58-64. Epub 2010 Oct 8.

Shigematsu Y, Hata I, Tajima G. Useful second-tier tests in expanded newborn screening of isovaleric acidemia and methylmalonic aciduria. J Inherit Metab Dis. 2010 Oct;33(Suppl 2):S283-8. Epub 2010 May 4.

Sitta A, Vanzin CS, Biancini GB, Manfredini V, de Oliveira AB, Wayhs CA, Ribas GO, Giugliani L, Schwartz IV, Bohrer D, Garcia SC, Wajner M, Vargas CR. Evidence that L-carnitine and selenium supplementation reduces oxidative stress in phenylketonuric patients. Cell Mol Neurobiol. 2011 Apr;31(3):429-36. Epub 2010 Dec 30.

Smith SJ, Diehl NN, Smith BD, Mohney BG. Urine catecholamine levels as diagnostic markers for neuroblastoma in a defined population: implications for ophthalmic practice. Eye (Lond). 2010 Dec;24(12):1792-6. Epub 2010 Sep 24.

Sniezawska A, Dorszewska J, Rozycka A, Przedpelska-Ober E, Lianeri M, Jagodzinski PP, Kozubski W. MTHFR, MTR, and MTHFD1 gene polymorphisms compared to homocysteine and asymmetric dimethylarginine concentrations and their metabolites in epileptic patients treated with antiepileptic drugs. Seizure. 2011 May 2. [Epub ahead of print]

Somaraju UR, Merrin M. Sapropterin dihydrochloride for phenylketonuria. Cochrane Database Syst Rev. 2010 Jun 16;(6):CD008005.

Strauss KA, Wardley B, Robinson D, Hendrickson C, Rider NL, Puffenberger EG, Shelmer D, Moser AB, Morton DH. Classical maple syrup urine disease and brain development: principles of management and formula design. Mol Genet Metab. 2010 Apr;99(4):333-45. Epub 2010 Jan 12.

Tan ES, Wiley V, Carpenter K, Wilcken B. Non-ketotic hyperglycinemia is usually not detectable by tandem mass spectrometry newborn screening. Mol Genet Metab. 2007 Apr;90(4):446-8. Epub 2007 Jan 4.

ten Hoedt AE, de Sonneville LM, Francois B, ter Horst NM, Janssen MC, Rubio-Gozalbo ME, Wijburg FA, Hollak CE, Bosch AM. High phenylalanine levels directly affect mood and sustained attention in adults with phenylketonuria: a randomised, double-blind, placebo-controlled, crossover trial. J Inherit Metab Dis. 2011 Feb;34(1):165-71. Epub 2010 Dec 10.

Trefz FK, Scheible D, Frauendienst-Egger G. Long-term follow-up of patients with phenylketonuria receiving tetrahydrobiopterin treatment. J Inherit Metab Dis. 2010 Mar 9. [Epub ahead of print]

Tu YF, Chen CY, Lin YJ, Chang YC, Huang CC. Neonatal neurological disorders involving the brainstem: neurosonographic approaches through the squamous suture and the foramen magnum. Eur Radiol. 2005 Sep;15(9):1927-33. Epub 2005 Apr 5.

Tuchman M, Lee B, Lichter-Konecki U, Summar ML, Yudkoff M, Cederbaum SD, Kerr DS, Diaz GA, Seashore MR, Lee HS, McCarter RJ, Krischer JP, Batshaw ML; Urea Cycle Disorders Consortium of the Rare Diseases Clinical Research Network. Cross-sectional multicenter study of patients with urea cycle disorders in the United States. Mol Genet Metab. 2008 Aug;94(4):397-402. Epub 2008 Jun 17.

Vaidyanathan K, Narayanan MP, Vasudevan DM. Organic acidurias: An updated review. Ind J Clin Biochem (Oct-Dec 2011) 26(4): 319 – 325.

Valentino F, Bivona G, Butera D, Paladino P, Fazzari M, Piccoli T, Ciaccio M, La Bella V. Elevated cerebrospinal fluid and plasma homocysteine levels in ALS. Eur J Neurol 2010 Jan, 17 (1): 84 – 9. Epub 2009 Jul 29.

van Spronsen FJ. Mild hyperphenylalaninemia: to treat or not to treat. J Inherit Metab Dis. 2011 Jun;34(3):651-6. Epub 2011 Feb 24.

Vara R, Turner C, Mundy H, Heaton ND, Rela M, Mieli-Vergani G, Champion M, Hadzic N. Liver transplantation for propionic acidemia in children. Liver Transpl. 2011 Jun;17(6):661-7.

Vernon HJ, Koerner CB, Johnson MR, Bergner A, Hamosh A. Introduction of sapropterin dihydrochloride as standard of care in patients with phenylketonuria. Mol Genet Metab. 2010 Jul;100(3):229-33. Epub 2010 Apr 3.

Wajner A, Burger C, Dutra-Filho CS, Wajner M, de Souza Wyse AT, Wannmacher CM. Synaptic plasma membrane Na(+), K (+)-ATPase activity is significantly reduced by the alpha-keto acids accumulating in maple syrup urine disease in rat cerebral cortex. Metab Brain Dis. 2007 Mar;22(1):77-88.

Wajner M, Coelho Dde M, Ingrassia R, de Oliveira AB, Busanello EN, Raymond K, Flores Pires R, de Souza CF, Giugliani R, Vargas CR. Selective screening for organic acidemias by urine organic acid GC-MS analysis in Brazil: fifteen-year experience. Clin Chim Acta. 2009 Feb;400(1-2):77-81. Epub 2008 Nov 1.

Walter JH, Patterson A, Till J, Besley GT, Fleming G, Henderson MJ. Bloodspot acylcarnitine and amino acid analysis in cord blood samples: efficacy and reference data from a large cohort study. J Inherit Metab Dis. 2009 Feb;32(1):95-101. Epub 2009 Jan 13.

Wasant P, Liammongkolkul S, Kuptanon C, Vatanavicharn N, Sathienkijakanchai A, Shinka T. Organic acid disorders detected by urine organic acid analysis: twelve cases in

Thailand over three-year experience. Clin Chim Acta. 2008 Jun;392(1-2):63-8. Epub 2008 Feb 23.

Weigel C, Kiener C, Meier N, Schmid P, Rauh M, Rascher W, Knerr I. Carnitine status in early-treated children, adolescents and young adults with phenylketonuria on low phenylalanine diets. Ann Nutr Metab. 2008;53(2):91-5. Epub 2008 Oct 22.

Yang Y, Sun F, Song J, Hasegawa Y, Yamaguchi S, Zhang Y, Jiang Y, Qin J, Wu X. Clinical and biochemical studies on Chinese patients with methylmalonic aciduria. J Child Neurol. 2006 Dec;21(12):1020-4.

Zhang Y, Song JQ, Liu P, Yan R, Dong JH, Yang YL, Wang LF, Jiang YW, Zhang YH, Qin J, Wu XR. Clinical studies on fifty-seven Chinese patients with combined methylmalonic aciduria and homocysteinemia. Zhonghua Er Ke Za Zhi. 2007 Jul;45(7):513-7.

Zhuo JM, Pratico D. Normalization of hyperhomocysteinemia improves cognitive deficits and ameliorates brain amyloidosis of a transgenic mouse model of Alzheimer's disease. FASEB J. 2010 Oct;24(10):3895-902. Epub 2010 Jun 2.

Zinnanti WJ, Lazovic J, Griffin K, Skvorak KJ, Paul HS, Homanics GE, Bewley MC, Cheng KC, Lanoue KF, Flanagan JM. Dual mechanism of brain injury and novel treatment strategy in maple syrup urine disease. Brain. 2009 Apr;132(Pt 4):903-18. Epub 2009 Mar 17.

Zwickler T, Lindner M, Aydin HI, Baumgartner MR, Bodamer OA, Burlina AB, Das AM, DeKlerk JB, Gokcay G, Grunewald S, Guffon N, Maier EM, Morava E, Geb S, Schwahn B, Walter JH, Wendel U, Wijburg FA, Muller E, Kolker S, Horster F. Diagnostic work-up and management of patients with isolated methylmalonic acidurias in European metabolic centres. J Inherit Metab Dis. 2008 Jun;31(3):361-7. Epub 2008 May 27.

4

Demonstration of Subclinical Organ Damage to the Central Nervous System in Essential Hypertension

Alina González-Quevedo[1], Sergio González García[1], Otman Fernández Concepción[1], Rosaralis Santiesteban Freixas[1], Luis Quevedo Sotolongo[2], Marisol Peña Sánchez[1], Rebeca Fernández Carriera[1] and Zenaida Hernández[1]

[1]Institute of Neurology and Neurosurgery, Havana,
[2]Central Clinic "Cira García", Havana,
Cuba

1. Introduction

Hypertension is a common condition, which affects approximately 25% of the adult population, with a higher prevalence in black (African origin) people. Presently it is considered to affect 1 billion people worldwide. Essential or primary hypertension, also known as hypertension of unknown cause, constitutes approximately 90-95% of cases of hypertension. It is a major risk factor for cardiovascular and cerebrovascular diseases and is responsible for most deaths worldwide. Risk factors for hypertension include family history, ageing, lifestyle (e.g. stress, diet, alcohol), and obesity.

The prevalence of hypertension in Cuba according to the 2010 statistics of the Ministry of Health is 202.7/1000 (http://files.sld.cu/hta/files/2011/09/prevalencia-de-hta.pdf), but it is considered to be underestimated. An epidemiological study conducted in 1995 in urban areas had revealed a prevalence of 30.6%.

As the population ages, the prevalence of hypertension is expected to increase even further, making it very important to establish more effective preventive measures. The Framingham Heart Study has implied that individuals who are normotensive at age 55 have a 90 percent lifetime risk for developing hypertension. It has been well established that the relationship between blood pressure (BP) and risk of cardiovascular events is continuous, consistent, and independent of other risk factors. The higher the BP, the greater the chance to suffer from heart attack, heart failure, stroke, and kidney disease (Chobanian et al, 2003).

Primary hypertension results from the interplay of internal derangements (primarily in the kidney) and the external environment. Sodium, the main extracellular cation, has long been considered the pivotal environmental factor in the disorder. Many pathophysiologic factors have been implicated in the genesis of essential hypertension: increased sympathetic nervous system activity, perhaps related to heightened exposure or response to psychosocial stress; overproduction of sodium-retaining hormones and vasoconstrictors; long-term high sodium intake; inadequate dietary intake of potassium and calcium; increased or inappropriate renin secretion with resultant increased production of angiotensin II and aldosterone; deficiencies of vasodilators, such as prostacyclin, nitric oxide, and the natriuretic peptides; alterations in expression of the kallikrein-kinin system that affect vascular tone and renal salt handling; abnormalities of resistance vessels, including selective lesions in the renal microvasculature; diabetes mellitus; insulin resistance; obesity; increased activity of vascular growth factors; alterations in adrenergic receptors that influence heart rate, iontropic properties of the heart, and vascular tone; and altered cellular ion transport. The concept that structural and functional abnormalities in the vasculature, including endothelial dysfunction, increased oxidative stress, vascular remodeling, and decreased compliance, may antedate hypertension and contribute to its pathogenesis has gained support in recent years (Adrogue & Madias, 2007; Oparil et al, 2003).

Hypertension has been extensively recognized as a highly prevalent risk factor for cardiovascular disease, becoming an increasingly common health problem worldwide because of increasing longevity and prevalence of contributing factors such as obesity, physical inactivity and an unhealthy diet. The current prevalence in many developing countries, particularly in urban societies, is already as high as those seen in developed countries. It also plays a major etiologic role in the development of cerebrovascular disease and renal failure.

In the 2007 European Guidelines for the management of arterial hypertension, it is recognized that although cardiovascular morbidity and mortality bear a continuous relationship with both systolic and diastolic blood pressures; the relationship has been reported to be less steep for coronary events than for stroke, which has been labelled as the most important "hypertension related" complication. The fact that hypertension is considered a major risk factor for an array of cardiovascular and related diseases, and the wide prevalence of high BP in the population, led to the World Health Organization (WHO) listing high BP as the first cause of death worldwide (Mancia et al, 2007).

Taking into account the very high prevalence of hypertension in the general population and its deleterious consequences, signs of organ involvement are sought carefully, and a large body of evidence is now available on the crucial role of subclinical organ damage. For cardiovascular and renal diseases this has been well established, as the techniques applied are widely available; but the detection of initial brain deterioration, requires the use of imaging techniques, whose availability and costs do not allow indiscriminate use by general medical practitioners.

In this chapter we present an update on the current status of markers employed for the early detection of brain damage in essential hypertension, and our experience in relation to the use of serum biochemical markers of brain injury.

2. Target organ damage in hypertension

The consequences of hypertension have been in constant debate since the mid 20th century. The most renowned consequences are probably those related with its role as a risk factor for myocardial infarction, heart failure, stroke and kidney disease, although it has also been involved in the development of vascular cognitive impairment and vascular dementia [Mancia et al, 2007; Chobanian et al, 2003; Henskens et al, 2009]. Chronic hypertension affects the cardiac and vascular systems, and various organs, especially the brain, kidney, and retina.

Table 1 shows the Position Statement of the 2007 European Guidelines for the Management of Arterial Hypertension concerning the detection of subclinical organ damage in hypertensive patients.

Organ damage	Techniques for detection
Heart • Left ventricular hypertrophy • Angina or prior myocardial infarction • Prior coronary revascularization • Heart failure	Electrocardiography should be part of all routine assessment of subjects with high BP in order to detect left ventricular hypertrophy, patterns of "strain", ischemia and arrhythmias. Echocardiography is recommended when a more sensitive detection of left ventricular hypertrophy is considered useful. Geometric patterns can be defined echocardio-graphically, of which concentric hypertrophy carries the worse prognosis. Diastolic dysfunction can be evaluated by transmitral Doppler.
Brain • Stroke or transient ischemic attack • White matter hyperintensities (WMH)	Silent brain infarcts, lacunar infarctions, microbleeds and white matter lesions are not infrequent in hypertensives, and can be detected by MRI or CT. Availability and costs do not allow indiscriminate use of these techniques. In elderly hypertensives, cognitive tests may help to detect initial brain deterioration.
Chronic kidney disease GFR below 60 ml/min per 1.73 m2 (corresponding approximately to a creatinine of >1.5 mg/dL in men or >1.3 mg/dL in women), 20 or (2) the presence of albuminuria (>300 mg/day or 200 mg albumin/g creatinine)	Diagnosis of hypertension-related renal damage is based on a reduced renal function or an elevated urinary excretion of albumin. Estimation from serum creatinine of glomerular filtration rate (MDRD formula, requiring age, gender, race) or creatinine clearance (Cockroft–Gault formula, requiring also body weight) should be routine procedure. Urinary protein should be sought in all hypertensives by dipstick. In dipstick negative patients low grade albuminuria (microalbuminuria) should be determined in spot urine and related to urinary creatinine excretion.
Peripheral arterial disease	Ultrasound scanning of carotid arteries is recommended when detection of vascular hypertrophy or asymptomatic atherosclerosis is deemed useful. Large artery stiffening (leading to isolated systolic hypertension in the elderly) can be measured by pulse wave velocity. It might be more widely recommended if its availability were greater. A low ankle-brachial BP index signals advanced peripheral artery disease.
Retinopathy	Fundoscopy – Examination of eye grounds is recommended in severe hypertensives only. Mild retinal changes are largely non-specific except in young patients. Hemorrhages, exudates and papilloedema, only present in severe hypertension, are associated with increased CV risk.

Table 1. Detection of subclinical organ damage in hypertensive patients

The brain is an early target for organ damage due to high BP, which is the major modifiable risk factor in men and women for ischemic and hemorrhagic stroke, as well as small vessel disease predisposing to lacunar infarction, white matter lesions (WML), and cerebral microbleeds, which are frequently silent. Arterial hypertension has been related to the development of brain damage, dementia, other CNS dysfunctions and even to milder forms of brain injury (Al-Sarraf and Philip, 2003; Amenta et al, 2003). The mechanisms underlying brain damage are thought to be a consequence of oxidative stress, inflammation and a defect in blood-brain barrier permeability (Al-Sarraf & Philip, 2003, Ishida et al, 2006; Poulet et al, 2006; Ueno et al, 2004).

Currently, hypertension guidelines mainly recognize the heart and kidneys as the crucial target organs affected by high blood pressure. Nevertheless, recently Henskens et al (2009) showed that silent cerebrovascular disease (identified with brain MRI) is a more frequent finding in hypertensive patients than cardiorenal damage. On the other hand, cardiovascular risk in these patients equaled that of patients with cardiorenal involvement and was significantly higher than that observed in patients without any hypertensive target-organ damage. This work suggested that the addition of silent cerebrovascular disease as a marker of hypertensive target-organ damage, apart from measures of cardiorenal involvement, refined the identification of patients at increased risk of cardiovascular and cerebrovascular complications. Thus, extending the search for hypertensive target-organ damage to other organs such as the brain might not only refine risk stratification, but might also optimize antihypertensive therapy. According to the results obtained by Henskens et al, 35% of the patients free of organ damage had actually silent brain damage. If we take into account that in the current guidelines for the management of arterial hypertension, the decision of drug intervention depends largely on the presence of target-organ involvement, these patients would be receiving suboptimal treatment.

The Reappraisal of the European Guidelines on hypertension management (Mancia et al, 2009) reports that, in a group of 192 untreated hypertensive patients (aged 18–90 years) without overt cardiovascular disease, silent cerebrovascular lesions (WML, lacunar infarcts, cerebral microbleeds) were more prevalent (44%) than cardiac (21%) and renal (26%) subclinical damage and frequently occur in the absence of other signs of organ damage. On the other hand, 58% of patients with demonstrable cardiac or renal damage or both had silent cerebrovascular lesions.

Stroke is the main neurological cause of mortality and the third most common cause of death worldwide, and hypertension is still it´s most important risk factor. In clinical trials, antihypertensive therapy has been associated with 35–40 percent reductions in stroke incidence [Chobanian et al, 2003].

Ohira et al (2006) studied a cohort of more than 14 000 men and women aged 45 to 64 years (free of clinical stroke) from the ARIC study (Atherosclerosis Risk in Communities), who were followed during an average of 13.4 years. They found that during the follow-up period, 531 incident ischemic strokes occurred (105 lacunar, 326 nonlacunar, and 100 cardioembolic strokes), and hypertension was the most powerful predictor for all ischemic stroke subtypes.

The evaluation of the consequences of hypertension on the heart and kidney has become a mainstay in routine clinical practice for years. Nevertheless, target organ damage to the brain is currently a research issue, and little has been accomplished in relation to introducing effective and low cost evaluation methods to be used by the medical practitioner.

3. Biomarkers for brain damage in hypertension

During the last decade research efforts have increased trying to demonstrate subclinical organ damage to the central nervous system as a consequence of essential hypertension. The most important evidence has been obtained employing imaging techniques (MRI, CT and positron emission tomography), as microvascular disease results in chronic ischemic changes affecting mainly the white matter.

Neuropsychological methods have demonstrated impairment of different cognitive domains (attention, memory, executive function) in hypertensive patients. Although the effect of anti-hypertensive treatment on cognitive function and dementia onset is controversial, a meta-analysis of randomized clinical trials suggested that anti-hypertensive treatment is beneficial for the prevention of cognitive decline, particularly in elderly high risk patients (O'Sullivan et al, 2003).

Another line of investigation has been brain electrical activity in hypertension. A recent study in neurologically asymptomatic hypertensive patients showed that quantitative EEG revealed altered spontaneous brain activity, mainly in the frontal and midline regions of the left hemisphere, which they infer as probably associated with brain hypoperfusion (De Quesada, 2010).

There is ongoing research into the association of blood pressure variability over the daytime and night-time periods (e.g.dipping status, early morning surge) with early brain deterioration in hypertension. To date it remains unknown whether and to what extent monitoring ambulatory blood pressure could prove useful for detecting subclinical damage of the central nervous system in hypertensive patients (Sierra, 2011).

There are many published reports indicating that serum molecular markers for neuronal damage are useful for estimating the timing and extent of cerebral injury, as well as for long term clinical outcome in several conditions, such as cardiopulmonary bypass, cardiac arrest, stroke, traumatic brain injury and others. For many years research has been directed toward the identification of biomarkers for establishing the differential diagnosis, aetiology and prognosis, which have gone from the application of clinical scores to more complex imaging techniques. In between these two methods, blood based biomarkers have received an important attention, especially during the last decade.

3.1 Imaging techniques

There is strong evidence that cerebral white matter hyperintensities (WMH) in hypertensive patients should be considered a silent early marker of brain damage. MRI and positron emission tomography (PET) techniques have shown signs of hypertensive target organ damage in the brain of asymptomatic hypertensive patients. WMHs or leukoaraiosis have been extensively documented in hypertensive patients, but silent lacunar infarcts and microbleeds can also be found, and recently dilated Virchow-Robin spaces have been considered as indicative of vascular damage (Angelini et al, 2009; Kitagawa, 2010; Lindgren et al, 1997; Mancia et al, 2007).

Hypertension is associated with the risk of subclinical brain damage noticed on cerebral MRI, particularly in elderly individuals. The most common types of brain lesions are WMH, which can be seen in almost all elderly individuals with hypertension and silent infarcts, the frequency of which varies between 10% and 30% according to different studies. Both lesions are characterized by high signal on T2-weighted images. Another type of lesion, more recently identified, are microbleeds, which are seen in about 5% of individuals on MRI Gradient echo (GRE) T2* images (Tzourio et al, 2010).

Several studies have suggested that sustained or uncontrolled hypertension is associated with a greater WMH load. The level of blood pressure also seems to play a role, higher blood pressure values being associated with higher grades of WMH. These dose-dependent effects provide strong support for a causal relationship between high BP and WMH.

Older age and hypertension are constantly reported to be the main risk factors for cerebral WMH. Hypertensive patients have a higher rate and extension of cerebral WMHs compared with normotensives (Sierra et al, 2011).

In humans, long term hypertension has been associated with the presence of periventricular and subcortical white matter lesions, and a subsequent cognitive decline has been demonstrated in certain settings (De Leeuw et al, 2002; Lindgren et al, 1997). Henskens et al (2009) described a continuous relationship between the volume of WMHs and ambulatory BP levels, while successfully controlled hypertension had a lower risk of WMHs (De Leeuw et al, 2002; Kuller et al, 2010). White matter lesions may arise from factors associated with brain hypoperfusion and breakdown of the blood-brain barrier, leading to decreased cerebral blood flow and consequent cerebral ischemia (De Leeuw et al, 2002; Henskens et al, 2009).

The clinical significance and pathological substrate of WMH are incompletely understood. It is known that they are an important prognostic factor for stroke, cognitive impairment, dementia and death. Cerebral WMH are more common and extensive in patients with cardiovascular risk factors, such as hypertension and diabetes mellitus, heart disease, and symptomatic cerebrovascular disease (Sierra el al, 2011).

Kitagawa (2010) studied the association between cerebral blood flow (CBF) and cognitive decline in hypertensive patients. They enrolled 27 cognitively intact patients with lacunar infarction or cerebral white matter lesions in MRI and measured CBF and cerebral vascular reactivity (CVR) with PET. Their results strongly suggest that cerebral hypoperfusion is associated with later cognitive decline in hypertensive patients with cerebral small vessel disease.

The pathogenesis of WMH remains unclear, but the main current hypothesis concerning the association between high BP and WMH is that long-standing hypertension causes lipohyalinosis of the media and thickening of the vessel walls, with narrowing of the lumen of the small perforating arteries and arterioles that nourish the deep white matter. On the other hand, low BP has also been reported to be a risk factor for WMH (Sierra, 2011).

3.2 Retinal microvascular abnormalities

The retina offers a unique, noninvasive, and easily accessible window to study the microvascular etiology of cerebrovascular disease. Retinal and cerebral small vessels share similar embryological origins, anatomical features, and physiological properties. The hypertensive retinal changes defined qualitatively from a fundus examination have been traditionally classified into four grades of retinopathy (Scheie, 1953); nevertheless, most hypertensive patients today present early in the process of their illness, and hemorrhages and exudates (grade 3), not to mention papilloedema (grade 4), are observed very rarely. The milder degrees of retinopathy appear to be largely non-specific arteriolar alterations (Grades 1 and 2) and their usefulness for prognosis has been questioned (Mancia et al, 2007), except for young patients. Thus, more selective methods for objectively investigating ocular damage in hypertension have been developed and studied. Digitized retinal photographs can be analyzed by a semiautomated program to quantify geometric and topological properties of arteriolar and venular trees. This method has identified hypertension-related topological alterations of retinal vasculature and showed that retinal arteriolar and venular narrowing may precede the development of hypertension (Grassi & Schmieder, 2011).

Cheung et al (2011) provided interesting data on the quantitative and qualitative assessment of retinal microvascular abnormalities in a general population and their relationships with blood pressure values. These authors developed new quantitative parameters which describe the retinal branching pattern (retinal vascular branching angle, the retinal vascular branching asymmetry ratio and the retinal vascular fractal dimension), as well as qualitative parameters (focal arteriolar narrowing, arteriovenous nicking, opacification of the arteriolar wall and retinopathy signs). These innovative parameters allow the investigators to improve the sensitivity and specificity of the approach in detecting retinal microcirculatory alterations.

Recently the presence of WMHs was said to be related not only to elevated brachial systolic BP, pulse pressure and arterial stiffness, but also to retinal arterial narrowing (Scuteri et al, 2011).

Studies have shown that retinal microvascular flow is reduced in persons with WMH and lacunar infarction. In a cohort of 1684 asymptomatic people aged 51–72 years from the ARIC study, individuals with WMH were more likely to have retinal microvascular abnormalities (Sierra et al, 2011). Retinal microvascular abnormalities measured at baseline were prospectively associated with a long-term risk of subclinical cerebrovascular disease on MRI, independent of conventional risk factors in this population-based cohort of middle-aged persons without clinical stroke. The authors suggested that retinal microvascular abnormalities are early and, possibly, more sensitive markers of subclinical cerebral small-vessel disease before radiological and clinical manifestations become apparent.

3.3 Cognitive tests

The role of hypertension as a risk factor for cognitive impairment is known from cross-sectional and longitudinal studies. The outcome of chronic microvascular damage is a continuous progression from mild cognitive alterations to overt vascular dementia. Semplicini et al (2011) reported the time course of cognitive changes in a cohort of long-term treated hypertensives, who never met the clinical criteria for dementia. At basal observation, the executive functions (the most affected cognitive domains) correlated with attention and cerebrovascular damage, but not with BP. They found that attention was positively correlated to BP (the higher the BP, the better attention performance). After 6-year follow-up, attention and executive functions improved, in spite of the minor BP changes, memory decline and progression of cerebrovascular damage. Based on these findings they suggested that short-term BP lowering negatively affected executive performance through unfavorable effects on attention. During long-term treatment, attention improved, probably because of adaptation of the cerebral circulation to lower BP, and this would also account for improvement of executive functions, in spite of the similar BP control and greater cerebrovascular damage.

Cognitive tests may help to detect initial brain deterioration in hypertension. It has been established that microvascular brain damage electively and predominantly affects executive function, with a slower information processing, impairments in the ability to shift from one task to another, and deficits in the ability to hold and manipulate information (i.e., working memory). Ideally, neuropsychological evaluation should include tests exploring multiple cognitive domains (executive function and activation, language, visuospatial ability, memory), in addition to neurobehavioral symptoms and mood. It has been put forward that future clinical guidelines should make clear that cognitive impairment has to be considered as target-organ damage in hypertensive patients, although it has been mentioned in the 2007 Guidelines from European Society of Hypertension (Scuteri et al, 2011).

The mechanisms underlying hypertension-related cognitive changes are complex and are not yet fully understood. It has been suggested that increased BP may explain the deterioration in cognitive functions in hypertensive individuals involving small vessel disease, white-matter lesions and endothelial dysfunction. An association was encountered between the presence of WMH and poorer performance on neuropsychological tests in middle-aged, asymptomatic, never-treated essential hypertensive patients (Sierra, 2011).

3.4 Physiological and neurophysiological methods

3.4.1 Ambulatory blood pressure monitoring

There is ongoing research into the association of blood pressure variability over the daytime and night-time periods (e.g. dipping status, early morning surge) with early brain deterioration in hypertension. To date it remains unknown whether and to what extent ambulatory blood pressure monitoring (ABPM) could prove useful for detecting subclinical damage of the central nervous system in hypertensive patients.

In essential hypertension, the presence of WMH has been associated with an exaggerated decline in nocturnal BP; however, this finding has not been replicated in subsequent studies. Steady and pulsatile components of daytime, night time and 24-h BP have gained increased interest in the prediction of WMH, lacunar infarctions and stroke. Van Boxtel et al (2006) reported no association between night time dipping of BP and WMH load, whereas daytime and 24-h pulse pressure averages were associated with pWMH, and systolic BP and mean arterial pressure for all periods were higher in patients with lacunar infarctions. They concluded that there was no relationship between diurnal BP rhythm and evidence of structural or functional cerebral damage in a population of newly diagnosed hypertensive individuals, but that the ABP profile may predict lesion type in early asymptomatic cerebral abnormalities.

Although in the Japanese population, nondipping and extreme dipping have repeatedly been associated with silent cerebrovascular disease (WMH and lacunar infarctions), the consequences of diurnal BP variations on the brain remain to be elucidated in Caucasian populations. Several reasons have been adduced: limitations in study size; different considerations for lesion description; classification of dipping (no consensus on what BP variable to use: systolic BP, diastolic BP or mean arterial pressure); optimal cutoff values; presentation of data (relative dipping or dipping status); duration of hypertension and treatment history (Van Boxtel et al, 2006). In advanced old age, hypertension was found to be associated with evidence of target-organ damage; ABPM was positively associated with cerebral periventricular hyperintensities on MRI, and was more effective than conventional BP measurement in predicting HT target-organ damage (O'Sullivan et al, 2003).

Very recently Sierra (2011) extensively reviewed the association between ABP parameters and WMH, and concluded that although ABPM 24-hour values are related to the presence and severity of cerebral WMH, the direction of this association still remains speculative and that larger, longitudinal studies will be required to establish causality.

3.4.2 Brain electrical activity

Another line of investigation has been brain electrical activity in hypertension. A study conducted in neurologically asymptomatic hypertensive patients showed that quantitative EEG revealed altered spontaneous brain activity, mainly in the frontal and midline regions of the left hemisphere, which they infer as probably associated with brain hypoperfusion (De Quesada et al, 2005). More recently De Quesada-Martínez & Reyes Moreno (2010) investigated the localization of paroxysmal activity employing Low Resolution Electromagnetic Tomography (LORETA) in 84 patients with high BP and no history of neurological diseases. They found that the generators for the paroxysmal activity were mainly localized on the right Brodmannn´s 17 and 37 areas, and on the left Brodmannn´s 6, 39 and 10 areas. These regions are very sensitive to hypoperfusion caused by arterial hypertension.

3.5 Blood biomarkers

There are many published reports indicating that serum molecular markers for neuronal damage are useful for estimating the timing and extent of cerebral injury, as well as for long term clinical outcome in several conditions, such as cardiopulmonary bypass, cardiac arrest, stroke, traumatic brain injury and others (Dassan et al, 2009; Gottesman & Wityk, 2006; Marchi et al, 2006; Selakovic et al, 2005; Shinozaki et al, 2009).

Nevertheless, to our best knowledge attempts to demonstrate silent brain damage in hypertension employing serum biochemical markers have only been made in two settings:

1. Schmidt et al. in 2004 provided preliminary evidence demonstrating that increased S100B was associated with eclampsia, but not with preeclampsia or chronic hypertension in pregnant women, conditions very dissimilar to essential hypertension. They hypothesized that increased S100B could be secondary to cerebral vascular changes leading to overperfusion, edema, and ischemia, as well as to seizures themselves, although they deemed the latter less plausible.
2. Al-Rawi and Atiyah (2009) measured salivary and serum levels of neuron specific enolase (NSE) in 25 hypertensive patients. Although they did not attain statistical significance, they observed higher mean serum NSE levels in hypertensive patients than in healthy controls, with values ranging between those obtained in ischemic stroke patients and healthy controls. The object of their study was not hypertension, and no associations were made with clinical variables related to the severity of hypertension.

For decades, researchers have sought for clinically useful blood biomarkers of nervous system injury, and these efforts have intensified in the past few years. Although the ideal biomarker remains elusive, several molecules have received attention (CK-BB, glial fibrillary acidic protein, S100B, NSE, among others) (Laskowitz et al, 2009; Mayer & Linares, 2009). Of these, NSE and S100B are the ones which have been studied most often in clinical settings (Dassan et al, 2009; Kleine et al, 2003; Konstantinou et al, 2008; Selakovic et al, 2005; Van Munster et al, 2009). NSE has been recognized in the guidelines developed by the American Academy of Neurology as a useful prognostic indicator in comatose patients with global hypoxic-ischemic brain injury.

Following we present our experience in relation to the serum biochemical markers (NSE and S100B) as early predictors of brain damage in essential hypertension (González-Quevedo et al, 2011).

Fifty patients with essential arterial hypertension, who had been referred by the general practitioner to the Department of Ophthalmology for evaluation of retinopathy were recruited. The hypertension status of the study sample was assessed using standard criteria formulated by Joint National Committee VII (Chobanian et al, 2003). The mean (±SD) age was 57.6±11.6 years, and 38% were males. Ninety six % of the patients had a diagnosis of essential hypertension that dated back from over 5 years (5 to 35 years); only 2 of them had less than five years of disease duration. All patients completed an interview aimed to ascertain their personal pathological history and medication used. Forty seven patients (94%) were receiving antihypertensive drugs. Those with clinical evidence of known neurological disease, malignancies, chronic degenerative or inflammatory diseases, recent infection or trauma were not included.

The control group was comprised of 42 apparently healthy subjects who volunteered to be included in this study - mean (±SD) age was 52.4±12.5 years, and 42.9% were males. Hypertension was excluded by clinical history and blood pressure (BP) measurement taken before blood extraction, no retinopathy was detected at fundoscopic examination, and no known history of neurological, cardiovascular, liver, renal, inflammatory or malignant diseases was reported. Those referring recent infection or trauma were not included.

Before blood extraction, BP was measured in patients and controls in the right arm and in the seated position after a 5-min rest period, following the recommendations of Perloff et al (1993). Hypertensive patients were classified in four groups according to BP measurements: <120/80; 120-139/80-89; 140-159/90-99 and > 160/100 (Chobanian et al, 2003). Fundoscopic examination to evaluate hypertensive retinopathy was carried out in all patients and controls and they were classified according to Scheie (1953).

Brain MRI scanning was conducted in 23 of the 50 hypertensive patients. Both groups of patients (with and without MRI) had a similar composition with respect to demographic and clinical variables. The degree of WMH severity was rated visually on axial FLAIR images using the Fazekas scale (Fazekas et al, 1987), and patients were classified in two groups:

- Group 0-I: Included Grade 0 (no hyperintense lesions) and Grade I (slight changes: only one lesion < 10 mm or grouped lesion areas < 20 mm for any diameter).
- Group II-III: Included Grade II (only one hyperintense lesion from 10 - 20 mm or grouped hyperintense areas > 20 mm for any diameter), and Grade III (severe changes: confluent hyperintense areas on both sides ≥ 20 mm for any diameter).

Lacunes were defined as hypointense foci of <3 mm on MPRAGE that were surrounded by white matter or subcortical gray matter and not located in areas with a high prevalence of widened perivascular spaces (eg, anterior commissure, vertex). The number of lacunes was recoded into none, few (1 to 3 lacunes), and many (4 lacunes or more).

Dilated Virchow Robin spaces (> 2 mm) were identified and classified in 3 groups: None (no dilated Virchow spaces); Few (1 to 3); Many (4 or more).

Serum S100B and NSE were determined employing the immunoassay kits CanAg S100 EIA (708-10) and CanAg NSE EIA (420-10) from CanAg Diagnostics AB (Sweden).

Table 2 shows the mean serum concentrations for S-100B and NSE in hypertensive patients and controls. Both proteins displayed significantly higher levels in patients with respect to controls, while no differences were detected with gender and age. No correlation was observed between NSE and S-100B levels.

Serum proteins	Control n=42	Hypertension n=50	Student´s t- test	P
S-100B (ng/L)	72.3 ± 29.5	108.6 ± 53.1	t = 3.944	p = 0.0002
NSE (µg/L)	8.6 ± 4.2	12.5 ± 7.9	t = 2.749	p = 0.002

Table 2. Mean ± SD of serum S-100B and NSE levels in controls and hypertensive patients

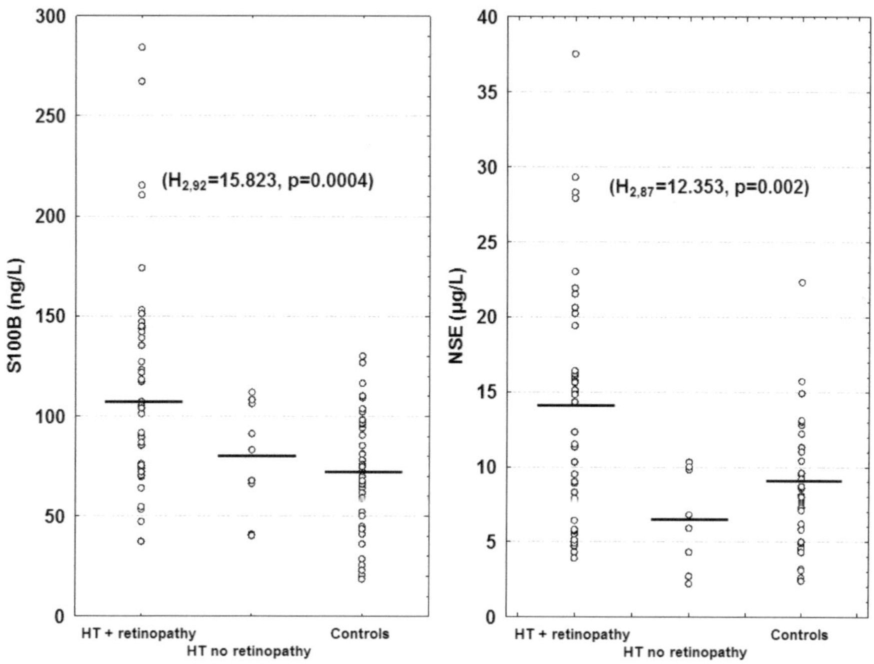

HT: hypertension
Results for Kruskal-Wallis test shown in the figure.
Pos hoc analysis for S-100B: HT + retinopathy *vs* control (p=0.0003)
Pos hoc analysis for NSE: HT + retinopathy *vs* HT no retinopathy (p=0.02)
HT + retinopathy *vs* control (p=0.01)

Fig. 1. Scatter plot of serum S-100B (A) and NSE (B) concentrations in controls and hypertensive patients with and without retinopathy.

Diastolic BP (DBP), but not systolic BP (SBP) taken immediately before blood extraction correlated with NSE levels (r=0.325, p = 0.023), while no correlation was found between S-100B concentration and SBP or DBP.

When patients were classified as having or not having retinopathy and compared with controls (Figure 1), higher NSE and S-100B levels were found to be associated with the presence of retinopathy (p=0.0004 and p=0.0022 respectively). For NSE a significant increase was demonstrated in patients exhibiting retinopathy with respect to those without retinopathy (p=0.029), while for S-100B, a similar tendency was observed, but it did not reach statistical significance. It should be pointed out that hypertensive patients without retinopathy displayed serum S-100B and NSE concentrations (means: 83 and 6.3 respectively) very similar to controls (means: 72.3 and 8.6 respectively).

The association with the grade of retinopathy could be further confirmed when patients were distributed according to NSE and S100B cut off levels. Figure 2 shows how the frequency of patients with NSE>14 µg/L and S100B>130 ng/L significantly increased with the grade of retinopathy. The X^2 test was conducted considering two groups of retinopathy: lower severity (0 – I) and higher severity (II – III) to avoid empty cells. It is noteworthy that NSE>14 µg/L and S100B>130 ng/L were not observed in hypertensive patients without retinopathy.

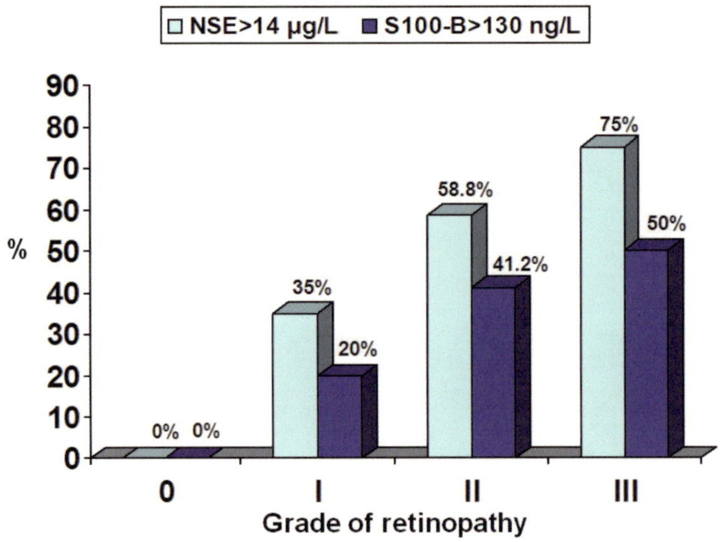

NSE: χ^2=6.766, p=0.009; S100B: χ^2=5.347, p=0.021

Fig. 2. Percentage of patients with increased serum NSE and S100B levels according to grade of retinopathy.

The independent variables included in the multivariate regression analysis (SBP, DBP, grade of retinopathy and years of hypertension), with NSE as the dependent variable, fitted the whole generalized regression model (multiple R=0.547; F=4.335, p=0.005). NSE was independently associated with diastolic blood pressure and grade of retinopathy, but not with systolic blood pressure and duration of hypertension; whereas no associations were observed for S-100B.

As brain MRI scans were performed in 23 of the hypertensive patients, the results were evaluated with respect to NSE and S-100B levels (Table 3). Distribution of the patients according to the Fazekas Scale revealed some degree of WMHs in 17 (73.9%), while only 6 patients displayed no hyperintense lesions (Grade 0). Eight patients classified as Grade I, seven as Grade II and 2 patients as grade III. Non parametric statistical analysis assembling Grades 0-I and Grades II-III, showed that patients with more severe WMHs had higher serum NSE levels than those with no hyperintensities or slight changes ($p < 0.05$), while S-100B levels did not differ. Hyperintensities were not associated with other risk factors (smoking, alcohol, diabetes).

Dilated Virchow Robin spaces and lacunes were detected in 11 and 5 patients respectively. No significant differences for S-100B or NSE levels were encountered when analyzing the presence of dilated Virchow spaces or of lacunes.

Brain MRI variables		n	S-100B (ng/L)	NSE (μg/L)
WMH (Fazekas scale)	Grades 0 - I	14	124.3 (53.2 – 210.4)	10.6 (3.9 – 16.4)
	Grades II - III	9	107.0 (53.6 – 215.3)	20.6 * (4.3 - 29.3)
Dilated Virchow Robin spaces	None	12	117.0 (53.2 – 151.0)	9.1 (4.3 – 20.2)
	Few	1	121.7	12.3
	Many	10	114.8 (63.7 – 241.3)	16.1 (4.6 – 28.8)
Presence of lacunes	None	18	131.1 (53.2 – 215.3)	13.3 (3.9 – 28.3)
	Few	5	103.8 (73.8 – 121.7)	12.3 (4.9 – 20.6)
	Many	0	-	-

WMH: white matter hyperintensities
Medians and 10-90 percentiles of NSE and S-100B are presented
* Mann-Whitney U test: Z = 1.980, p= 0.049 (Fazekas scale 0-I *vs* II-III)

Table 3. Brain MRI variables and serum concentrations of S-100B and NSE in hypertensive patients.

To rule out the effect of antihypertensive treatment on blood levels of S-100B and NSE, two analyses were carried out: 1) effect of one or two antihypertensive drugs *vs* joint administration of more than two drugs (polytherapy) and 2) effect of individual groups of antihypertensive drugs (ACE inhibitors, calcium channel blockers, β-blockers, diuretics). No significant differences were observed when patients treated with polytherapy were compared with those receiving one or two drugs. None of the individual groups of antihypertensive drugs increased the serum concentrations of S-100B and NSE.

3.5.1 Discussion of blood markers in hypertension

In the present study we examined the status of serum NSE and S-100B in patients with essential arterial hypertension, and their possible implication as early markers of brain damage. We found that both markers were significantly higher in hypertensive patients than in controls and the multivariate analysis revealed that NSE was independently associated with two variables expressing severity of hypertension: diastolic blood pressure (but not systolic) and grade of retinopathy; while S-100B was not associated with any of the clinical variables analyzed. Furthermore, seeking for a neuroanatomical support to the serum concentration of these brain specific proteins, brain MRI studies performed in a group of hypertensive patients, denoted a relationship between increased serum NSE levels (but not S-100B) and more severe white matter lesions. This is the first study demonstrating raised NSE levels related to severity in essential hypertension, and suggesting that it may be a marker of early brain damage accompanying the hypertensive syndrome.

MRI and positron emission tomography (PET) techniques have shown signs of hypertensive target organ damage in the brain of asymptomatic hypertensive patients as we explained with more details in previous sections of this chapter. Although this study is limited by the fact that brain MRI could only be performed in half of the cohort, a relationship between increased serum NSE levels and severity of WMHs was observed.

The fact that NSE and S-100B are elevated in hypertensive patients with respect to controls does not necessarily denote early signs of brain damage. It is important to take into account that although S100B and NSE are highly specific for brain tissue, they are also expressed in other cell types under physiological and pathological conditions. S-100B is found in adipocytes, bladder and colon cells, and elevated serum levels have been reported in patients with bone fractures, thoracic contusions, burns and melanoma (Dassan et al, 2009; Kleine et al, 2003). NSE is also present in erythrocytes and platelets; while high serum levels have been reported with malignant tumors such as neuroblastomas, small cell carcinoma of the lung and seminomas (Kleine et al, 2003; Shinozaki et al, 2009). Although the issue of contamination of these serum proteins with extracerebral sources was strictly controlled in this study, it cannot be absolutely ruled out.

Our results indicate that NSE is independently associated with the severity of hypertension (specifically expressed through increased DBP and the grade of retinopathy) and the brain MRI studies suggest that NSE increase could be in relation to the severity of white matter lesions. The fact that non-nervous tissue NSE content is so low with respect to brain that it is not liable to increase serum levels - with the exception of malignancies of the neuroendocrine system and some other tumors (Kleine et al, 2003) -, could point to a certain degree of silent brain damage in a subset of hypertensive patients.

In the case of S-100B, the lack of association with variables related to the severity of hypertension after multivariate analysis, and with MRI findings, strongly suggests that this increase is probably not originating in the nervous system. Nevertheless, this issue remains an open question that should be addressed in the future.

An additional cause leading to elevation of S-100B and NSE could have been the antihypertensive treatment that more than 90% of the patients were receiving. Nevertheless, the analysis carried out indicates that no specific group of antihypertensive drugs was associated with increased serum S-100B or NSE in our study, nor did we find any reference in the literature in this respect.

Our results provide preliminary evidence suggesting that raised NSE and S100B could be the result of silent brain damage in a group of hypertensive patients; however, inflammation is an important coexisting factor that must be considered, especially in the case of S100B, where no clear association could be established with severity of hypertension or of WMHs. The possibility that increased NSE and/or S100B could be related to the systemic inflammatory process clearly demonstrated in hypertension cannot be ruled out, and will be the object of future work in our laboratory.

Since the observation made by Sesso et al in 2003 that increasing levels of C-reactive protein were associated with an increased risk of developing hypertension, scientists have been trying to unravel the mechanisms linking chronic low-grade systemic inflammation with high blood pressure. Independent associations between inflammatory biomarkers (C-reactive protein, interleukins 6 and 18, tumor necrosis factor-α) and measures of arterial stiffness and wave reflections (Schnabel et al, 2008; Vlachopoulos et al, 2010) and in essential hypertension (Bautista et al, 2005) have been established.

There are some reports linking S100B with inflammation. Depending on its concentration, S100B has two opposing effects, trophic and toxic. At nanomolar concentrations, S100B stimulates neurite outgrowth and enhances survival of neurons. However, at micromolar concentrations, S100B stimulates the expression of proinflammatory cytokines such as IL-6 and induces apoptosis (Steiner et al, 2011).

In experimental animals, overproduction of S100B in the astrocytes of stroke-prone spontaneously hypertensive rats has been demonstrated, while treatment with arundic acid prevented hypertension-induced stroke and inhibited the enlargement of the stroke lesion by preventing the inflammatory changes caused by overproduction of the S100B protein in the astrocytes (Higashino et al, 2009). On the other hand, in a clinical setting, the degree of systemic inflammation was found to be associated with S100B concentration in acute ischemic stroke, independent of the size of the ischemic lesion (Beer et al, 2010).

Very recently Steiner et al (2011) provided solid evidence showing that $CD3^+$ $CD8^+$ T cells and $CD3^-$ $CD56^+$ NK cells express S100B, and that stimulated $CD8^+$ T cells release S100B which could lead to activation of granulocytes and monocytes. This could indicate a novel regulatory mechanism of innate immune functions by S100B+ T cells distinct from cytokine- and chemokine-mediated pathways. Due to the emerging role of S100B as an interface with the immune system, the results provide the ground for a wide array of future studies in physiological and pathological conditions that have been associated with increased S100B levels (Steiner et al, 2011).

Thus, the association of raised S100B levels in hypertensive patients -where low level chronic inflammation has been well established- could gain new meaning in view of the above described and formerly unknown close interactions between S100B and the immune system. Overall, at this point all these considerations are hypothetical and require additional research.

In conclusion, in the present study we have shown that serum NSE and S-100B are elevated in hypertensive patients, and furthermore that NSE (but not S-100B) is associated with the severity of hypertension and white matter lesions. Our findings provide for the first time preliminary evidence suggesting that raised NSE could be the result of silent brain damage in a subset of hypertensive patients. Additional research is needed involving larger cohorts, more sensitive imaging techniques and the use of other biochemical, electrophysiological and neurocognitive methods in order to consistently confirm this hypothesis.

4. Conclusion

Contrary to the subclinical detection of cardiovascular and renal target organ damage, which is very well established in clinical practice for the management of hypertension, brain target organ damage to date has no readily available technique to be used by the medical practitioner. From the evidence previously presented, it is obvious that at this moment, the only method that can be reliably employed for this purpose is brain MRI. Nevertheless, MRI is not as widely accessible as it would be needed, to screen such a highly prevalent disease, and is furthermore, very costly. On the other hand, it should be taken into account that several studies have alerted on the high frequency of subclinical brain target organ damage, as compared to cardiorenal damage. Thus there is no doubt that the search for effective, less expensive and available methods is urgently required. In this respect blood biomarkers of brain damage are a promising and practically unexplored avenue that needs to be more deeply investigated.

What could be the clinical relevance of our preliminary findings? The use of serum S-100B and NSE as early and quantitative markers could prove important as a potential tool in the hands of clinicians for the detection and prevention of initial brain deterioration in hypertensive patients. On the other hand, the longitudinal study of this cohort could also offer important information on their usefulness as prognostic factors.

5. References

Adrogue HJ & Madias NE. Sodium and potassium in the pathogenesis of hypertension. (2007). *N Engl J M*, 356,1966-78. ISSN: 0028-4793

Al-Sarraf H & Philip L. Effect of hypertension on the integrity of blood brain and blood CSF barriers, cerebral blood flow and CSF secretion in the rat. (2003). *Brain Res*, 975,179-88.

Amenta F, Di Tullio MA & Tomassoni D. Arterial Hypertension and Brain Damage—Evidence from Animal Models (2003). *Clin Exp Hypertens*,25,359–380. ISSN: 1064-1963.

Bautista LE, Vera LM, Arenas IA & Gamarra G. Independent association between inflammatory markers (C-reactive protein, interleukin-6, and TNF-α) and essential hypertension. (2005). *J Hum Hypertens*,19,149–54. ISSN: 0950-9240

Beer C, Blacker D, Bynevelt M, Hankey GJ & Puddey IB. Systemic markers of inflammation are independently associated with S100B concentration: results of an observational study in subjects with acute ischaemic stroke. (2010). *J Neuroinflammation*, 7,(Oct 29),71. ISSN: 1742-2094

Cheung CY, Tay WT, Mitchell P, Wang JJ, Hsu W, et al. Quantitative and qualitative retinal microvascular characteristics and blood pressure. (2011).*J Hypertens*,29,1380–91. ISSN: 0263-6352.

Chobanian AV, Bakris GL, Black HR, Cushman WC, Green LA, et al. The Seventh Report of the Joint National Committee on Prevention, Detection, Evaluation, and Treatment of High Blood Pressure: the JNC 7 Report. (2003). *JAMA*,289, 19 (May 21),2560-72. ISSN: 0098-7484

Dassan P, Keir G & Brown M. Criteria for a clinically informative serum biomarker in acute ischaemic stroke: A review of S100B. (2009). *Cerebrovasc Dis*,27, 295–302.

de Leeuw FE, De Groot JC, Oudkerk M, Witteman JC, Hofman A, van Gijn J & Breteler MM. Hypertension and cerebral WML in a prospective cohort study. (2002). *Brain*. 2002,125 (Apr 125),765-72. ISSN 0006-8950.

De Quesada Martínez ME & Reyes Moreno M. Localización de la actividad paroxística en pacientes con hipertensión arterial con el uso de la tomografía electromagnética de baja resolución (LORETA). (2010). VITAE. Academia Biomédica Digital. Octubre-Diciembre, N°44. ISSN 1317-987X ISSN 1317-987X. ISSN: 1317-987

De Quesada-Martínez ME, Blanco-García M, Díaz-De Quesada L. Early functional disorders of the brain in uncomplicated hypertensive patients. (2005). Rev Neurol;40:199–209. ISSN 0210-0010,

Fazekas F, Chawluk JB, Alavi A, Hurtig HI & Zimmerman RA. MR signal abnormalities at 1.5 T in Alzheimer's dementia and normal aging. (1987). *AJR Am J Roentgenol*,149,351–56. ISSN: 0361-803X

Gottesman RF & Wityk RJ. Brain Injury from Cardiac Bypass Procedures. (2006). *Semin Neurol*. 26,4,432-39. ISSN: 0271-8235.

Grassi G & Schmieder RE. The renaissance of the retinal microvascular network assessment in hypertension: new challenges. (2011). J Hypertens, 29:1289–1291. ISSN: 0263-6352.

Grubb NR, Simpson C, Sherwood RA, Abraha HD, Cobbe SM, O'Carroll RE, Deary I & Fox KA. Prediction of cognitive dysfunction after resuscitation from out-of-hospital cardiac arrest using serum neuron-specific enolase and protein S-100. (2007). *Heart*. 93(Oct),10,1268-73. ISSN 1468-201X.

Henskens LH, Kroon AA, van Oostenbrugge RJ, Gronenschild EH, Hofman PA, Lodder J & de Leeuw PW. Associations of ambulatory blood pressure levels with white matter hyperintensity volumes in hypertensive patients. (2009). *J Hypertens*, 27 (Jul),7,1446–52. ISSN: 0263-6352.

Henskens LH, van Oostenbrugge RJ, Kroon AA, Hofman PA, Lodder J & de Leeuw PW. Detection of silent cerebrovascular disease refines risk stratification of hypertensive patients. (2009). *J Hypertens*,27,846–53. ISSN: 0263-6352.

Higashino H, Niwa A, Satou T, Ohta Y, Hashimoto S, Tabuchi M, Ooshima K. Immunohistochemical analysis of brain lesions using S100B and glial fibrillary acidic protein antibodies in arundic acid- (ONO-2506) treated stroke-prone spontaneously hypertensive rats. (2009). J Neural Transm 116:1209–1219. ISSN 0033-2909

Ishida H, Takemori K, Dote K & Ito H. Expression of glucose transporter-1 and aquaporin-4 in the cerebral cortex of stroke-prone spontaneously hypertensive rats in relation to the blood-brain barrier function. (2006). *Am J Hypertens*. 19,33-9. ISSN: 0895-7061.

Kandiah P, Ortega S & Torbey MT. Biomarkers and Neuroimaging of Brain Injury after Cardiac Arrest. (2006). *Semin Neurol.* 26.413-21. ISSN: 0271-8235.

Kearney PM, Whelton M, Reynolds K,Muntner P, Whelton PK & He J. Global burden of hypertension: analysis of worldwide data. (2005). *Lancet.*365.217-23. ISSN: 0140-6736.

Kitagawa K. Cerebral blood flow measurement by PET in hypertensive subjects as a marker of cognitive decline. (2010). *Journal of Alzheimer's Disease.*20.855–859. ISSN: 1387-2877.

KleineTO, Benes L & Zöfel P. The Clinical Usefulness of a Biomarker-Based Diagnostic Test for Acute Stroke: Studies of the brain specificity of S100B and neuron-specific enolase (NSE) in blood serum of acute care patients. (2003). *Brain Res Bull.*61.265–79. ISSN: 0361-9230.

Konstantinou EA, Venetsanou K, Mitsos AP, et al. Neuron Specific Enolase (NSE): A Valuable Prognostic Factor of Central Nervous System Dysfunction Following Cardiac Surgery. (2008). *Brit J Anaesth Recov Nurs.*9.22–28. ISSN: 1742-6456.

Kuller LH, Karen L, Margolis, Gaussoin SA & Bryan NR. Relationship of hypertension, blood pressure, and blood pressure control with white matter abnormalities in the Women's Health Initiative Memory Study (WHIMS)—MRI Trial. (2010). *J Clin Hypertens.* 12.3(March).203–12. ISSN: 1751-7176.

Laskowitz DT, Kasner SE, Saver J, Remmel KS, Jauch EC and BRAIN Study Group. Biomarker Rapid Assessment in Ischemic Injury (BRAIN) Study. (2009). *Stroke.*40.77-85. ISSN: 0039-2499.

Lindgren A, Roijer A, Rudling O, Norrving B, Larsson EM, Eskilsson J, Wallin L, Olsson B & Johansson BB. Cerebral lesions on magnetic resonance imaging, heart disease, and vascular risk factors in subjects without stroke. A population-based study. (1994). *Stroke.* 25.5(May).929–34. ISSN: 0039-2499.

Mancia G, De Backer G, Dominiczak A, Cifkova R, Fagard R, Germano G, et al. Guidelines for the Management of Arterial Hypertension. The Task Force for the Management of Arterial Hypertension of the European Society of Hypertension (ESH) and of the European Society of Cardiology (ESC). (2007). *J Hypertens.* 25.6(Jun).1105–87. ISSN: 0263-6352.

Mancia G, Laurent S, Agabiti-Rosei E, Ambrosioni E, Burnier M, Caulfield MJ, et al. Reappraisal of European guidelines on hypertension management: a European Society of Hypertension Task Force documental. (2009). *Blood Press.* 18(6):308-47. ISSN: 0803-7051.

Marchi N, Rasmussen P, Kapural M, Fazio V, Kight K, Mayberg MR, et al. Peripheral markers of brain damage and blood-brain barrier dysfunction. (2003). *Restor Neurol Neurosci.* 21.3-4.109-21. ISSN: 0922-6028.

Mayer SA & Linares G. Can a simple blood test quantify brain injury? (2009). *Crit Care.*13.4(July 15). 166-67. ISSN: 1364-8535.

Moritz S, Warnat J, Bele S, Graf BM & Woertgen C. The prognostic value of NSE and S100B from serum and cerebrospinal fluid in patients with spontaneous subarachnoid hemorrhage. (2010). *J Neurosurg Anesthesiol.* 22.1.21-31. ISSN: 0898-4921.

O'Sullivan C, Duggan J, Lyons S, Thornton J, Lee M, O'Brien E. Hypertensive target-organ damage in the very elderly. (2003). Hypertension 42 (2): 130-135. ISSN: 0194-911X.

Oertel M, Schumacher U, McArthur DL, Kästner S, Böker D-K. S-100B and NSE: markers of initial impact of subarachnoid haemorrhage and their relation to vasospasm and outcome. (2006). J Clin Neurosci, 13:834–40. ISSN 0090-5550.

Ohira T, Shahar E, Chambless LE, Rosamond WD, Mosley TH & Folsom AR. Risk factors for ischemic stroke subtypes the Atherosclerosis Risk in Communities Study. (2006). *Stroke*.37.2493-98.

Oparil S, Amin Zaman M & Calhoun DA. Pathogenesis of Hypertension. 2003. *Ann Intern Med.* 39.761-76. ISSN: 0003-4819.

Perloff D, Grim C, Flack J, Frohlich ED, Hill M, McDonald M & Morgenstern BZ. Human blood pressure determination by sphygmomanometry. (1993). *Circulation*. 88(5Pt 1). Nov.2460-70. ISSN: 0009-7322.

Pham N, Fazio V, Cucullo L, Teng Q, Biberthaler P, et al. Extracranial sources of S100B do not affect serum levels. (2010). *PLoS ONE*. 5(9).e12691. ISSN-1932-6203.

Poulet R, Gentile MT, Vecchione C, Distaso M, Aretini A, Fratta L, et al. Acute hypertension induces oxidative stress in brain tissues. (2006). *J Cereb Blood Flow Metab*. 26.2. (Feb).253-62. ISSN: 0271-678X

Scheie HG. Evaluation of ophthalmoscopic changes of hypertension and arteriolar sclerosis. (1953). *AMA Arch Ophthalmol*.49.117-38. ISSN 0003-9950.

Schmidt AP, Tort AB, Amaral OB, Schmidt AP, Walz R, et al. Serum S100B in Pregnancy-Related Hypertensive Disorders: A Case–Control Study. (2004). *Clin Chem*.50.2(Feb).435-38.

Schnabel R, Larson MG, Dupuis J, Lunetta KL, Lipinska I, Meigs JB, et al. Relations of inflammatory biomarkers and common genetic variants with arterial stiffness and wave reflection. (2008). *Hypertension*. 51.6 (Jun).1651-7. ISSN: 0194-911X.

Scuteri A, Nilsson PM, Tzourio PM, Redon J & Laurent S. Microvascular brain damage with aging and hypertension: pathophysiological consideration and clinical implications. (2011). J Hypertens 29:1469–1477. ISSN: 0263-6352.

SelakovicV, Raicevic R & Radenovic L. The increase of neuron-specific enolase in cerebrospinal fluid and plasma as a marker of neuronal damage in patients with acute brain infarction (2005). *J Clin Neurosci*.12.542–47. ISSN: 0967-5868.

Semplicini A, Inverso G, Realdi R, Macchini L, Maraffon M et al. Blood pressure control has distinct effects on executive function, attention, memory and markers of cerebrovascular damage Relevance for evaluating the effect of antihypertensive treatment on cognitive domains. (2011). J Hum Hypert 25, 80–87. ISSN: 0950-9240.

Sesso HD, Buring JE, Rifai N, Blake GJ, Gaziano JM & Ridker PM. C-reactive protein and the risk of developing hypertension. (2003). *JAMA*. 290.2945–51. ISSN: 0098-7484.

Shinozaki K, Oda S, Sadahiro T, Nakamura M, Hirayama Y, Abe R, et al. S-100B and neuron-specific enolase as predictors of neurological outcome in patients after cardiac arrest and return of spontaneous circulation: a systematic review. (2009). *Crit Care*. 13.4.R121. ISSN: 1364-8535.

Sierra C, de La Sierra A, Mercader J, Gomez-Angelats E, Urbano-Marquez A, Coca A. Silent cerebral white matter lesions in middle-aged essential hypertensive patients. (2002). Hypertens, 20: 519–524. ISSN: 0263-6352.

Sierra C, López-Soto A & Coca A. Connecting cerebral white matter lesions and hypertensive target organ damage (2011). *Journal of Aging Research* doi:10.4061/2011/438978. ISSN:2090-2204.

Sierra C. Associations between ambulatory blood pressure parameters and cerebral white matter lesions. (2011). Int J Hypertens, doi:10.4061/2011/478710. ISSN: 20900384

Steiner J, Marquardt N, PaulsI, SchiltzK, RahmouneH, BahnS et al. Human CD8+ T cells and NK cells express and secrete S100B upon stimulation. (2011). *Brain Behav Immun.* 25 (6):1233-41. ISSN: 0889-1591.

Tzourio C, Nilsson P, Scuteri A & Laurent S.Subclinical brain damage and hypertension. European Society of Hypertension Scientific Newsletter: Update on Hypertension Management 2010.11.45.

Ueno M, Sakamoto H, Liao YJ, Onodera M, Huang CL, Miyanaka H, Nakagawa T. Blood-brain barrier disruption in the hypothalamus of young adult spontaneously hypertensive rats. (2004). *Histochem Cell Biol.*122. 2(Aug).131-37. ISSN 0948-6143.

Ueno M, Sakamoto H, Tomimoto H, Akiguchi I, Onodera M, Huang CL & Kanenishi K. Blood-brain barrier is impaired in the hippocampus of young adult spontaneously hypertensive rats. (2004). *Acta Neuropathol.*107.6 (Jun).532-38. ISSN 0001-6322.

van Boxtel MPJ, Henskens LHG, Kroon AA, Hofman PAM , Gronenschild EHBM, Jolles J & de Leeuw PW. Ambulatory blood pressure, asymptomatic cerebrovascular damage and cognitive function in essential hypertension. (2006). *J Hum Hypert.*20.5–13. ISSN: 0950-9240.

Vlachopoulos C, Ioakeimidis N, Aznaouridis K, Bratsas A, Baou K, Xaplanteris P, Lazaros G & Stefanadis C. Association of Interleukin-18 levels with global arterial function and early structural changes in men without cardiovascular disease. (2010). Am J Hypertens. 23.4.(Apr).351-7. ISSN: 0895-7061.

Weber T. Low-grade systemic inflammation, arterial structure and function, and hypertension. (2010). Am J Hypert. 23.4.346. ISSN: 0895-7061.

Whiteley W. Identifying blood biomarkers to improve the diagnosis of stroke. (2011). J R Coll Physicians Edinb.41.152–4. ISSN 0035-8819.

Wong TY & Mitchell P. Hypertensive Retinopathy. (2004). NEJM.351.2310-17. ISSN: 0028-4793.

5

Pathology of Neurodegenerative Diseases

YoungSoo Kim[1], Yunkyung Kim[1], Onyou Hwang[2] and Dong Jin Kim[1]
[1]*Korea Institute of Science and Technology*
[2]*University of Ulsan College of Medicine, Republic of Korea*

1. Introduction

As the average life expectancy has been extended by the current state-of-art medical technologies, the elderly population is increasing rapidly. The world is now facing the 'ageing era', which comes with social issues like neurodegenerative diseases. Neurodegenerative diseases are progressive neurological disorders highly linked to brain injuries from which there is no recovery. Selective neuronal loss in particular regions of our brain causes different types of neurodegenerative diseases such as Alzheimer's disease (AD), Parkinson's disease (PD), stroke, amyotrophic lateral sclerosis (ALS), and many others. Two of the most common forms are AD and PD, and currently there are no fundamental cure available.

AD is a lethal disorder associated with progressive neuronal cell death beginning in hippocampus and cortex regions. Typical indications of AD are gradual memory loss, cognitive impairment and behavior dysfunction to death. Owing to the complex pathological cascade, the cause of AD is not yet clearly understood. Among the numerous pathological causes of AD in dispute, cumulative neurotoxicity induced by misfolded β-amyloid (Aβ) and phosphorylated tau proteins is strongly supported by genetic and clinical evidences. At present, there is no cure available to treat AD patients for recovery.

Parkinson's disease (PD) is a progressive neurodegenerative movement disorder associated with a selective loss of the dopamine(DA)rgic neurons in the substantia nigra pars compacta and the degeneration of projecting nerve fibers in the striatum. Currently, there is no therapy clinically available that delays the neurodegenerative process, and therefore modification of the disease course via neuroprotective therapy is an important unmet clinical need. Increasing evidence suggests that oxidative stress has a major impact on the pathogenesis of PD. Studies have demonstrated both in vivo and in vitro that the metabolism of DA itself contributes to oxidative stress, resulting in modification of intracellular macromolecules whose functions are important for cell survival. Mitochondrial dysfunction and the consequent increase in reactive oxygen species (ROS) also trigger a sequence of events that leads to cell demise. In addition, activated microglia produce nitric oxide and superoxide during neuroinflammatory responses, and this is aggravated by the molecules released by DAergic neurons such as α-synuclein, neuromelanin and matrix metalloproteinase-3. A number of proteins whose gene mutation is linked to familial forms of PD have been found, and analyses of their normal cellular functions as well as dysfunctions as consequences of oxidative stress have shed light to understanding the pathogenesis of PD.

We will review in this chapter the current understanding of the etiology and pathogenesis of AD and PD, with an emphasis on protein abnormalities, and efforts that are being made toward development of disease-modifying therapy.

2. Alzheimer's disease (AD)

Alzheimer's disease (AD) is the most common and fatal neurodegenerative disorder with disastrous effects on the senior population (Maslow, 2008). About 10% of people over 65 years old and half of those over 85 suffer from AD. Prevalence of this progressive disorder increases with ageing, affecting 3% of people between 60-69-year-olds, 5% of those between 70-79 and 30-50% of those between 80-89. Typical symptoms of AD are memory loss, cognitive impairment and behavior dysfunction to death. In many cases, AD patients develop physiological dysfunctions such as swallowing, balance and bladder control. Psychological symptoms such as depression are often associated with the disorder. According to the progression of the disorder, patients are categorized into seven stages; no impairment, very mild decline, mild decline, moderate decline, moderately severe decline, severe decline and very severe decline.

At present, there are five FDA-approved medications (donepezil, galantamine, memantine, rivastigmine and tacrine) to treat symptoms of AD. However, they can only slow down the progression or temporarily increase cognitive functions by enhancing neuronal communications. These commercially available drugs target secondary symptoms such as memory loss (cholinesterase inhibitors and memantine), behavior (antidepressants, anxiolytics and antipsychotics) and sleep changes (antidepressants, benzodiazepines, sleeping pills and antipsychotics). Therefore, current AD patients lack a fundamental therapy to stop neurodegeneration. Not only is there no fundamental drug to stop or reverse AD, but also no quantitative diagnostic system has been developed yet. At this time, the only confident method to determine AD is a postmortem diagnosis. For living patients, a series of neuropsychological and medical assessment is used for primary diagnosis and dementia-like symptoms are ruled out via brain scans or blood, urine and spinal fluid test. Thus, increasing interests on early detection of the disease highlight a need for simpler and reliable diagnostic tools and robust biological markers. As a result, molecular imaging pathological hallmarks of AD, senile plaque (SP) and intracellular neurofibrillary tangles (NFT), in living brain tissues are currently on focus by many researchers and physicians. Among a wide variety of brain imaging technologies, development of radiolabeled imaging probes for single photon emission computed tomography (SPECT) and positron emission tomography (PET) are mainly studied due to several advantages; real time targeted molecular imaging with very low concentration of imaging probes and possible quantification of target molecule (Klunk et al., 1994; Skovronsky et al., 2000). Hence, development of SP and NFT binding probes for direct marking in living AD brains is urgently desired for early diagnosis and monitoring of the disease progression

2.1 Pathology

The etiology of AD is not clearly understood yet. However, backtracking anatomical and biochemical signs allow us to postulate etiology in the upstream of the disorder. Typical indications from autopsy are brain shrinkage, blood-brain barrier damage and synaptic loss due to neuronal cell death. A wide variety of neurotoxic candidates have been suggested such as increased concentration of aggregated proteins, mitochondria dysfunction, reduced synthesis of neurotransmitters, inflammation and oxidative stress in AD brain. Among them, genetic and clinical evidences strongly support that the most dominant etiologic paradigm of Alzheimer's pathology is Aβ and tau hypotheses (J.A. Hardy and Higgins, 1992). Interestingly, these two proteins were already found as biomarkers of AD when a German psychiatrist, Dr. Alois Alzheimer reported the first documented case on his fifty-year-old female patient in 1907. During the brain autopsy of the patient, he discovered two pathological hallmarks in the hippocampus and neocortex regions of the postmortem brain tissue (Alzheimer, 1991; J.A. Hardy and Higgins, 1992). The former is consisted of misfolded Aβ proteins surrounded by dystrophic neurites and abnormal synapses, and the latter is made of abnormally hyperphosphorylated tau proteins of paired helical filaments. Activated microglia and neuropil threads are also known as positive findings. Significant loss of neurons and synapses has been found as highly associated with these four biomarkers.

Given the prominence of two major hallmarks, SP and NFT, there have been considerable arguments on Aβ and tau hypotheses concerning the primary element of the pathogenesis and their pathological order. According to clinical observation of temporal ordering of biomarker abnormalities based on decreased CSF Aβ(1-42) level, increased CSF tau level, decreased fluorodeoxyglucose level, increased Aβ plaque level and structural MRI measurements, deposition of Aβ leads NFT formation of tau begin simultaneously (Jack et al., 2010). Jack Jr. and colleagues also proposed SP as a target for early diagnosis and NFT for disease severity, because Aβ plaque formation almost reaches its saturation level by the time clinical symptoms appear and p-tau tangle forms in parallel to the progress of neuronal injury, dysfunction and degeneration. However, it is still debatable if abnormalities of both proteins are obligatory for AD progression.

2.2 Amyloidogenesis

2.2.1 APP processing and the generation of Aβ

Aβ is a 39 to 43 amino acid long peptide generated through abnormal sequential proteolysis of amyloid precursor protein (APP) by β- and γ-secretases (Fig. (1)). Various Aβ isoforms (Aβ39, Aβ40, Aβ41, Aβ42 and Aβ43) are determined by cleavage within the transmembrane domain of APP by γ-secretase. Because the Aβ domain of APP, in general, is cleaved by α-secretase, Aβ is rarely produced in normal human brain (R.K. Lee et al., 1995). However, when Aβ are generated, it misfolds into β-sheet conformation in the brain and induces neurodegeneration in hippocampus and cortex. Among the several isoforms, Aβ40 and Aβ42 peptides are the most common constituents of the neurotoxic soluble oligomers (Kayed et al., 2003; Kuo et al., 1996; Roher et al., 1996) and insoluble fibrils (Blanchard et al., 1997; Shoji et al., 2000), which damage neuronal cells in AD brains. Even though Aβ40 is the most abundant isomer (90%), Aβ42 is the more fibrillogenic and toxic among all and highly related to the development of AD (Selkoe and Schenk, 2003). It was previously reported that a slight increase of Aβ42 in the brain induced symptoms of AD (Hartmann et al., 1997). In addition, Aβ42 is known to misfold into fibrils in a short period of time. Aβ40, on the other hand, is the most abundant specie with a significant role in the initiation of amyloidogenesis in AD brains (Bitan et al., 2003; Jan et al., 2008; Y. Kim et al., 2009). In addition, oxidative stress and inflammatory damage have shown high correlation with Aβ deposition, stimulating neuronal cell death (J.A. Hardy and Higgins, 1992). Aβ40 and Aβ42 were reported to play critical roles in redox catalysis and formation of metal chelated clusters providing strong momentum to AD investigators (Balakrishnan et al., 1998; Butterfield and Kanski, 2002; S.T. Liu et al., 1999; Schoneich et al., 2003). Therefore, regulation of amyloidognesis is an excellent target for the protection of neurotoxic brain damage and holds promise in the precise understanding of the prevention or progression of AD. To this end, interpretation of the *in vivo* amyloidogenic mechanism is the key to the cure for AD.

2.2.2 Aβ misfolding cascade (monomer, oligomer, protofilbril, fibril)

According to previous researches on amyloidogenesis, there are three significant states of Aβ misfolding; monomers, soluble oligomers and insoluble fibrils. In addition, it was found that neurotoxic effects of Aβ are driven by misfolding (Blanchard et al., 1997; Kayed et al., 2003; Kuo et al., 1996; Roher et al., 1996; Shoji et al., 2000). Recent studies proved that soluble oligomers are commonly observed in human AD cerebrospinal fluid (Pitschke et al., 1998) and highly correlated with the severity of the disorder than insoluble fibrils (Kuo et al., 1996). In addition, APP metabolism pathway resulting in neutoxic Aβ oligomerization is observed to be related with oxidative stress and inflammatory damage in central nervous system (CNS) (Klein et al., 2004; Stine et al., 2003)Amyloidogenesis is a nucleation-dependent process and characterized by two phases; slow nucleation and fast extension phases (Jarrett and Lansbury, 1993; Lomakin et al., 1997; Naiki and Gejyo, 1999; Naiki and Nakakuki, 1996). Due to the pathological responsibility of soluble oligomers (J. Hardy and Selkoe, 2002), investigation of Aβ oligomers has become a critical target in AD research for the past three decades. However, oligomer study is challenging due to its instability and inaccessibility. Oligomers, particularly in solution, tend to quickly aggregate into larger species.

Although amyloidogenesis occurs favorably and solely within Aβ peptides, numbers of studies reported external inducers of amyloid aggregation such as metal, proteoglycan (PG) and tau. A wide variety of glycosaminoglycans (GAGs), expressed on the cell surface, are co-localized with Aβ aggregates in AD brain (Snow et al., 1994; Su et al., 1992; Wilhelmus et al., 2007). The electrostatic interactions of Aβ and GAG might result in facilitation of protein conformational changes that induce fibril formation, stabilization of the β-sheet amyloid structure, and inhibition of proteolysis (Fraser et al., 1992; McLaurin and Fraser, 2000). In addition, it was reported that the interactions between Aβ and GAGs were the result from the binding affinity of GAGs as potent accelerators or stabilizers of Aβ fibril formation (Castillo et al., 1999; McLaurin, Franklin, Kuhns, et al., 1999; McLaurin, Franklin, Zhang, et al., 1999; Verbeek et al., 1997). Particularly, highly sulfated GAGs such as heparin, heparan sulfate (HS), keratan sulfate (KS), and chondroitin sulfate (CS) are universally associated with diverse amyloidogenesis cascades, suggesting that they play a critical role in *in vivo* Aβ fibril formation (Brunden et al., 1993; Castillo et al., 1999; Kisilevsky et al., 2007; McLaurin, Franklin, Kuhns, et al., 1999; McLaurin, Franklin, Zhang, et al., 1999; Multhaup et al., 1995; Snow et al., 1995; Snow et al., 1994). Among them, HS and CS interact with the 13-16 Aβ residues (HHQK domain) that promote Aβ fibril formation and stabilize formed fibrils (Defelice and Ferreira, 2002; Motamedi-Shad et al., 2009). Thus, negatively charged sulfate moieties of GAGs are believed to bind to various forms of Aβ including preexisting fibrils and to induce a conformational switch to β-sheet structures (Castillo et al., 1999). Therefore, GAG-induced amyloidogenesis derived from previous observations has been then confirmed by positive/negative effects to amyloidogenesis as low molecular weight (LMW) GAG derivatives and mimetics (Castillo et al., 1997; Miller et al., 1997; Santa-Maria et al., 2007; Wright, 2006).

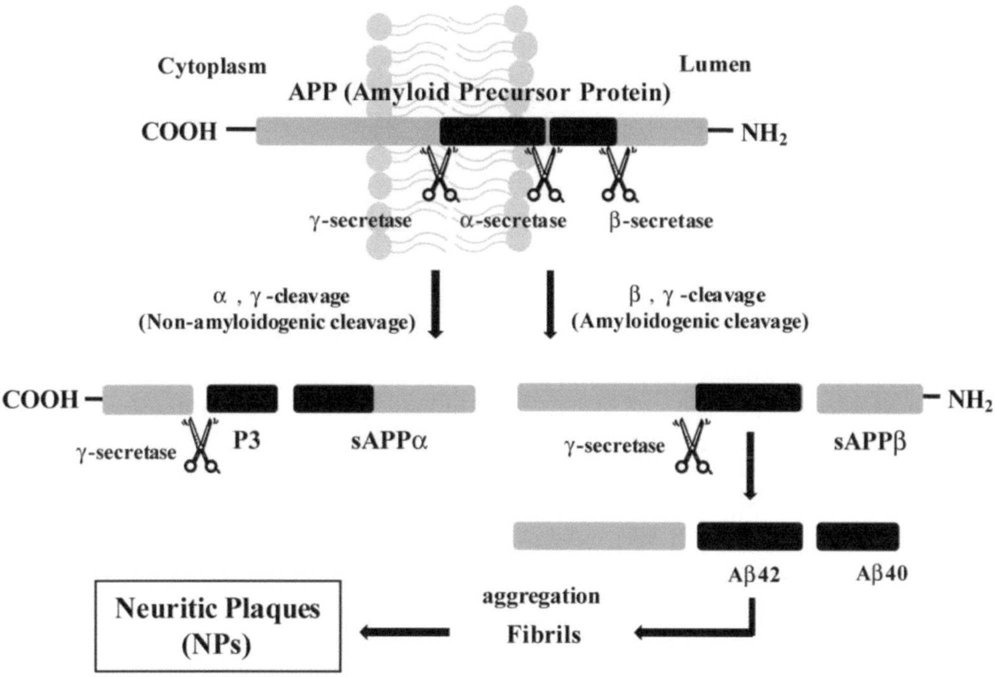

Fig. 1. APP processing and the generation of Aβ (taken from Y. Kim et al., 2009)

2.3 Taoupathy

2.3.1 Tau pathology in AD and tauopathies

Since Alois Alzheimer discovered the presence of abnormal fibrous inclusions within neurons in a patient's brain, the inclusions, called neurofibrillary tangles (NFTs) are considered one of the key requirements for making the pathological diagnosis of AD (Perl, 2010). The major component of neurofibrillary tangles is tau, which is a microtubule-associated protein that plays a important role in the development of neuronal polarity and neuronal processes (Mazanetz and Fischer, 2007). In normal adult brain, tau binds to microtubules, promoting microtubule assembly and facilitating axonal dynamics in a neuron (Brandt et al., 2005). When pathologically hyperphosphorylated, tau molecules are dissociated from microtubules and become insoluble fibrous tangles (Figure 3). NFTs are accumulated in neuronal perikarya or dystrophic neurites in axons and dendrites, causing degeneration of tangle-bearing neurons. The density of NFTs in a brain correlates fairly well with regional and global aspects of cognitive decline during the progression of AD (Binder et al., 2005).

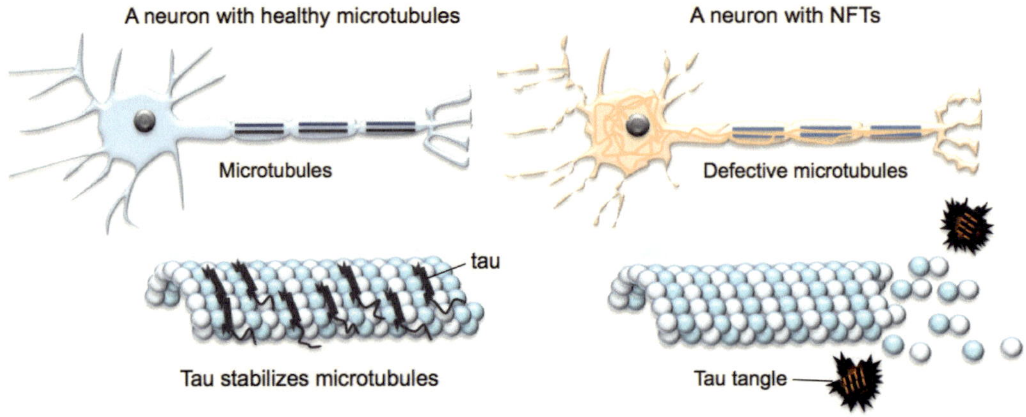

Fig. 2. The formation of NFTs and microtubule disruption (adapted from Brunden et al., 2009).

Tau and NFT pathology are not only specific for AD, but are part of the pathology in a number of neurodegenerative disorders, collectively called 'tauopahies'(Gendron and Petrucelli, 2009). In a number of tauopathies, the formation of NFTs is the primary cause of neurodegeneration (Iqbal et al., 2005). In AD pathology, however, the formation of NTFs in considered to be secondary events following Amyloidogenesis (Perl, 2010). Hence, both plaques and tangles are required to establish a definite diagnosis of AD. Regardless of whether NTFs occurs early or later in the disease pathology, it is clear that the formation of NFTs directly correlates with neurodegeneration. In this section, we will look for the genetic, biochemical and pathological mechanism of tau aggregation.

2.3.2 Neurofilamentary tangle (NFT) formation and neurotoxicity

NFTs are predominantly composed of paired helical filaments which appear to be made up of 10-nm filaments helically twisted each other (Perry et al., 1985). To aggregate into a paired helical filament, tau molecules undergo a series of abnormal modifications and conformational changes (Garcia-Sierra et al., 2003). Numerous studies have suggested that it is initiated by phosphorylation of tau molecules. Tau hyperphosphorylation induces a conformational shift of the molecule into a compact structure, called "Alz50 state"(Mandelkow et al., 1996). (Figure 4) In this state, a proline-rich region of a tau molecule contacts to microtubule binding region of the same molecule. In this state that tau first forms aggregates into filaments. The further filamentalization is accompanied or facilitated with proteolytic cleavages of tau (Binder et al., 2005). Many reports suggested that caspases, activated by amyloid plagues, cleave tau (Fasulo et al., 2000; Gamblin et al., 2003). The truncated tau molecule, named tau-66, assembles much faster and to a greater extent than its native form (Wischik, 1989).

The deposition of NFT is one of the most significant pathological signatures in AD and tauopathies; hence, there has been great effort to understand how the deposition of NFT cause neurodegeneration. NFT may damage neurons and glial cells in a number of ways (Gendron and Petrucelli, 2009). NFTs may be toxic to neurons by acting as physical barriers in the cytoplasm or NFT may also cause neuronal toxicity by reducing normal tau function stabilizing microtubules. In addition, protein aggregates are not inert end-products but actively influence diverse cell metabolism, like proteasomal activity.

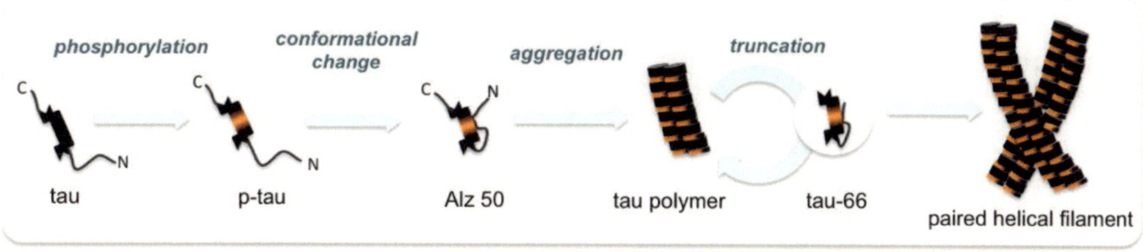

Fig. 3. Diagrammatic representation of tau conformation and NFT formation

Prior to or during NFT formation, tau undergoes numerous, and potentially harmful, modifications as shown in figure 4. The presence of these intermediates may play diverse roles in the onset and progression of disease prior to the development NFT-induced neurotoxicity. There are several mechanisms that suggest how non-fibril tau species could induce neuronal degeneration (Alonso et al., 1994). Especially hyperphosphorylated tau before NFT formation leads to microtubule disassembly, impairment of axonal transport, and organelle dysfunctions in neurons, leading to the neuronal cell apoptosis (Reddy, 2011).

2.3.3 Tau isoforms and mutations

The human tau gene is located on chromosome 17 and consisted of 16 exons. In an adult human brain, six isoforms of tau are produced from the single gene by alternative splicing (Iqbal et al., 2005). (Figure 5) The most striking feature of tau isoforms comes from the alternative splicing of exon 10. As the exon 9-12 encode tandem repeats that serve as microtubule binding domains, the alternative splicing of exon 10 generates tau isoforms containing three or four microtubule binding domains, respectively as Tau 3R or Tau 4R (Andreadis, 2005). In vitro studies have suggested that Tau 4R has greater affinity to microtubule and is more efficient at promoting microtubule assembly (Goedert and Jakes, 1990; Goedert et al., 1989). The splicing of tau mRNA is keenly controlled during development; tau 3R forms are predominantly expressed in a fetal brain, but the ratio of 3R and 4R tau transcripts becomes equal in adult brain. The disruption of this delicate balance is known to cause tauopathy (Kar et al., 2005). The expression levels of tau proteins in AD brains are approximately eight-fold higher than in age-matched controls, and this initiates hyperphosphorylation of tau, either polymerized into NFTs (Kopke et al., 1993).

Growing evidences also suggested that some of the missense mutations directly increase the tendency of tau to aggregate into NFTs (Nacharaju et al., 1999). There are two major types of mutations; coding mutations and intronic mutations (Hutton, 2000). Most coding mutations occur in exons 9-13 encoding microtubule binding regions, and produce tau proteins with a reduced ability in binding to microtubules (Hasegawa et al., 1998). In addition, intronic mutations that affect the splicing of exon 10, increase the proportion of 4R tau transcripts (Dayanandan et al., 1999; Hong et al., 1998; Hutton et al., 1998). As a result of the mutation, the ratio of 4R over 3R tau isoforms increases about two folds and it induces neurodegeneration (Hutton et al., 1998).

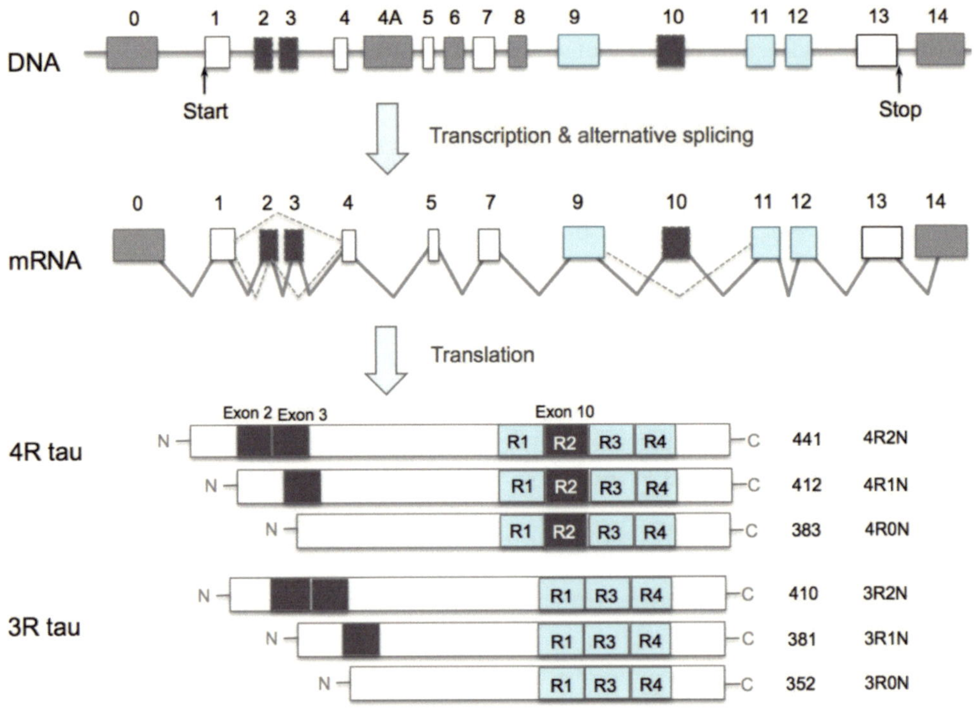

Fig. 4. Illustration represents human tau gene, mRNA, and six isoforms (adapted from Gendron and Petrucelli, 2009).

2.3.4 Tau hyperphosphorylation

In addition to isoform variation, phosphorylation of tau is an important factor in microtubule-binding of tau. Tau isolated from adult brain, is partially phosphorylated with an average of about 2 moles of phosphate per mole of protein, and this promotes association with tubulin, which leads to stabilization of microtubules and facilitates axonal transport (Drechsel et al., 1992; Mazanetz and Fischer, 2007). In contrast, tau isolated from the AD patient's brain (mostly NFTs) contains 6 to 8 moles of phosphate per mole of protein (Mazanetz and Fischer, 2007). The hyperphosphorylation changes tau conformation (Buee-Scherrer et al., 1995) leading to decrease in the microtubule-binding affinity (Braak and Braak, 1987).

The longest form of tau isoforms contains 79 serine or threonine residues and 5 tyrosine residues. Among these, about 30 residues are known as actual phosphorylation sites under normal physiological conditions. Of the sites that are phosphorylated in tau, 13 sites are followed by proline residues. Therefore proline-directed kinases such as GSK3β (glycogen synthase kinase 3β), CDK5 (cyclin-dependent kinase 5) and ERK2 (extracellular signal-regulated kinase 2) have received the most attention as the responsible kinases of tau (Dhavan and Tsai, 2001; Perry et al., 1999; Shelton and Johnson, 2004; Spittaels et al., 2000). In addition, non-proline-directed kinases such as microtubule affinity-regulating kinase (MARK) (Ferrer et al., 2001; Sawamura et al., 2001), and tyrosine kinases such as FYN have also been suggested to be relevant to neurodegeneration (Chin et al., 2005; G. Lee et al., 2004).

Evidences have showed that CDK5 colocalized with NFTs and its elevated activity was observed in AD brains (K.Y. Lee et al., 1999). Moreover, the association of CDK5 with pre-tangles (Augustinack et al., 2002; Tseng et al., 2002) suggested that CDK5 might be involved in the early stage of NFT formation during AD progression. GSK3β highly expressed in the brain is associated with a variety of neurodegenerative disease including AD (Bhat et al., 2004). In AD, GSK3β contributes in the generation β-amyloid and the phosphorylation of tau proteins to form NFTs. The inhibition of GSK3β efficiently reduces tau phosphorylation (Hong et al., 1997; Munoz-Montano et al., 1997). ERK2 is known to regulate microtubule-assembly of tau as tau-phosphorylation by ERK2 significantly decreases the affinity of tau to microtubules. These kinases are potential target candidates for tauopathy drug discovery.

2.4 Diagnosis of AD

Current clinical test of AD is mostly conducted via non-histochemical approaches like mini-mental state exam (MMSE), which are often difficult, unreliable and unfeasible as a diagnosis tool. Therefore, growing unmet needs on early detection of the disorder highlight development of simple and reliable diagnostic tools and robust biological markers. Accordingly, visualizing pathological hallmarks of AD such as SPs and NFTs in living brain is on focus. Among a wide variety of brain imaging technologies, radiolabeled imaging probes for single photon emission computed tomography (SPECT) or positron emission tomography (PET) are mainly studied for AD diagnosis due to numeral advantages; real time targeted molecular imaging with very low concentration of imaging probes and possible quantification of target molecule (Klunk et al., 1994; Skovronsky et al., 2000). Therefore, development of Aβ and phosphorylated tau binding probes for targeted molecular imaging in AD brains is urgently desired for early diagnosis and monitoring of AD progression (Fig (2)). Particularly, a probe soluble Aβ oligomer is extremely promising since oligomers are find in brains years earlier than actual AD symptoms start to occur. [^{11}C]PIB (Pittsburgh Compound-B, [^{11}C]6-OH-BTA-1) and [^{18}F]FDDNP (2-(1-(6-((2-[^{18}F]fluoroethyl)(methyl)amino)-2-naphthyl)ethylidene)malononitrile) which bind to Aβ fibrils in brain are presently available in vivo for early diagnosis of AD (Agdeppa et al., 2003; Klunk et al., 2004; Mathis et al., 2002). While [^{11}C]PIB is very specific to Aβ with short half life, [^{18}F]FDDNP can bind to both SP and NFT with approximate half life of two hours. Lately pharmaceutical companies and FDA search for molecular imaging probes which can visualize both SP and NFT, because each hallmarks is also found in other types of brain disease as described above. Amyvid™ ([^{18}F]AV-45), unable to bind to tau protein and recently refused by FDA, was useful in ruling out the presence of pathologically significant levels of Aβ in the brain, but insufficient to determine AD patients.

2.5 Therapeutic strategies of AD

At present, there is no commercially available cure for AD patients. NMDA antagonist, memantine, and acetylcholinesterase (AChE) inhibitors, Aricept, are the only available treatments in the market for AD, even though they can only decelerate the progression of the disease and provide temporal cognitive enhancement. Thus, regulation of Aβ cascade is pursued by researchers to prevent neurodegenerative progression of AD (J. Hardy and Selkoe, 2002). Among several anti-amyloidogenesis strategies, β- and γ-secretase inhibitors, Aβ protease regulators, Aβ aggregation inhibitors, metal chelators, RAGE inhibitors and immunotherapy are promising therapeutic targets (D.S. Choi et al., 2006; Hamaguchi et al., 2006; Schenk et al., 1999). There are several drug candidates in development such as small molecule Aβ aggregation inhibitors, copper-zinc chelators and Aβ specific antibodies.

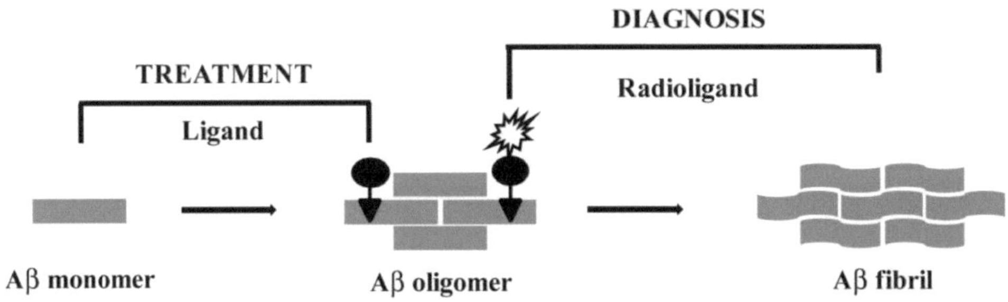

Fig. 5. Targets for amyloid treatment and diagnosis (taken from Y. Kim et al., 2009)

2.5.1 Anti-amyloidogenesis

For last two decades, AD drug discovery has targeted amyloidogenesis and there have been various types of drug candidates such as small molecules, peptides, natural products and antibodies. Monomeric Aβ has been considered as the precursor to neurotoxic species such as soluble oligomers and insoluble protofibrils (Barrow and Zagorski, 1991; Lazo et al., 2005; Xu et al., 2005) and induced R&D of aggregation inhibitors to prevent amyloidogenesis and to reduce neurotoxicity. Toxic oligomers and protofibrils are interesting targets for anti-inflammatory research (Finder and Glockshuber, 2007). Aβ oligomer of molecular weight 56 kDa (Aβ*56) is one of the well-known neurotoxic species (Reed et al., 2009).

Tramiprosate (Alzhemed), 3-amino-1-propanesulfonic acid, was a small molecule targeting Aβ aggregation (Gervais et al., 2007), which was unfortunately dropped in clinical trial III. It was reported to bind to soluble Aβ and to maintain the peptide in a α-helical rich conformation to inhibit Aβ deposition. It was also claimed that it might interrupt GAG from stabilizing amyloidogenesis. Tramiprosate decreased Aβ-induced neuronal cell death and crossed the BBB. An AD transgenic mouse model study resulted in significant reduction of Aβ fibrils and decrease in the levels of soluble and insoluble Aβ in the brain (Sullivan, 2007). A type of NSAIDs, Flurizan ((*R*)-flurbiprofen) (Black, 2007), by Myriad Genetics was also dropped in clinical study as an Aβ lowering drug candidate. The immunotherapeutic approach is based on the function of antibodies binding to Aβ or lowering Aβ aggregates in AD brains. Clinical trial of AN-1792 (Patton et al., 2006), a drug candidate to induce an immune response against Aβ, was stopped after severe symptoms of aseptic meningoencephalitis. Bapineuzumab (AAB-001) (Melnikova, 2007), a humanized monoclonal antibody against Aβ, is currently in final stage of clinical trial.

2.5.2 RAGE inhibitors

The receptor for advanced glycation end products (RAGE) is an influx transporter of Aβ monomer across the blood-brain barrier (BBB) into the brain from plasma, while the low-density lipoprotein receptor-related protein (LRP-1) regulates efflux of Aβ out of the brain. Given the critical role of RAGE in AD development, RAGE is considered as a potent target for AD therapy. RAGE inhibitors have a significant advantage in R&D because they do not have to cross BBB even though their role is to treat a brain disease. Pfizer's PF-04494700 (TTP488) was the most advanced inhibitor of RAGE activation in clinical trial until the company discontinued its development at the end of 2011.

2.5.3 Secretase modulators

Preventing proteolysis of APP from Aβ release has been a promising therapeutic target. β-Secretase cleaves extracellular domain of APP to form a cell membrane-bound fragment, C99, of which transmembrane domain is then sequentially cleaved by γ-secretase to produce Aβ. The physiological function of β-secretase cleavage of APP is unknown. Numbers of secretase inhibitors have been developed and entered clinical trials by many global drug industries, but none of them received FDA approval yet.

2.5.4 Mitochondria dysfunction

Rediscovery of an anti-histamine drug, Dimebon (3,6-dimethyl-9-(2-methyl-pyridyl-5)-ethyl-1,2,3,4-tetrahydro-γ-carboline dihydrochloride), as an Alzheimer effective drug triggered high interests in mitochondria-mediated apoptosis in AD brain. Mitochondrial permeability transition pore (mPTP) is consisted of three major components, adenine nucleotide translocase (ANT), cyclophilin D (CypD) and the voltage-dependent anion channel (VDAC). Recent studies revealed direct interaction between Aβ and CypD and suggested mPTP opening as a promising therapeutic target for AD. Because mPTP regulates apoptosis in many cells, it is a common drug target for a wide variety of disorders.

2.5.5 Neurotransmitters

In AD brains, cholinergic neurons and neurotransmitters such as acetylcholine (ACh) are significantly reduced (Bartus et al., 1982; Bowen et al., 1992; Davies and Maloney, 1976). Thus, enhancement of central cholinergic neurotransmission has been a therapeutic strategy (Bartus et al., 1982; Camps and Muñoz-Torrero, 2002). Currently available major drugs to treat AD are AChE inhibitors, such as tacrine (Cognex) (Knapp et al., 1994), rivastigmine (Exelon) (Jann, 2000), donepezil (Aricept) (Rogers et al., 1998) and galantamine (Reminyl) (Wilcock et al., 2000) and used for mild to moderate AD. However, the AChEI approach is only for temporal symptomatic improvements of cognition (Ibach and Haen, 2004).

2.5.6 Anti-oxidants and metal chelators

Studies on neurotoxic Aβ aggregates suggested that excess generation of radical oxygen species (ROS) can be led by amyloidogenesis and induce neuronal cell death (Butterfield et al., 2001; Frank and Gupta, 2005; Tabner et al., 2001). The ROS hypothesis is supported by numbers of clinical evidences in AD brains such as increased level of neurotoxic trace elements (Fe, Al, and Hg), lipid peroxidation, protein oxidation, DNA oxidation, and decreased energy metabolism/cytochrome c oxidation (Markesbery, 1997). Thus, anti-oxidant protection strategy to reduce neuronal oxidative injuries can contribute to attenuate neurodegeneration (Behl, 1999). It was revealed that formation of oxygen free radicals needs to be potentiated by Fe^{II}, Cu^{II}, and Zn^{II} (Behl et al., 1994; Bush et al., 2003; Butterfield et al., 2001; Doraiswamy and Finefrock, 2004; Gaggelli et al., 2006; Smith et al., 1997). Studies on metal chelators showed chemical interference of ROS formation and neuronal cell protection from Aβ-induced neurotoxicity. It was found anti-oxidants inhibited amyloidogenesis both *in vitro* and *in vivo* (Ono et al., 2006).

2.5.7 Anti-inflammation

Neuro-inflammation has been recognized as one of the most critical factors in many neurodegenerative diseases (Halliday et al., 2000; McGeer and McGeer, 1999). Inflammatory activity is often found co-localized with Aβ fibrils in AD patients and such correlation suggested non-steroidal anti-inflammatory drugs (NSAIDs) to treat AD (Bullock, 2002; Hull et al., 1999). Significantly declined risk of AD development in rheumatoid arthritis patients administered NSAIDs brought attentions of AD researchers on anti-inflammation via inhibition of COX-1 and COX-2 pathways (McGeer et al., 1996; Pasinetti, 2001; Stewart et al., 1997)(X. Liang et al., 2005).

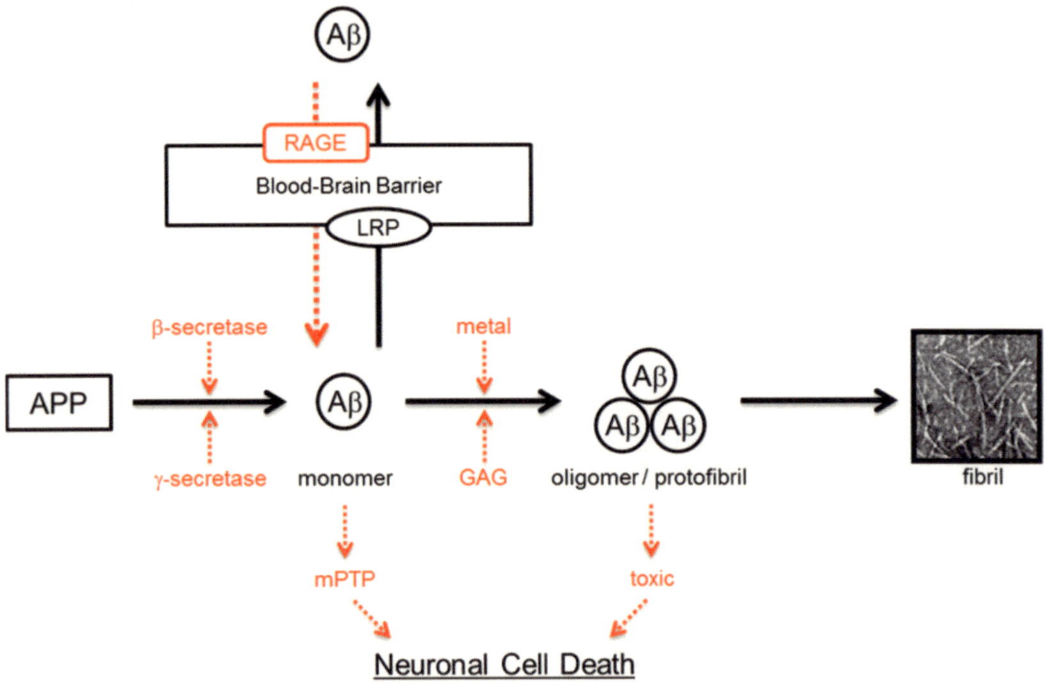

Fig. 6. Drug targets in amyloid cascade

2.5.8 Anti-tau phosphrylation

Prevention of tau pathology has begun to emerge as a feasible approach to prevent neurodegeneration, although efforts in this area lag behind the anti-amyloid research. The current tau-oriented therapies are focused on preventing tau phosphorylation. Recent data have implicated both GSK3β and CDK5 in aberrant tau phosphorylation and association with microtubules (Spittaels et al., 2000), and growing evidences also suggest that ERK2 is one of the key regulators of neurofilamentary degeneration (Perry et al., 1999). Currently, these three kinases, GSK3β, CDK5, and ERK2, are the major drug targets for tau-oriented therapeutics.

3. Parkinson's disease (PD)

PD is the second most common neurodegenerative disease, accompanied by extrapyramidal motor dysfunction. It is a progressive disease, and the prevalence increases with age, affecting 1 % of people over 60 years of age, 3.4 % of those over 70, and 4% of those over 80 (de Lau and Breteler, 2006; Olanow et al., 2009). The primary symptoms of PD include resting tremor, bradykinesia, rigidity and postural stability, and as the disease progresses, other symptoms such as depression, dementia, sleep abnormalities and autonomic failure also become evident (Chaudhuri and Schapira, 2009).

Because the primary symptoms of PD are related to the deficiency in the neurotransmitter DA, the current treatment of PD involves administration of drugs that will facilitate DAergic neurotransmission. This includes the DA precursor L-3,4-dihydroxyphenylalanine (L-DOPA), monoamine oxidase inhibitors, and DA receptor agonists. Deep brain stimulation following surgical manipulation is also being utilized in patients with severe motor fluctuations. None of the currently available therapies, however, can delay the degeneration itself, and chronic treatment with L-DOPA often causes motor and psychiatric side effects (Fahn, 1989). Currently, ways to modify the disease course by neuroprotection are actively being sought for.

3.1 Pathology

PD is associated with a selective loss of the neurons in the midbrain area called the substantia nigra pars compacta. These neurons contain the neurotransmitter DA, and their projecting nerve fibers reside in the striatum. Two pathological hallmarks of the postmortem brains of PD patients are the presence of proteinacious inclusion bodies called Lewy bodies and the presence of a reactive microgliosis in the affected areas.

While the majority of PD cases are sporadic (90–95%), rare familial forms involving mutations in a number of genes have been described. Although the familial forms represent only a small fraction of PD cases, the mechanism by which mutation of these genes lead to degeneration of DAergic neurons have shed light to understanding of the pathophysiology of PD. Gene multiplication or missense mutations in the α-synuclein gene have been linked to PD (Farrer, 2006). In two genome-wide association studies, the α-synuclein gene locus has been identified as a major risk factor for PD (Satake et al., 2009; Simon-Sanchez et al., 2009). Aggregated α-synuclein is a major constituent of the Lew bodies (Spillantini et al., 1998). Gene knockout of α-synuclein gene renders mice resistant to a DAergic cytotoxin (Dauer et al., 2002). Mutations of the parkin or PINK1 genes are causes of autosomal recessive PD. Their gene products are mitochondrial proteins, and mutations in the respective genes lead to mitochondrial defects, free radical formation, and consequently cell demise (Gandhi et al., 2009; Gegg et al., 2009; Grunewald et al., 2009). Mutations in the LRRK2 gene represent the most common cause among the familial cases of PD. The LRRK2 gene product is a large multidomain protein with a kinase domain (Paisan-Ruiz et al., 2004; Zimprich et al., 2004).

Mutations in the DJ- 1 gene are associated with an early onset autosomal recessive PD.(Bonifati et al., 2003) The loss of DJ-1 renders the cells vulnerable to oxidative stress, whereas overexpression of DJ-1 provides protection, suggesting the DJ-1 may be an antioxidant protein. Indeed, DJ-1 has been shown to have an atypical peroxiredoxin-peroxidase activity (Andres-Mateos et al., 2007). High temperature requirement A2 (HtrA2/Omi) is a serine protease that is present predominantly in the intermembrane space of mitochondria, where it is thought to be involved in protein quality control, and its heterozygous missense mutations have been found in sporadic cases of PD (Strauss et al., 2005).

As the majority of PD cases are sporadic, environmental factors play a critical role in the etiology of PD. Occupational uses of herbicides or pesticides increase the risk of PD (Barbeau et al., 1987; Kamel et al., 2007; Semchuk et al., 1992; Tanner et al., 2009). In animals, the pesticide rotenone and the broad-spectrum herbicide paraquat reproduce the PD phenotype in animals (Betarbet et al., 2000; Przedborski et al., 2004). In addition, exposure to organic solvents, carbon monoxide, and carbon disulfide (Corrigan et al., 1998) are thought to play roles, and more generally, industrialization, rural environment, well water, plant-derived toxins, and bacterial and viral infection (Schapira and Jenner, 2011). Interestingly, caffeine intake and cigarette smoking reduce the risk of PD, although the mechanism is not understood (Ascherio et al., 2001; Warner and Schapira, 2003). Aging is an obvious factor associated with the onset of PD, and it is generally speculated that failure of normal cellular processes that occurs with aging causes increased vulnerability of DAergic neurons (Obeso et al., 2010).

3.2 Oxidative stress

Oxidative stress occurs when an imbalance is formed between production of reactive oxygen species (ROS) and cellular antioxidant activity. Oxidative stress is thought to be the underlying mechanism that leads to cellular dysfunction and demise in PD (Andersen, 2004; Jenner, 2003). The substantia nigra of PD patients exhibit increased levels of oxidized lipids (Bosco et al., 2006), proteins and DNA (Nakabeppu et al., 2007) and decreased levels of reduced glutathione (GSH) (Zeevalk et al., 2008). Because of the presence of ROS-generating enzymes such as tyrosine hydroxylase, monoamine oxidase and tyrosinase, the DAergic neurons are particularly prone to oxidative stress. In addition, the nigral DAergic neurons contain iron, which catalyzes the Fenton reaction, in which superoxide radicals and hydrogen peroxide can create further oxidative stress (Halliwell, 1992). Because of this intrinsic sensitivity to reactive species, a moderate oxidative stress can trigger a cascade of events that lead to cell demise. The major sources of such oxidative stress generated for the nigral DAergic neurons are thought to be the ROS produced during DA metabolism, mitochondrial dysfunction, and inflammation, as discussed below in more detail.

Oxidative stress is generated from DA metabolism, mitochondrial dysfunction and microglial activation. Mitochondrial dysfunction can occur as a result of environmental factors such as dopaminergic toxins, as well as mutation of genes whose gene products are important for mitochondrial function, such as Parkin, PINK1, DJ-1, and HtrA2. Mitochondrial dysfunction leads to accumulation of ROS and release of cytochrome c and HtrA2, both of which lead to apoptosis.

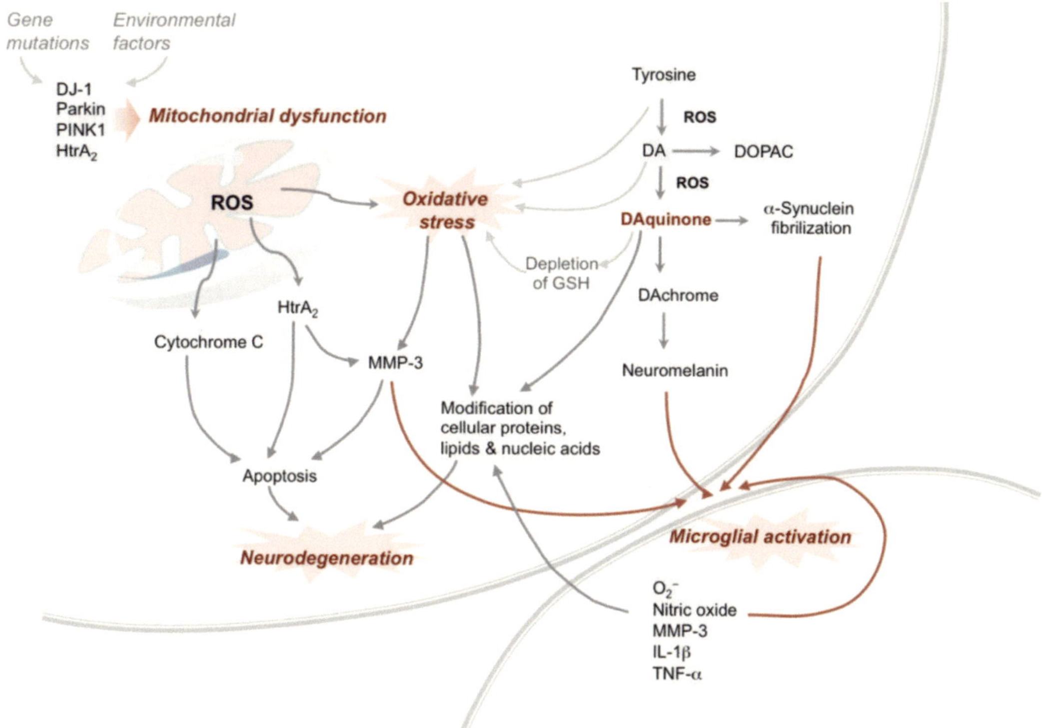

Fig. 7. Molecular cascades of DAergic neurodegeneration in the pathophysiology of PD.

3.3 DA metabolism

The neurotransmitter DA itself can be a source of oxidative stress. Lines of evidence suggest oxidation of DA and consequent quinone modification and oxidative stress as a major factor contributing to the vulnerability of DAergic cells (Asanuma et al., 2003; H.J. Choi et al., 2003; Hastings and Zigmond, 1997). Although DA is normally stored in vesicles, excess cytosolic DA is easily oxidized both spontaneously (Hastings and Zigmond, 1997) and enzymatically (Maker et al., 1981) to produce DA quinone.

The DA quinone species are capable of covalently modifying cellular nucleophiles, including low molecular weight sulfhydryls such as GSH and protein cysteinyl residues (Graham, 1978), whose normal functions are important for cell survival. Notably, DA quinone has been shown to modify a number of proteins whose dysfunctions have been linked to PD pathophysiology, such as α-synuclein, parkin, DJ-1, and ubiquitin C-terminal hydrolase L1 (UCH-L1). DA quinone covalently modifies α-synuclein monomer (Dunnett and Bjorklund, 1999) and promotes the conversion of α-synuclein to the cytotoxic protofibril form (Conway et al., 2001). The DA quinone-modified α-synuclein is not only poorly degraded but also inhibits the normal degradation of other proteins by chaperone-mediated autophagy (Martinez-Vicente et al., 2008). Conversely, α-synuclein can bind to and permeabilize the vesicle membrane, causing leakage of DA into the cytosol (Lotharius and Brundin, 2002). Parkin is also covalently modified by DA and becomes insoluble, which leads to inactivation of its E2 ubiquitin ligase activity (LaVoie et al., 2005). Catechol-mofieid parkin has been detected in the substantia nigra but not other regions of human brain, and parkin insolubility is observed in PD brain (LaVoie et al., 2005). In addition, DA quinone modification of UCH-L1, the enzyme whose gene mutation leads to autosomal dominant PD, and DJ-1 have also been observed both in brain mitochondrial preparations and DAergic cells (Van Laar et al., 2009). Since both UCH-L1 and DJ-1 contain a cysteine residue that is important for their activity (Nishikawa et al., 2003; Qu et al., 2009) and their oxidative modification at cysteine has been observed in PD(J. Choi et al., 2004; J. Choi et al., 2006), the DA quinone modification is likely the cause of inactivation of these enzymes.

DA quinone has also been shown to cause inactivation of the DA transporter and tyrosine hydroxylase (Kuhn et al., 1999). In addition, it leads to mitochondrial dysfunction (C.S. Lee et al., 2002) and swelling of brain mitochondria (Berman and Hastings, 1999). Accordingly, the subunits of Complex I and Complex III of the electron transport chain in the mitochondria, whose dysfunction can affect mitochondrial respiration and ROS production, were also shown to be targets of DA quinone modification (Van Laar et al., 2009). In addition, ER-60/GRP58/ERp57 and protein disulfide isomerase-5, the proteins involved in protein folding in the endoplasmic reticulum, are also modified by DA quinone (Van Laar et al., 2009).

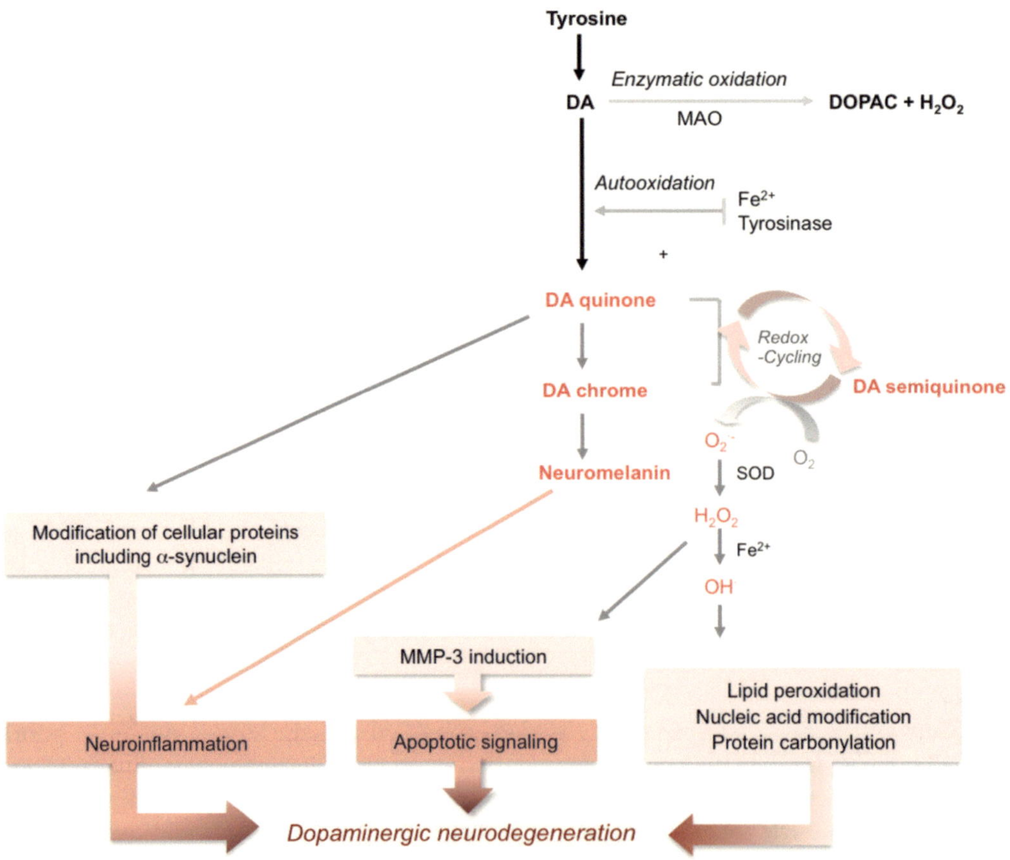

Fig. 8. Dopaminergic neurodegeneration.

In addition, when in excess, DA quinone cyclizes to become the highly reactive aminochrome, whose redox-cycling leads to generation of superoxide and depletion of cellular NADPH and ultimately polymerize to form neuromelanin (Jenner and Olanow, 1996). Neuromelanin in turn can exacerbate the neurodegenerative process by triggering neuroinflammation (Zecca et al., 2008), as described below. Furthermore, hydrogen peroxide is generated during DA metabolism by monoamine oxidase (Maker et al., 1981) and is subsequently converted to the highly reactive hydroxyl radical in the presence of transition metal ions (Halliwell, 1992), which also contributes to oxidative stress. DA metabolites have been shown to induce proteosomal inhibition, which can lead the cells to undergo apoptosis (Zafar et al., 2007; Zafar, Inayat-Hussain, et al., 2006).

A line of evidence points to the existence of in vivo DA oxidation and its toxicity in human brain. Neuromelanin, the final product of DA oxidation, is accumulated in the nigral region (Zecca et al., 2003). Higher levels of cysteinyl-catechol derivatives are found in postmortem nigral tissues of PD patients compared to age-matched controls, suggesting cytotoxic nature of DA oxidation (Spencer et al., 1998). In animals, DA directly injected into the striatum caused selective toxicity to DAergic terminals that was proportional to the levels of DA oxidation and quinone-modified proteins (Rabinovic et al., 2000). Mice expressing a low level of ventricular monoamine transporter-2, presumably with increased cytosolic DA level, showed evidence of DA oxidation and the age-dependent loss of nigral DA neurons (Caudle et al., 2008). In addition, accumulation of cytosolic DA induced via expression of DA transporter rendered the striatal GABA neurons vulnerable (Chen et al., 2008).

DA is either enzymatically or spontaneously converted to the highly reactive DA quinone, which depletes cellular GSH, modifies cellular proteins at their sulfhydryl groups, and induces fibrilization of α-synuclein.

3.4 Mitochondrial dysfunction

Mitochondrial dysfunction and the resulting oxidative stress are associated with the pathogenesis of PD (Schapira and Gegg, 2011). Oxidative stress causes peroxidation of the mitochondria-specific lipid cardiolipin, which results in release of cytochrome c to the cytosol, triggering the apoptotic pathway. Neurons heavily depend on aerobic respiration for ATP, and hydrogen peroxide and superoxide radicals are normally produced during oxidative phosphorylation as byproducts in the mitochondria. Any pathological situation leading to mitochondrial dysfunction can cause a dramatic increase in ROS and overwhelm the cellular antioxidant mechanisms.

Because DAergic neurons are intrinsically more ROS-generating and vulnerable as described above, any event that triggers further oxidative stress can be harmful to the cell. Damage to Complex I in the electron transport chain is thought to be especially critical. The mitochondrial complex I inhibitors rotenone and 1-methyl-4-phenyl-1,2,3,6-tetrahydropyridine (MPTP), when injected intraperitoneally, exert preferential cytotoxicity to the DAergic neurons (Betarbet et al., 2002). Reduced Complex I activity has been found in tissues from subjects with PD (Benecke et al., 1993; Mizuno et al., 1989; Parker et al., 1989). Higher numbers of respiratory chain deficient DA neurons have been found in PD patients than in age-matched controls (Bender et al., 2006). Furthermore, mitochondrial density in the somatodendritic region of nigral neurons has been observed to be abnormally low (C.L. Liang et al., 2007).

Perhaps the strongest evidence for mitochondrial dysfunction in PD pathophysiology comes from the findings that mutations in genes of mitochondrial proteins Parkin, DJ-1, HtrA2/Omi, and PINK have all been linked to familial forms of PD. The Parkin protein is an E3 ligase (Y. Zhang et al., 2000) and is associated with the mitochondrial outer membrane (Darios et al., 2003). Cells derived from patients with Parkin gene mutation show decreased Complex I activity and ATP production (Grunewald et al., 2010; Mortiboys et al., 2008; Muftuoglu et al., 2004). Mice deficient in Parkin gene have show reduced striatal respiratory chain activity along with oxidative damage (Palacino et al., 2004). Drosophila with functional deletions of parkin has fragmented mitochondria (Greene et al., 2003).

PINK1 protein is a kinase that has been observed to be located in the mitochondria. Mutations in PINK1 induce mitochondrial dysfunction including reduced mitochondrial DNA, a deficiency of ATP, excess free radical formation and abnormal calcium handling (Gandhi et al., 2009; Gegg et al., 2009; Grunewald et al., 2009). Drosophila with functional deletions of PINK1 has fragmented mitochondria (I.E. Clark et al., 2006; Park et al., 2006).

DJ-1 is a mitochondrially enriched, redox-sensitive protein and an atypical peroxiredoxin-like peroxidase that scavenges H2O2 (Andres-Mateos et al., 2007; Canet-Aviles et al., 2004), and DJ-1 KO mice accumulate more ROS and exhibit fragmented mitochondrial phenotype (Andres-Mateos et al., 2007; Irrcher et al., 2010). Interestingly, this aberrant mitochondrial morphology could be rescued by the expression of PINK1 and parkin (Irrcher et al., 2010).

HtrA2/Omi is a mitochondrially located serine protease and has been associated with PD. HtrA2/Omi seems to promote survival under physiological conditions by maintaining homeostasis and serving as a protein quality control factor, and loss of its activity results in accumulation of unfolded mitochondrial proteins (Jones et al., 2003; Krick et al., 2008; Martins et al., 2004; Moisoi et al., 2009).

In addition, α-synuclein, although mostly cytosolic, seems to interact with mitochondrial membranes (Nakamura et al., 2008) and to inhibit complex I (Devi et al., 2008; G. Liu et al., 2009). Mice overexpressing mutant α-synuclein exhibit abnormalities in the mitochondrial structure and function (Martin et al., 2006). α-Synuclein has also been shown to inhibit mitochondrial fusion, and interestingly, this was rescued by PINK1, Parkin, and DJ-1 (Kamp et al., 2010), again suggesting the existence of a functional relationship among the products of these PD-related genes.

3.5 Neuroinflammation

Neuronal loss in PD is associated with chronic inflammation, which is controlled primarily by microglia, the resident innate immune cells and the main immune responsive cells in the central nervous system. Microglial reaction has been found in the SN of sporadic PD patients (Banati et al., 1998; Gerhard et al., 2006; Knott et al., 2000; McGeer et al., 1988) as well as familial PD patients (T. Yamada, 1993) and in the SN and/or striatum of PD animal models elicited by MPTP (Cicchetti et al., 2002; Francis et al., 1995; Kurkowska-Jastrzebska et al., 1999; T. Yamada, 1993).

Microglia are activated in response to injury or toxic insult as a self-defensive mechanism to remove cell debris and pathogens. When activated, microglia release free radicals such as nitric oxide and superoxide, as well as proinflammatory cytokines including IL-1β and TNF-α, and proteases. Overactivated and/or chronically activated state of microglia causes excessive and uncontrolled neuroinflammatory responses, leading to self-perpetuating vicious cycle of neurodegeneration (Qian et al., 2010). This is thought to be exacerbated by inflammatory signals from molecules released from damaged neurons, leading to induction of reactive microgliosis (Qian et al., 2010). Molecules that are released from damaged nigral DAergic neurons and induce microglial activation include neuromelanin, α-synuclein, and active form of MMP-3, as described below.

Neuromelanin is the dark insoluble polymer made from DAchrome and confers the dark pigmentation to the substantia nigra. Insoluble extraneuronal neuromelanin granules have been observed in patients of juvenile PD (Ishikawa and Takahashi, 1998) and idiopathic PD, as well as those with MPTP-induced parkinsonism (Langston et al., 1999). Addition of neuromelanin extracted from PD brain to microglia culture caused increases in proinflammatory cytokines and nitric oxide (Wilms et al., 2003). Intracerebral injection of neuromelanin caused strong microglia activation and a loss of DAergic neurons in the substantia nigra (Zecca et al., 2008). Together with the finding that neuromelanin remains for a very long time in the extracellular space (Langston et al., 1999), neuromelanin has been proposed to be one of the molecules that are released from the nigral DAergic neurons and induce chronic neuroinflammation in PD.

Cytoplasmic accumulation of fibrillar α-synuclein in Lewy bodies (Spillantini et al., 1997) is thought to be related to pathophysiology of PD. Although mostly intracellular, a fraction of this protein is released from neurons (H.J. Lee et al., 2005), and α-synuclein is found in the cerebrospinal fluid from PD patients and normal subjects (Borghi et al., 2000), and in human plasma (El-Agnaf et al., 2003). That the released α-synuclein participates in neuroinflammation was demonstrated by the finding that the addition of aggregated human α-synuclein to a primary mesencephalic neuron-glia culture caused activation of microglia and DAergic neurodegeneration and that this cytotoxicity did not occur in the absence of microglia (W. Zhang et al., 2005). In addition, neuron-derived α-synuclein stimulates astrocytes to produce inflammatory modulators that augment microglial chemotaxis, activation and proliferation. (Farina et al., 2007) Nitration of α-synuclein, presumably due to increased nitric oxide, facilitates the neuroinflammatory responses (Benner et al., 2008; Gao et al., 2008). More recently, it has been shown that transgenic mice expressing mutant α-synuclein developed persistent neuroinflammation and chronic progressive degeneration of the nigrostriatal DA pathway when inflammation was triggered by a low level of lipopolysaccharide (Gao et al., 2011).

The active form of MMP-3 is released from apoptotic DAergic cells, and the MMP-3 activity causes microglial activation as evidenced by increased production of superoxide, TNF-α, and IL-1β (Y.S. Kim et al., 2005). In addition, the MMP-3 activity is increased in DAergic neurons in response to cell stress and triggers apoptotic signaling (D.H. Choi et al., 2008; E.M. Kim and Hwang, 2011; E.M. Kim et al., 2010). In MMP-3 knockout mice, the microglial activation following exposure to MPTP is abrogated, and this is accompanied by a lower level of superoxide production compared to their wild type (Y.S. Kim et al., 2007). A recent study has demonstrated that MMP-3 causes cleavage of protease activated receptor-1 (PAR-1) (E.J. Lee et al., 2010), whose removal of N-terminal extracellular domain renders the remaining domain acting as a tethered ligand, subsequently triggering generation of intracellular signals (Vu et al., 1991) and activation of microglia (Suo et al., 2002).

Furthermore, the proform of IL-1β is cleaved by MMP-3 to yield the biologically active IL-1β (Schonbeck et al., 1998). In addition, MMP-3 expression is induced in activated microglial cells (Woo et al., 2008), and conversely, MMP-3 is induced by cytokines and free radicals in microglial cells (Jian Liu and Rosenberg, 2005). Therefore, a vicious cycle may exist, where MMP-3 released from DAergic neurons leads to production of cytokines and free radicals, and this in turn causes a further production of microglial MMP-3 and subsequent release. MMP-3 can also cause degradation of blood brain barrier and infiltration of neutrophils, which can further contribute to neuroinflammation (Gasche et al., 2001; Gurney et al., 2006).

3.6 Therapeutic strategies of PD

Currently, there is no therapy clinically available that delays the neurodegenerative process itself, and therefore modification of the disease course via neuroprotective therapy is an important unmet clinical need. Thus, understanding of the pathophysiology and etiology of the disease at cellular and molecular levels and finding molecular targets against which neuroprotective/disease-modifying therapy may be developed is the crucial issue in the field of PD research.

Because the clinical symptoms of PD does not manifest until more than 70% of the nigral DA neurons have degenerated (Marek K, 2009), ways to delay the degenerative progression in the presymptomatic, early stage of degeneration will prove to be highly beneficial. Early detection of PD is now available with the advances in brain imaging techniques such as positron emission tomography (PET) and functional magnetic resonance imaging (fMRI). Biomarkers that can be used for early diagnosis of PD as well as following disease progression are being actively sought for, and some promising biomarker candidates have been discussed (Gerlach et al., 2011). Once the presymptomatic PD patients have been identified, disease-modifying, neuroprotective therapy should be able to delay development of motor disabilities and prolong time to L-DOPA initiation, allowing the pre-symptomatic patients to lead a normal life for a longer period of time. In addition, the disease-modifying drugs administered in combination with the current therapy in patients with moderate-to-advanced stages of PD may also be beneficial in improving the quality of life.

As described above, oxidative stress derived from DA metabolism, inflammation and mitochondrial dysfunction is thought to be the hallmark of PD pathogenesis, and antioxidant mechanism should prove to an effective neuroprotective therapy for PD. However, no direct antioxidant, either administered alone or in combination, has been observed to completely halt the progression of PD. The direct antioxidants vitamin C and β-carotene have shown no neuroprotective effect on PD patients (Etminan et al., 2005). Supplemental vitamin E also did not delay the need to start levodopa therapy in patients with early untreated PD in the DATATOP study (Parker et al., 1989). Coenzyme Q10, which is both an antioxidant and an enhancer of mitochondrial function, did not show benefit (Investigators, 2007), and a 16-month phase III clinical trial in a large population (600 patients with early PD (The QE3 study) was dropped in May 2011, because an interim analysis revealed no futility to complete the study (Clinicaltrials.gov).

Attempts have been made to design disease-modifying neuroprotective therapies against neuroinflammation. The steroid dexamethasone has been reported to attenuate the degeneration of DA-containing neurons induced by MPTP (Kurkowska-Jastrzebska et al.,

1999) or lipopolysaccharide (Castano et al., 2002). However, steroids have limitations for long-term use in clinical situations due to side effects. Although non-steroidal anti-inflammatory drugs, such as salicylic acid, are able to attenuate the MPTP-induced striatal DA depletion (Sairam et al., 2003), there is no clinical evidence supporting their neuroprotective effect. In addition, the tetracycline derivatives minocycline (Du et al., 2001; Tikka et al., 2001; Wu et al., 2002) has shown to inhibit neuroinflammation both in vitro and in animal models. A pilot clinical study using minocycline as a potential disease-modifying drug for PD, however, has generated disappointing results. The drug, mainly due to the large dose required, led to unwanted side effects and a high drop-out rates among patients (Investigators., 2008).

We have shown that doxycycline, another tetracycline derivative that penetrates the blood brain barrier, downregulates the cell stress-induced MMP-3 expression and release and attenuates apoptosis in the DAergic CATH.a cells (Cho et al., 2009). It also suppresses the increase in MMP-3 gene expression as well as nitric oxide and inflammatory cytokines in microglial cells in culture, and provides protection of the nigral DAergic neurons and suppresses micorglial activation and astrogliosis in the MPTP-induced mouse PD model.

We have also synthesized a novel compound 7-hydroxy-6-methoxy-2-propionyl-1,2,3,4-tetrahydroisoquinoline (PTIQ) which effectively suppressed induction of MMP-3 in DAergic cells and prevented the resulting cell death. PTIQ was able to downregulate expression of MMP-3 along with IL-1β, TNF-α and cyclooxygenase-2 and blocked nuclear translocation of NF-κB in activated microglia (Son et al., 2011). In MPTP-elicited mouse model of PD, PTIQ attenuated the associated motor deficits, prevented neurodegeneration, and suppressed microglial activation in the substantia nigra. It has a good potential as a drug for central nervous system, because it entered the brain rather rapidly, and it was relatively stable against liver microsomal enzymes, showed no apparent inhibitory effect on the cytochrome p450 subtypes or hERG channel, exhibited little cytotoxicity on liver cells or lethality.

Other molecules that downregulate MMP-3 and neuroinflammation and provide DAergic neuroprotection have been reported. It has been observed that ghrelin, an endogenous ligand for growth hormone secretagogue receptor 1a (GHS-R1a), attenuates MMP-3 expression, nigrostriatal DAergic neuron loss, microglial activation, and subsequent release of TNF-α, IL-1β, and nitrite in mesencephalic neurons in MPTP mouse model of PD (Moon et al., 2009). Another group of investigators has reported that exendin-4, a naturally occurring and more potent and stable analog of glucagons-like peptide-1 (GLP-1) that selectively binds at the GLP-1 receptor, also downregulates MMP-3 expression along with attenuation of DAergic neuron loss and microglial activation (S. Kim et al., 2009).

3.6.1 NQO1 and its inducers as protective agents

The enzyme NAD(P)H:quinone reductase (DT-diaphorase; NAD(P)H-(quinone acceptor) oxidoreductase; EC 1.6.99.2; NQO1) catalyzes two-electron reduction of quinone to the redox-stable hydroquinone (Cavelier and Amzel, 2001; Joseph et al., 2000). Since DA and its metabolites have been implicated in the pathogenesis of PD, NQO1 may exert a protective effect against such conditions. Indeed, the toxic accumulation of the DA quinone (as well as L-DOPA quinone) can be prevented by the action of NQO1. NQO1 protected against damaging effects of cyclized quinones and oxidative stress induced during their redox cycling (Zafar, Inayat-Hussain, et al., 2006), and against DA (Zafar, Siegel, et al., 2006) and 6-hydroxyDA (Jia et al., 2008). Induction of NQO1 by sulforaphane, dimethyl fumarate, 3H-1,2-dithiole-3-thione, tert-butylhydroquinone (tBHQ), and butylated hydroxyanisole protected against neurocytotoxicity associated with DA quinone in vitro (H.J. Choi et al., 2003; Duffy et al., 1998; Han et al., 2007; Hara et al., 2003; Jia et al., 2009; Jia et al., 2008; Miyazaki et al., 2006; Siebert et al., 2009);; and against MPTP-elicited toxicity in vivo (Jazwa et al., 2011). In addition, NQO1 is known to maintain both α-tocopherol and coenzyme Q10 in their reduced, antioxidant state (Siegel et al., 1997).

While NQO1 is abundant in the liver where it participates in the phase II detoxification, the enzyme is also expressed in the brain (Stringer et al., 2004). In addition to its predominant expression in astrocytes (Flier et al., 2002), NQO1 is also expressed, albeit to a less degree, in DArgic neurons in the substantia nigra (van Muiswinkel et al., 2004). Moreover, a marked increase in the neuronal expression of NQO1 was consistently observed in the Parkinsonian substantia nigra (van Muiswinkel et al., 2004). Studies have shown that a polymorphism (C609T) of NQO1 that results in a decrease or total loss of its expression is associated with PD (Harada et al., 2001; Jiang et al., 2004), although another group reported no such association (Okada et al., 2005).

Pharmacological induction of NQO1 is achieved by the transcription factor Nrf-2 binding to a cis-acting enhancer sequence termed antioxidant response element (ARE). Therefore, Nrf-2 activation in DAergic neurons may be accompanied by coordinate elevation of expression of many other genes that also contain the ARE sequence. These include the enzymes that are known as cytoprotective proteins, such as glutathione S-transferase, epoxide hydrolase, heme oxygenase-1, catalase, and superoxide dismutase and glucuronosyltransferase, thioredoxin, glutathione peroxidase, the catalytic and modulatory subunits of gamma-glutamyl synthase (GCLM, GCLC), and thioredoxin reductase (J. Clark and Simon, 2009). Which of these proteins are actually expressed and induced in the nigral DArgic neurons needs to be experimentally sorted out. It is likely that the protective effect of the known NQO1 inducers is contributed by the other cytoprotective enzymes coordinately induced along with NQO. It should be noted, however, that the direct ability of NQO1 to catalyze the detoxification of DA quinone metabolites seems most important in cellular defense of DAergic cells (Dinkova-Kostova and Talalay, 2010). It has been shown that catalase, superoxide dismutase, and heme oxygenase-1 are not effective in providing neuroprotection against DA quinone (Innamorato et al., 2010; Zafar, Inayat-Hussain, et al., 2006; Zafar, Siegel, et al., 2006). Therefore, NQO1 and Nrf2 should serve as viable cellular targets for neuroprotective therapy for PD.

4. References

Aisen, P.S. (2003). Effects of rofecoxib or naproxen vs placebo on Alzheimer disease progression: a randomized controlled trial. *JAMA,* Vol. 289, pp. 2819-2826, ISSN 0098-7484

Alonso, A.C. (1994). Role of abnormally phosphorylated tau in the breakdown of microtubules in Alzheimer disease. *Proceedings of the National Academy of Sciences of the United States of America,* Vol. 91, pp. 5562-5566, ISSN 0027-8424

Alvarez, A. (1997). Acetylcholinesterase promotes the aggregation of amyloid-beta-peptide fragments by forming a complex with the growing fibrils. *J Mol Biol,* Vol. 272, pp. 348-361, ISSN 0022-2836

Alzheimer, A. (1991). A contribution concerning the pathological anatomy of mental disturbances in old age, 1899. *Alzheimer Dis Assoc Disord,* Vol. 5, pp. 69-70, ISSN 0893-0341

Andersen, J.K. (2004). Oxidative stress in neurodegeneration: cause or consequence? *Nat Med,* Vol. 10 Suppl, pp. S18-25, ISSN 1078-8956

Andreadis, A. (2005). Tau gene alternative splicing: expression patterns, regulation and modulation of function in normal brain and neurodegenerative diseases. *Biochimica et biophysica acta,* Vol. 1739, pp. 91-103, ISSN 0006-3002

Andres-Mateos, E. (2007). DJ-1 gene deletion reveals that DJ-1 is an atypical peroxiredoxin-like peroxidase. *Proc Natl Acad Sci U S A,* Vol. 104, pp. 14807-14812, ISSN 0027-8424

Asanuma, M. (2003). Dopamine- or L-DOPA-induced neurotoxicity: the role of dopamine quinone formation and tyrosinase in a model of Parkinson's disease. *Neurotox Res,* Vol. 5, pp. 165-176, ISSN 1029-8428

Ascherio, A. (2001). Prospective study of caffeine consumption and risk of Parkinson's disease in men and women. *Ann Neurol,* Vol. 50, pp. 56-63, ISSN 0364-5134

Augustinack, J.C. (2002). Colocalization and fluorescence resonance energy transfer between cdk5 and AT8 suggests a close association in pre-neurofibrillary tangles and neurofibrillary tangles. *Journal of neuropathology and experimental neurology,* Vol. 61, pp. 557-564, ISSN 0022-

Balakrishnan, R. (1998). Alzheimer's beta-amyloid peptide: affinity for metal chelates. *Journal of Peptide Research,* Vol. 51, pp. 91-95.

Banati, R.B. (1998). Glial pathology but absence of apoptotic nigral neurons in long-standing Parkinson's disease. *Mov Disord,* Vol. 13, pp. 221-227, ISSN 0885-3185

Barbeau, A. (1987). Ecogenetics of Parkinson's disease: prevalence and environmental aspects in rural areas. *Can J Neurol Sci,* Vol. 14, pp. 36-41, ISSN 0317-1671

Barrow, C.J., and Zagorski, M.G. (1991). Solution structures of beta peptide and its constituent fragments: relation to amyloid deposition. *Science,* Vol. 253, pp. 179-182, ISSN

Bartolini, M. (2003). beta-Amyloid aggregation induced by human acetylcholinesterase: inhibition studies. *Biochem Pharmacol,* Vol. 65, pp. 407-416, ISSN 0006-2952

Bartus, R.T. (1982). The cholinergic hypothesis of geriatric memory dysfunction. *Science,* Vol. 217, pp. 408-414, ISSN 0036-8075

Behl, C. (1999). Alzheimer's disease and oxidative stress: implications for novel therapeutic approaches. *Prog Neurobiol,* Vol. 57, pp. 301-323, ISSN 0301-0082

Behl, C. (1994). Hydrogen peroxide mediates amyloid beta protein toxicity. *Cell,* Vol. 77, pp. 817-827, ISSN 0092-8674

Bender, A. (2006). High levels of mitochondrial DNA deletions in substantia nigra neurons in aging and Parkinson disease. *Nat Genet,* Vol. 38, pp. 515-517, ISSN 1061-4036

Benecke, R. (1993). Electron transfer complexes I and IV of platelets are abnormal in Parkinson's disease but normal in Parkinson-plus syndromes. *Brain,* Vol. 116 (Pt 6), pp. 1451-1463, ISSN 0006-8950

Benner, E.J. (2008). Nitrated alpha-synuclein immunity accelerates degeneration of nigral dopaminergic neurons. *PLoS One,* Vol. 3, pp. e1376, ISSN 1932-6203

Berman, S.B., and Hastings, T.G. (1999). Dopamine oxidation alters mitochondrial respiration and induces permeability transition in brain mitochondria: implications for Parkinson's disease. *J Neurochem,* Vol. 73, pp. 1127-1137, ISSN 0022-3042

Betarbet, R. (2002). Animal models of Parkinson's disease. *Bioessays,* Vol. 24, pp. 308-318, ISSN 0265-9247

Betarbet, R. (2000). Chronic systemic pesticide exposure reproduces features of Parkinson's disease. *Nat Neurosci,* Vol. 3, pp. 1301-1306, ISSN 1097-6256

Bhat, R.V. (2004). Glycogen synthase kinase 3: a drug target for CNS therapies. *Journal of neurochemistry,* Vol. 89, pp. 1313-1317, ISSN 0022-3042

Binder, L.I. (2005). Tau, tangles, and Alzheimer's disease. *Biochimica et biophysica acta,* Vol. 1739, pp. 216-223, ISSN 0006-3002

Bitan, G. (2003). Amyloid beta -protein (Abeta) assembly: Abeta 40 and Abeta 42 oligomerize through distinct pathways. *Proc Natl Acad Sci U S A,* Vol. 100, pp. 330-335, ISSN

Black, S.E. (2007). S3-02-02: Flurizan. *Alzheimer's Dementia,* Vol. 3, pp. S199.

Blanchard, B.J. (1997). Mechanism and prevention of neurotoxicity caused by beta-amyloid peptides: relation to Alzheimer's disease. *Brain Research,* Vol. 776, pp. 40-50.

Bonifati, V. (2003). DJ-1(PARK7), a novel gene for autosomal recessive, early onset parkinsonism. *Neurol Sci,* Vol. 24, pp. 159-160, ISSN 1590-1874

Borghi, R. (2000). Full length alpha-synuclein is present in cerebrospinal fluid from Parkinson's disease and normal subjects. *Neurosci Lett,* Vol. 287, pp. 65-67, ISSN 0304-3940

Bosco, D.A. (2006). Elevated levels of oxidized cholesterol metabolites in Lewy body disease brains accelerate alpha-synuclein fibrilization. *Nat Chem Biol,* Vol. 2, pp. 249-253, ISSN 1552-4450

Bowen, D.M. (1992). Treatment strategies for Alzheimer's disease. *Lancet,* Vol. 339, pp. 132-133, ISSN 0140-6736

Braak, H., and Braak, E. (1987). Argyrophilic grains: characteristic pathology of cerebral cortex in cases of adult onset dementia without Alzheimer changes. *Neuroscience letters,* Vol. 76, pp. 124-127, ISSN 0304-3940

Brandt, R. (2005). Tau alteration and neuronal degeneration in tauopathies: mechanisms and models. *Biochimica et biophysica acta,* Vol. 1739, pp. 331-354, ISSN 0006-3002

Brunden, K.R. (1993). pH-dependent binding of synthetic beta-amyloid peptides to glycosaminoglycans. *J Neurochem,* Vol. 61, pp. 2147-2154, ISSN 0022-3042

Brunden, K.R. (2009). Advances in tau-focused drug discovery for Alzheimer's disease and related tauopathies. *Nature reviews. Drug discovery,* Vol. 8, pp. 783-793, ISSN 1474-1784

Buee-Scherrer, V. (1995). Neurofibrillary degeneration in amyotrophic lateral sclerosis/parkinsonism-dementia complex of Guam. Immunochemical characterization of tau proteins. *The American journal of pathology,* Vol. 146, pp. 924-932, ISSN 0002-9440

Bullock, R. (2002). New drugs for Alzheimer's disease and other dementias. *Br J Psychiatry,* Vol. 180, pp. 135-139, ISSN 0007-1250

Bush, A.I. (2003). Copper, beta-amyloid, and Alzheimer's disease: tapping a sensitive connection. *Proc Natl Acad Sci U S A,* Vol. 100, pp. 11193-11194, ISSN 0027-8424

Butterfield, D.A. (2001). Evidence of oxidative damage in Alzheimer's disease brain: central role for amyloid beta-peptide. *Trends Mol Med,* Vol. 7, pp. 548-554, ISSN 1471-4914

Butterfield, D.A., and Kanski, J. (2002). Methionine residue 35 is critical for the oxidative stress and neurotoxic properties of Alzheimer's amyloid beta-peptide 1-42. *Peptides,* Vol. 23, pp. 1299-1309.

Camps, P., and Muñoz-Torrero, D. (2002). Cholinergic drugs in pharmacotherapy of Alzheimer's disease. *Mini Rev Med Chem,* Vol. 2, pp. 11-25, ISSN 1389-5575

Canet-Aviles, R.M. (2004). The Parkinson's disease protein DJ-1 is neuroprotective due to cysteine-sulfinic acid-driven mitochondrial localization. *Proc Natl Acad Sci U S A,* Vol. 101, pp. 9103-9108, ISSN 0027-8424

Castano, A. (2002). The degenerative effect of a single intranigral injection of LPS on the dopaminergic system is prevented by dexamethasone, and not mimicked by rh-TNF-alpha, IL-1beta and IFN-gamma. *J Neurochem,* Vol. 81, pp. 150-157, ISSN 0022-3042

Castillo, G.M. (1999). The sulfate moieties of glycosaminoglycans are critical for the enhancement of beta-amyloid protein fibril formation. *J Neurochem,* Vol. 72, pp. 1681-1687, ISSN 0022-3042

Castillo, G.M. (1997). Perlecan binds to the beta-amyloid proteins (A beta) of Alzheimer's disease, accelerates A beta fibril formation, and maintains A beta fibril stability. *J Neurochem,* Vol. 69, pp. 2452-2465, ISSN 0022-3042

Caudle, W.M. (2008). Altered vesicular dopamine storage in Parkinson's disease: a premature demise. *Trends Neurosci,* Vol. 31, pp. 303-308, ISSN 0166-2236

Cavelier, G., and Amzel, L.M. (2001). Mechanism of NAD(P)H:quinone reductase: Ab initio studies of reduced flavin. *Proteins,* Vol. 43, pp. 420-432, ISSN 0887-3585

Chaudhuri, K.R., and Schapira, A.H. (2009). Non-motor symptoms of Parkinson's disease: dopaminergic pathophysiology and treatment. *Lancet Neurology,* Vol. 8, pp. 464-474, ISSN 1474-4422

Chen, L. (2008). Unregulated cytosolic dopamine causes neurodegeneration associated with oxidative stress in mice. *J Neurosci,* Vol. 28, pp. 425-433, ISSN 1529-2401

Cherny, R.A. (2001). Treatment with a copper-zinc chelator markedly and rapidly inhibits beta-amyloid accumulation in Alzheimer's disease transgenic mice. *Neuron,* Vol. 30, pp. 665-676, ISSN 0896-6273

Chin, J. (2005). Fyn kinase induces synaptic and cognitive impairments in a transgenic mouse model of Alzheimer's disease. *The Journal of neuroscience : the official journal of the Society for Neuroscience,* Vol. 25, pp. 9694-9703, ISSN 1529-2401

Cho, Y. (2009). Doxycycline is neuroprotective against nigral dopaminergic degeneration by a dual mechanism involving MMP-3. *Neurotox Res,* Vol. 16, pp. 361-371, ISSN 1476-3524

Choi, D.H. (2008). A novel intracellular role of matrix metalloproteinase-3 during apoptosis of dopaminergic cells. *J Neurochem,* Vol. 106, pp. 405-415, ISSN 1471-4159

Choi, D.S. (2006). PKCepsilon increases endothelin converting enzyme activity and reduces amyloid plaque pathology in transgenic mice. *Proc Natl Acad Sci U S A,* Vol. 103, pp. 8215-8220, ISSN 0027-8424

Choi, H.J. (2003). Dopamine-dependent cytotoxicity of tetrahydrobiopterin: a possible mechanism for selective neurodegeneration in Parkinson's disease. *J Neurochem,* Vol. 86, pp. 143-152, ISSN 0022-3042

Choi, J. (2004). Oxidative modifications and down-regulation of ubiquitin carboxyl-terminal hydrolase L1 associated with idiopathic Parkinson's and Alzheimer's diseases. *J Biol Chem,* Vol. 279, pp. 13256-13264, ISSN 0021-9258

Choi, J. (2006). Oxidative damage of DJ-1 is linked to sporadic Parkinson and Alzheimer diseases. *J Biol Chem,* Vol. 281, pp. 10816-10824, ISSN 0021-9258

Cicchetti, F. (2002). Neuroinflammation of the nigrostriatal pathway during progressive 6-OHDA dopamine degeneration in rats monitored by immunohistochemistry and PET imaging. *Eur J Neurosci,* Vol. 15, pp. 991-998, ISSN 0953-816X

Clark, I.E. (2006). Drosophila pink1 is required for mitochondrial function and interacts genetically with parkin. *Nature,* Vol. 441, pp. 1162-1166, ISSN 1476-4687

Clark, J., and Simon, D.K. (2009). Transcribe to survive: transcriptional control of antioxidant defense programs for neuroprotection in Parkinson's disease. *Antioxid Redox Signal,* Vol. 11, pp. 509-528, ISSN 1557-7716

Conway, K.A. (2001). Kinetic stabilization of the alpha-synuclein protofibril by a dopamine-alpha-synuclein adduct. *Science,* Vol. 294, pp. 1346-1349, ISSN 0036-8075

Corrigan, F.M. (1998). Diorthosubstituted polychlorinated biphenyls in caudate nucleus in Parkinson's disease. *Exp Neurol,* Vol. 150, pp. 339-342, ISSN 0014-4886

Darios, F. (2003). Parkin prevents mitochondrial swelling and cytochrome c release in mitochondria-dependent cell death. *Hum Mol Genet,* Vol. 12, pp. 517-526, ISSN 0964-6906

Darvesh, S. (2003). Neurobiology of butyrylcholinesterase. *Nat Rev Neurosci,* Vol. 4, pp. 131-138, ISSN 1471-003X

Dauer, W. (2002). Resistance of alpha -synuclein null mice to the parkinsonian neurotoxin MPTP. *Proc Natl Acad Sci U S A,* Vol. 99, pp. 14524-14529, ISSN 0027-8424

Davies, P., and Maloney, A.J. (1976). Selective loss of central cholinergic neurons in Alzheimer's disease. *Lancet,* Vol. 2, pp. 1403, ISSN 0140-6736

Dayanandan, R. (1999). Mutations in tau reduce its microtubule binding properties in intact cells and affect its phosphorylation. *FEBS letters,* Vol. 446, pp. 228-232, ISSN 0014-5793

De Ferrari, G.V. (2001). A structural motif of acetylcholinesterase that promotes amyloid beta-peptide fibril formation. *Biochemistry,* Vol. 40, pp. 10447-10457, ISSN 0006-2960

de Lau, L.M., and Breteler, M.M. (2006). Epidemiology of Parkinson's disease. *Lancet Neurology,* Vol. 5, pp. 525-535, ISSN 1474-4422

Defelice, F.G., and Ferreira, S.T. (2002). Physiopathological modulators of amyloid aggregation and novel pharmacological approaches in Alzheimer's disease. *An Acad Bras Cienc,* Vol. 74, pp. 265-284, ISSN 0001-3765

Devi, L. (2008). Mitochondrial import and accumulation of alpha-synuclein impair complex I in human dopaminergic neuronal cultures and Parkinson disease brain. *J Biol Chem,* Vol. 283, pp. 9089-9100, ISSN 0021-9258

Dhavan, R., and Tsai, L.H. (2001). A decade of CDK5. *Nature reviews. Molecular cell biology,* Vol. 2, pp. 749-759, ISSN 1471-0072

Diamant, S. (2006). Butyrylcholinesterase attenuates amyloid fibril formation in vitro. *Proc Natl Acad Sci U S A,* Vol. 103, pp. 8628-8633, ISSN 0027-8424

Dinkova-Kostova, A.T., and Talalay, P. (2010). NAD(P)H:quinone acceptor oxidoreductase 1 (NQO1), a multifunctional antioxidant enzyme and exceptionally versatile cytoprotector. *Arch Biochem Biophys,* Vol. 501, pp. 116-123, ISSN 1096-0384

Doraiswamy, P.M., and Finefrock, A.E. (2004). Metals in our minds: therapeutic implications for neurodegenerative disorders. *Lancet Neurol,* Vol. 3, pp. 431-434, ISSN 1474-4422

Drechsel, D.N. (1992). Modulation of the dynamic instability of tubulin assembly by the microtubule-associated protein tau. *Molecular biology of the cell,* Vol. 3, pp. 1141-1154, ISSN 1059-1524

Du, Y. (2001). Minocycline prevents nigrostriatal dopaminergic neurodegeneration in the MPTP model of Parkinson's disease. *Proc Natl Acad Sci U S A,* Vol. 98, pp. 14669-14674, ISSN 0027-8424

Duffy, S. (1998). Activation of endogenous antioxidant defenses in neuronal cells prevents free radical-mediated damage. *J Neurochem,* Vol. 71, pp. 69-77, ISSN 0022-3042

Dunnett, S.B., and Bjorklund, A. (1999). Prospects for new restorative and neuroprotective treatments in Parkinson's disease. *Nature,* Vol. 399, pp. A32-39, ISSN 0028-0836

El-Agnaf, O.M. (2003). Alpha-synuclein implicated in Parkinson's disease is present in extracellular biological fluids, including human plasma. *FASEB J,* Vol. 17, pp. 1945-1947, ISSN 1530-6860

Etminan, M. (2005). Intake of vitamin E, vitamin C, and carotenoids and the risk of Parkinson's disease: a meta-analysis. *Lancet Neurology,* Vol. 4, pp. 362-365, ISSN 1474-4422

Fahn, S. (1989). Adverse effects of levodopa in Parkinson's disease. In Handb Exp Pharmacol, Calne, D.B.,(Ed.) pp. 386-409, Berlin

Farina, C. (2007). Astrocytes are active players in cerebral innate immunity. *Trends Immunol,* Vol. 28, pp. 138-145, ISSN 1471-4906

Farrer, M.J. (2006). Genetics of Parkinson disease: paradigm shifts and future prospects. *Nat Rev Genet,* Vol. 7, pp. 306-318, ISSN 1471-0056

Fasulo, L. (2000). The neuronal microtubule-associated protein tau is a substrate for caspase-3 and an effector of apoptosis. *Journal of neurochemistry,* Vol. 75, pp. 624-633, ISSN 0022-3042

Ferrer, I. (2001). Phosphorylated map kinase (ERK1, ERK2) expression is associated with early tau deposition in neurones and glial cells, but not with increased nuclear DNA vulnerability and cell death, in Alzheimer disease, Pick's disease, progressive supranuclear palsy and corticobasal degeneration. *Brain pathology,* Vol. 11, pp. 144-158, ISSN 1015-6305

Finder, V.H., and Glockshuber, R. (2007). Amyloid-beta aggregation. *Neurodegener Dis,* Vol. 4, pp. 13-27, ISSN 1660-2854

Flier, J. (2002). The neuroprotective antioxidant alpha-lipoic acid induces detoxication enzymes in cultured astroglial cells. *Free Radic Res,* Vol. 36, pp. 695-699, ISSN 1071-5762

Francis, J.W. (1995). Neuroglial responses to the dopaminergic neurotoxicant 1-methyl-4-phenyl-1,2,3,6-tetrahydropyridine in mouse striatum. *Neurotoxicol Teratol,* Vol. 17, pp. 7-12, ISSN 0892-0362

Frank, B., and Gupta, S. (2005). A review of antioxidants and Alzheimer's disease. *Ann Clin Psychiatry,* Vol. 17, pp. 269-286, ISSN 1040-1237

Fraser, P.E. (1992). Effects of sulfate ions on Alzheimer beta/A4 peptide assemblies: implications for amyloid fibril-proteoglycan interactions. *J Neurochem,* Vol. 59, pp. 1531-1540, ISSN 0022-3042

Gaggelli, E. (2006). Copper homeostasis and neurodegenerative disorders (Alzheimer's, prion, and Parkinson's diseases and amyotrophic lateral sclerosis). *Chem Rev,* Vol. 106, pp. 1995-2044, ISSN 0009-2665

Gamblin, T.C. (2003). Caspase cleavage of tau: linking amyloid and neurofibrillary tangles in Alzheimer's disease. *Proceedings of the National Academy of Sciences of the United States of America,* Vol. 100, pp. 10032-10037, ISSN 0027-8424

Gandhi, S. (2009). PINK1-associated Parkinson's disease is caused by neuronal vulnerability to calcium-induced cell death. *Mol Cell,* Vol. 33, pp. 627-638, ISSN 1097-4164

Gao, H.M. (2008). Neuroinflammation and oxidation/nitration of alpha-synuclein linked to dopaminergic neurodegeneration. *J Neurosci,* Vol. 28, pp. 7687-7698, ISSN 1529-2401

Gao, H.M. (2011). Neuroinflammation and alpha-synuclein dysfunction potentiate each other, driving chronic progression of neurodegeneration in a mouse model of Parkinson's disease. *Environ Health Perspect,* Vol. 119, pp. 807-814, ISSN 1552-9924

Garcia-Sierra, F. (2003). Conformational changes and truncation of tau protein during tangle evolution in Alzheimer's disease. *Journal of Alzheimer's disease : JAD,* Vol. 5, pp. 65-77, ISSN 1387-2877

Gasche, Y. (2001). Matrix metalloproteinase inhibition prevents oxidative stress-associated blood-brain barrier disruption after transient focal cerebral ischemia. *J Cereb Blood Flow Metab,* Vol. 21, pp. 1393-1400, ISSN 0271-678X

Gegg, M.E. (2009). Silencing of PINK1 expression affects mitochondrial DNA and oxidative phosphorylation in dopaminergic cells. *PLoS One,* Vol. 4, pp. e4756, ISSN 1932-6203

Gendron, T.F., and Petrucelli, L. (2009). The role of tau in neurodegeneration. *Molecular neurodegeneration,* Vol. 4, pp. 13, ISSN 1750-1326

Gerhard, A. (2006). In vivo imaging of microglial activation with [11C](R)-PK11195 PET in idiopathic Parkinson's disease. *Neurobiol Dis,* Vol. 21, pp. 404-412, ISSN 0969-9961

Gerlach, M. (2011). Biomarker candidates of neurodegeneration in Parkinson's disease for the evaluation of disease-modifying therapeutics. *J Neural Transm,* Vol. 1435-1463

Gervais, F. (2007). Targeting soluble Abeta peptide with Tramiprosate for the treatment of brain amyloidosis. *Neurobiol Aging,* Vol. 28, pp. 537-547, ISSN 1558-1497

Giacobini, E. (2002). Inhibition of acetyl- and butyryl-cholinesterase in the cerebrospinal fluid of patients with Alzheimer's disease by rivastigmine: correlation with cognitive benefit. *J Neural Transm,* Vol. 109, pp. 1053-1065, ISSN 0300-9564

Goedert, M., and Jakes, R. (1990). Expression of separate isoforms of human tau protein: correlation with the tau pattern in brain and effects on tubulin polymerization. *The EMBO journal,* Vol. 9, pp. 4225-4230, ISSN 0261-4189

Goedert, M. (1989). Multiple isoforms of human microtubule-associated protein tau: sequences and localization in neurofibrillary tangles of Alzheimer's disease. *Neuron,* Vol. 3, pp. 519-526, ISSN 0896-6273

Graham, D.G. (1978). Oxidative pathways for catecholamines in the genesis of neuromelanin and cytotoxic quinones. *Mol Pharmacol,* Vol. 14, pp. 633-643, ISSN 0026-895X

Greene, J.C. (2003). Mitochondrial pathology and apoptotic muscle degeneration in Drosophila parkin mutants. *Proc Natl Acad Sci U S A,* Vol. 100, pp. 4078-4083, ISSN 0027-8424

Greig, N.H. (2001). A new therapeutic target in Alzheimer's disease treatment: attention to butyrylcholinesterase. *Curr Med Res Opin,* Vol. 17, pp. 159-165, ISSN 0300-7995

Grunewald, A. (2009). Differential effects of PINK1 nonsense and missense mutations on mitochondrial function and morphology. *Exp Neurol,* Vol. 219, pp. 266-273, ISSN 1090-2430

Grunewald, A. (2010). Mutant Parkin impairs mitochondrial function and morphology in human fibroblasts. *PLoS One,* Vol. 5, pp. e12962, ISSN 1932-6203

Gurney, K.J. (2006). Blood-brain barrier disruption by stromelysin-1 facilitates neutrophil infiltration in neuroinflammation. *Neurobiol Dis,* Vol. 23, pp. 87-96, ISSN 0969-9961

Halliday, G. (2000). Alzheimer's disease and inflammation: a review of cellular and therapeutic mechanisms. *Clin Exp Pharmacol Physiol,* Vol. 27, pp. 1-8, ISSN 0305-1870

Halliwell, B. (1992). Reactive oxygen species and the central nervous system. *J Neurochem,* Vol. 59, pp. 1609-1623, ISSN 0022-3042

Hamaguchi, T. (2006). Anti-amyloidogenic therapies: strategies for prevention and treatment of Alzheimer's disease. *Cell Mol Life Sci,* Vol. 63, pp. 1538-1552, ISSN 1420-682X

Han, J.M. (2007). Protective effect of sulforaphane against dopaminergic cell death. *J Pharmacol Exp Ther,* Vol. 321, pp. 249-256, ISSN 0022-3565

Hara, H. (2003). Increase of antioxidative potential by tert-butylhydroquinone protects against cell death associated with 6-hydroxydopamine-induced oxidative stress in neuroblastoma SH-SY5Y cells. *Brain Res Mol Brain Res,* Vol. 119, pp. 125-131, ISSN 0169-328X

Harada, S. (2001). An association between idiopathic Parkinson's disease and polymorphisms of phase II detoxification enzymes: glutathione S-transferase M1 and quinone oxidoreductase 1 and 2. *Biochem Biophys Res Commun,* Vol. 288, pp. 887-892, ISSN 0006-291X

Hardy, J., and Selkoe, D.J. (2002). The amyloid hypothesis of Alzheimer's disease: progress and problems on the road to therapeutics. *Science,* Vol. 297, pp. 353-356, ISSN 1095-9203

Hardy, J.A., and Higgins, G.A. (1992). Alzheimer's disease: the amyloid cascade hypothesis. *Science,* Vol. 256, pp. 184-185, ISSN 0036-8075

Hartmann, T. (1997). Distinct sites of intracellular production for Alzheimer's disease A beta40/42 amyloid peptides. *Nat Med,* Vol. 3, pp. 1016-1020, ISSN 1078-8956

Hasegawa, M. (1998). Tau proteins with FTDP-17 mutations have a reduced ability to promote microtubule assembly. *FEBS letters,* Vol. 437, pp. 207-210, ISSN 0014-5793

Hastings, T.G., and Zigmond, M.J. (1997). Loss of dopaminergic neurons in parkinsonism: possible role of reactive dopamine metabolites. *J Neural Transm Suppl,* Vol. 49, pp. 103-110, ISSN 0303-6995

Hong, M. (1997). Lithium reduces tau phosphorylation by inhibition of glycogen synthase kinase-3. *The Journal of biological chemistry,* Vol. 272, pp. 25326-25332, ISSN 0021-9258

Hong, M. (1998). Mutation-specific functional impairments in distinct tau isoforms of hereditary FTDP-17. *Science,* Vol. 282, pp. 1914-1917, ISSN 0036-8075

Hull, M. (1999). Anti-inflammatory substances - a new therapeutic option in Alzheimer's disease. *Drug Discovery Today,* Vol. 4, pp. 275-282, ISSN 1359-6446

Hutton, M. (2000). Molecular genetics of chromosome 17 tauopathies. *Annals of the New York Academy of Sciences,* Vol. 920, pp. 63-73, ISSN 0077-8923

Hutton, M. (1998). Association of missense and 5'-splice-site mutations in tau with the inherited dementia FTDP-17. *Nature,* Vol. 393, pp. 702-705, ISSN 0028-0836

Ibach, B., and Haen, E. (2004). Acetylcholinesterase inhibition in Alzheimer's Disease. *Curr Pharm Des,* Vol. 10, pp. 231-251, ISSN 1381-6128

Inestrosa, N.C. (1996). Acetylcholinesterase accelerates assembly of amyloid-beta-peptides into Alzheimer's fibrils: possible role of the peripheral site of the enzyme. *Neuron,* Vol. 16, pp. 881-891, ISSN 0896-6273

Innamorato, N.G. (2010). Different susceptibility to the Parkinson's toxin MPTP in mice lacking the redox master regulator Nrf2 or its target gene heme oxygenase-1. *PLoS One,* Vol. 5, pp. e11838, ISSN 1932-6203

Investigators, T.N.N.-P. (2007). A randomized clinical trial of coenzyme Q10 and GPI-1485 in early Parkinson disease. *Neurology,* Vol. 68, pp. 20-28, ISSN 1526-632X

Investigators., N.N.-P. (2008). A pilot clinical trial of creatine and minocycline in early Parkinson disease: 18-month results. *Clin Neuropharmacol,* Vol. 31, pp. 141-150, ISSN 1537-162X

Iqbal, K. (2005). Tau pathology in Alzheimer disease and other tauopathies. *Biochimica et biophysica acta,* Vol. 1739, pp. 198-210, ISSN 0006-3002

Irrcher, I. (2010). Loss of the Parkinson's disease-linked gene DJ-1 perturbs mitochondrial dynamics. *Hum Mol Genet,* Vol. 19, pp. 3734-3746, ISSN 1460-2083

Ishikawa, A., and Takahashi, H. (1998). Clinical and neuropathological aspects of autosomal recessive juvenile parkinsonism. *J Neurol,* Vol. 245, pp. P4-9, ISSN 0340-5354

Jack, C.R. (2010). Hypothetical model of dynamic biomarkers of the Alzheimer's pathological cascade. *Lancet Neurology,* Vol. 9, pp. 119-128, ISSN 1474-4422

Jan, A. (2008). The ratio of monomeric to aggregated forms of Abeta40 and Abeta42 is an important determinant of amyloid-beta aggregation, fibrillogenesis, and toxicity. *J Biol Chem,* Vol. 283, pp. 28176-28189, ISSN 0021-9258

Jann, M.W. (2000). Rivastigmine, a new-generation cholinesterase inhibitor for the treatment of Alzheimer's disease. *Pharmacotherapy,* Vol. 20, pp. 1-12, ISSN 0277-0008

Jarrett, J.T., and Lansbury, P.T., Jr. (1993). Seeding "one-dimensional crystallization" of amyloid: a pathogenic mechanism in Alzheimer's disease and scrapie? *Cell,* Vol. 73, pp. 1055-1058, ISSN 0092-8674

Jazwa, A. (2011). Pharmacological targeting of the transcription factor Nrf2 at the basal ganglia provides disease modifying therapy for experimental parkinsonism. *Antioxid Redox Signal,* Vol. 14, pp. 2347-2360, ISSN 1557-7716 (Electronic)

Jenner, P. (2003). Oxidative stress in Parkinson's disease. *Ann Neurol,* Vol. 53 Suppl 3, pp. S26-36; discussion S36-28, ISSN 0364-5134

Jenner, P., and Olanow, C.W. (1996). Oxidative stress and the pathogenesis of Parkinson's disease. *Neurology,* Vol. 47, pp. S161-170, ISSN 0028-3878

Jia, Z. (2009). Cruciferous nutraceutical 3H-1,2-dithiole-3-thione protects human primary astrocytes against neurocytotoxicity elicited by MPTP, MPP(+), 6-OHDA, HNE and acrolein. *Neurochem Res,* Vol. 34, pp. 1924-1934, ISSN 1573-6903 (Electronic)

Jia, Z. (2008). Potent induction of total cellular GSH and NQO1 as well as mitochondrial GSH by 3H-1,2-dithiole-3-thione in SH-SY5Y neuroblastoma cells and primary human neurons: protection against neurocytotoxicity elicited by dopamine, 6-hydroxydopamine, 4-hydroxy-2-nonenal, or hydrogen peroxide. *Brain Res,* Vol. 1197, pp. 159-169, ISSN 0006-8993

Jian Liu, K., and Rosenberg, G.A. (2005). Matrix metalloproteinases and free radicals in cerebral ischemia. *Free Radic Biol Med,* Vol. 39, pp. 71-80, ISSN 0891-5849

Jiang, X.H. (2004). [A study on the relationship between polymorphism of human NAD(P)H: quinone oxidoreductase and Parkinson's disease in Chinese]. *Zhonghua Yi Xue Yi Chuan Xue Za Zhi,* Vol. 21, pp. 120-123, ISSN 1003-9406

Jones, J.M. (2003). Loss of Omi mitochondrial protease activity causes the neuromuscular disorder of mnd2 mutant mice. *Nature,* Vol. 425, pp. 721-727, ISSN 1476-4687 (Electronic)

Joseph, P. (2000). Role of NAD(P)H:quinone oxidoreductase 1 (DT diaphorase) in protection against quinone toxicity. *Biochem Pharmacol,* Vol. 60, pp. 207-214, ISSN 0006-2952

Kamel, F. (2007). Pesticide exposure and self-reported Parkinson's disease in the agricultural health study. *Am J Epidemiol,* Vol. 165, pp. 364-374, ISSN 0002-9262

Kamp, F. (2010). Inhibition of mitochondrial fusion by alpha-synuclein is rescued by PINK1, Parkin and DJ-1. *EMBO J,* Vol. 29, pp. 3571-3589, ISSN 1460-2075 (Electronic)

Kar, A. (2005). Tau alternative splicing and frontotemporal dementia. *Alzheimer disease and associated disorders,* Vol. 19 Suppl 1, pp. S29-36, ISSN 0893-0341

Kayed, R. (2003). Common structure of soluble amyloid oligomers implies common mechanism of pathogenesis. *Science,* Vol. 300, pp. 486-489, ISSN

Kim, E.M., and Hwang, O. (2011). Role of matrix metalloproteinase-3 in neurodegeneration. *J Neurochem,* Vol. 116, pp. 22-32, ISSN 1471-4159

Kim, E.M. (2010). Matrix metalloproteinase-3 is increased and participates in neuronal apoptotic signaling downstream of caspase-12 during endoplasmic reticulum stress. *J Biol Chem,* Vol. 285, pp. 16444-16452, ISSN 1083-351X

Kim, S. (2009). Exendin-4 protects dopaminergic neurons by inhibition of microglial activation and matrix metalloproteinase-3 expression in an animal model of Parkinson's disease. *J Endocrinol,* Vol. 202, pp. 431-439, ISSN 1479-6805

Kim, Y. (2009). Multivalent & multifunctional ligands to beta-amyloid. *Curr Pharm Des,* Vol. 15, pp. 637-658, ISSN 1873-4286

Kim, Y.S. (2007). A pivotal role of matrix metalloproteinase-3 activity in dopaminergic neuronal degeneration via microglial activation. *FASEB J,* Vol. 21, pp. 179-187, ISSN 1530-6860

Kim, Y.S. (2005). Matrix metalloproteinase-3: a novel signaling proteinase from apoptotic neuronal cells that activates microglia. *J Neurosci,* Vol. 25, pp. 3701-3711, ISSN 1529-2401

Kisilevsky, R. (2007). Heparan sulfate as a therapeutic target in amyloidogenesis: prospects and possible complications. *Amyloid,* Vol. 14, pp. 21-32, ISSN 1350-6129

Klein, W.L. (2004). Small assemblies of unmodified amyloid beta-protein are the proximate neurotoxin in Alzheimer's disease. *Neurobiol Aging,* Vol. 25, pp. 569-580, ISSN 0197-4580

Klunk, W.E. (1994). Development of small molecule probes for the beta-amyloid protein of Alzheimer's disease. *Neurobiol Aging,* Vol. 15, pp. 691-698, ISSN 0197-4580

Knapp, M.J. (1994). A 30-week randomized controlled trial of high-dose tacrine in patients with Alzheimer's disease. The Tacrine Study Group. *JAMA,* Vol. 271, pp. 985-991, ISSN 0098-7484

Knott, C. (2000). Inflammatory regulators in Parkinson's disease: iNOS, lipocortin-1, and cyclooxygenases-1 and -2. *Mol Cell Neurosci,* Vol. 16, pp. 724-739, ISSN 1044-7431

Kopke, E. (1993). Microtubule-associated protein tau. Abnormal phosphorylation of a non-paired helical filament pool in Alzheimer disease. *The Journal of biological chemistry,* Vol. 268, pp. 24374-24384, ISSN 0021-9258

Krick, S. (2008). Mpv17l protects against mitochondrial oxidative stress and apoptosis by activation of Omi/HtrA2 protease. *Proc Natl Acad Sci U S A,* Vol. 105, pp. 14106-14111, ISSN 1091-6490

Kuhn, D.M. (1999). Tyrosine hydroxylase is inactivated by catechol-quinones and converted to a redox-cycling quinoprotein: possible relevance to Parkinson's disease. *J Neurochem,* Vol. 73, pp. 1309-1317, ISSN 0022-3042

Kuo, Y.M. (1996). Water-soluble Abeta (N-40, N-42) oligomers in normal and Alzheimer disease brains. *J Biol Chem,* Vol. 271, pp. 4077-4081, ISSN 0021-9258

Kurkowska-Jastrzebska, I. (1999). The inflammatory reaction following 1-methyl-4-phenyl-1,2,3, 6-tetrahydropyridine intoxication in mouse. *Exp Neurol,* Vol. 156, pp. 50-61, ISSN 0014-4886

Langston, J.W. (1999). Evidence of active nerve cell degeneration in the substantia nigra of humans years after 1-methyl-4-phenyl-1,2,3,6-tetrahydropyridine exposure. *Ann Neurol,* Vol. 46, pp. 598-605, ISSN 0364-5134 0364-5134

LaVoie, M.J. (2005). Dopamine covalently modifies and functionally inactivates parkin. *Nat Med,* Vol. 11, pp. 1214-1221, ISSN 1078-8956

Lazo, N.D. (2005). On the nucleation of amyloid beta-protein monomer folding. *Protein Sci,* Vol. 14, pp. 1581-1596, ISSN 0961-8368

Lee, C.S. (2002). Differential effect of catecholamines and MPP(+) on membrane permeability in brain mitochondria and cell viability in PC12 cells. *Neurochem Int,* Vol. 40, pp. 361-369, ISSN 0197-0186

Lee, E.J. (2010). Alpha-synuclein activates microglia by inducing the expressions of matrix metalloproteinases and the subsequent activation of protease-activated receptor-1. *J Immunol,* Vol. 185, pp. 615-623, ISSN 1550-6606 (Electronic)

Lee, G. (2004). Phosphorylation of tau by fyn: implications for Alzheimer's disease. *The Journal of neuroscience : the official journal of the Society for Neuroscience,* Vol. 24, pp. 2304-2312, ISSN 1529-2401

Lee, H.J. (2005). Intravesicular localization and exocytosis of alpha-synuclein and its aggregates. *J Neurosci,* Vol. 25, pp. 6016-6024, ISSN 1529-2401

Lee, K.Y. (1999). Elevated neuronal Cdc2-like kinase activity in the Alzheimer disease brain. *Neuroscience research,* Vol. 34, pp. 21-29, ISSN 0168-0102

Lee, R.K. (1995). Amyloid precursor protein processing is stimulated by metabotropic glutamate receptors. *Proc Natl Acad Sci U S A,* Vol. 92, pp. 8083-8087, ISSN 0027-8424

Liang, C.L. (2007). Mitochondria mass is low in mouse substantia nigra dopamine neurons: implications for Parkinson's disease. *Exp Neurol,* Vol. 203, pp. 370-380, ISSN 0014-4886

Liang, X. (2005). Deletion of the prostaglandin E2 EP2 receptor reduces oxidative damage and amyloid burden in a model of Alzheimer's disease. *J Neurosci,* Vol. 25, pp. 10180-10187, ISSN 1529-2401 (Electronic)

Lim, G.P. (2000). Ibuprofen suppresses plaque pathology and inflammation in a mouse model for Alzheimer's disease. *J Neurosci,* Vol. 20, pp. 5709-5714, ISSN 0270-6474

Liu, G. (2009). alpha-Synuclein is differentially expressed in mitochondria from different rat brain regions and dose-dependently down-regulates complex I activity. *Neurosci Lett,* Vol. 454, pp. 187-192, ISSN 1872-7972 (Electronic)

Liu, S.T. (1999). Histidine-13 is a crucial residue in the zinc ion-induced aggregation of the A beta peptide of Alzheimer's disease. *Biochemistry,* Vol. 38, pp. 9373-9378, ISSN

Lomakin, A. (1997). Kinetic theory of fibrillogenesis of amyloid beta-protein. *Proc Natl Acad Sci U S A,* Vol. 94, pp. 7942-7947, ISSN 0027-8424

Lotharius, J., and Brundin, P. (2002). Pathogenesis of Parkinson's disease: dopamine, vesicles and alpha-synuclein. *Nat Rev Neurosci,* Vol. 3, pp. 932-942, ISSN 1471-003X

Maker, H.S. (1981). Coupling of dopamine oxidation (monoamine oxidase activity) to glutathione oxidation via the generation of hydrogen peroxide in rat brain homogenates. *J Neurochem,* Vol. 36, pp. 589-593, ISSN 0022-3042

Mandelkow, E.M. (1996). Structure, microtubule interactions, and phosphorylation of tau protein. *Annals of the New York Academy of Sciences,* Vol. 777, pp. 96-106, ISSN 0077-8923

Marek K, J.D. (2009). Can we image premotor Parkinson disease? *Neurology,* Vol. S21-26,

Markesbery, W.R. (1997). Oxidative Stress Hypothesis in Alzheimer's Disease. *Free Radical Biol Med,* Vol. 23, pp. 134-147,

Martin, L.J. (2006). Parkinson's disease alpha-synuclein transgenic mice develop neuronal mitochondrial degeneration and cell death. *J Neurosci,* Vol. 26, pp. 41-50, ISSN 1529-2401

Martinez-Vicente, M. (2008). Dopamine-modified alpha-synuclein blocks chaperone-mediated autophagy. *J Clin Invest,* Vol. 118, pp. 777-788, ISSN 0021-9738

Martins, L.M. (2004). Neuroprotective role of the Reaper-related serine protease HtrA2/Omi revealed by targeted deletion in mice. *Mol Cell Biol,* Vol. 24, pp. 9848-9862, ISSN 0270-7306

Maslow, K. (2008). 2008 Alzheimer's disease facts and figures. *Alzheimer's Dementia,* Vol. 4, pp. 110-133, ISSN 1552-5260

Mazanetz, M.P., and Fischer, P.M. (2007). Untangling tau hyperphosphorylation in drug design for neurodegenerative diseases. *Nature Reviews Drug Discovery,* Vol. 6, pp. 464-479, ISSN 1474-1776

McGeer, P.L. (1988). Reactive microglia are positive for HLA-DR in the substantia nigra of Parkinson's and Alzheimer's disease brains. *Neurology,* Vol. 38, pp. 1285-1291, ISSN 0028-3878

McGeer, P.L., and McGeer, E.G. (1999). Inflammation of the brain in Alzheimer's disease: implications for therapy. *J Leukoc Biol,* Vol. 65, pp. 409-415, ISSN 0741-5400

McGeer, P.L. (1996). Arthritis and anti-inflammatory agents as possible protective factors for Alzheimer's disease: a review of 17 epidemiologic studies. *Neurology,* Vol. 47, pp. 425-432, ISSN 0028-3878

McLaurin, J. (1999). A sulfated proteoglycan aggregation factor mediates amyloid-beta peptide fibril formation and neurotoxicity. *Amyloid,* Vol. 6, pp. 233-243, ISSN 1350-6129

McLaurin, J. (1999). Interactions of Alzheimer amyloid-beta peptides with glycosaminoglycans effects on fibril nucleation and growth. *Eur J Biochem,* Vol. 266, pp. 1101-1110, ISSN 0014-2956

McLaurin, J., and Fraser, P.E. (2000). Effect of amino-acid substitutions on Alzheimer's amyloid-beta peptide-glycosaminoglycan interactions. *Eur J Biochem,* Vol. 267, pp. 6353-6361, ISSN 0014-2956

Melnikova, I. (2007). Therapies for Alzheimer's disease. *Nat Rev Drug Discovery,* Vol. 6, pp. 341-342, ISSN 1474-1776

Miller, J.D. (1997). Localization of perlecan (or a perlecan-related macromolecule) to isolated microglia in vitro and to microglia/macrophages following infusion of beta-amyloid protein into rodent hippocampus. *Glia,* Vol. 21, pp. 228-243, ISSN 0894-1491

Miyazaki, I. (2006). Methamphetamine-induced dopaminergic neurotoxicity is regulated by quinone-formation-related molecules. *FASEB J,* Vol. 20, pp. 571-573, ISSN 1530-6860

Mizuno, Y. (1989). Deficiencies in complex I subunits of the respiratory chain in Parkinson's disease. *Biochem Biophys Res Commun,* Vol. 163, pp. 1450-1455, ISSN 0006-291X

Moisoi, N. (2009). Mitochondrial dysfunction triggered by loss of HtrA2 results in the activation of a brain-specific transcriptional stress response. *Cell Death Differ,* Vol. 16, pp. 449-464, ISSN 1476-5403

Moon, M. (2009). Neuroprotective effect of ghrelin in the 1-methyl-4-phenyl-1,2,3,6-tetrahydropyridine mouse model of Parkinson's disease by blocking microglial activation. *Neurotox Res,* Vol. 15, pp. 332-347, ISSN 1476-3524

Mortiboys, H. (2008). Mitochondrial function and morphology are impaired in parkin-mutant fibroblasts. *Ann Neurol,* Vol. 64, pp. 555-565, ISSN 1531-8249

Motamedi-Shad, N. (2009). Kinetic analysis of amyloid formation in the presence of heparan sulfate: faster unfolding and change of pathway. *J Biol Chem,* Vol. 284, pp. 29921-29934, ISSN 1083-351X

Muftuoglu, M. (2004). Mitochondrial complex I and IV activities in leukocytes from patients with parkin mutations. *Mov Disord,* Vol. 19, pp. 544-548, ISSN 0885-3185

Multhaup, G. (1995). Characterization of the high affinity heparin binding site of the Alzheimer's disease beta A4 amyloid precursor protein (APP) and its enhancement by zinc(II). *J Mol Recognit,* Vol. 8, pp. 247-257, ISSN 0952-3499

Muñoz, F.J., and Inestrosa, N.C. (1999). Neurotoxicity of acetylcholinesterase amyloid beta-peptide aggregates is dependent on the type of Abeta peptide and the AChE concentration present in the complexes. *FEBS Lett,* Vol. 450, pp. 205-209, ISSN 0014-5793

Munoz-Montano, J.R. (1997). Lithium inhibits Alzheimer's disease-like tau protein phosphorylation in neurons. *FEBS letters,* Vol. 411, pp. 183-188, ISSN 0014-5793

Nacharaju, P. (1999). Accelerated filament formation from tau protein with specific FTDP-17 missense mutations. *FEBS letters,* Vol. 447, pp. 195-199, ISSN 0014-5793

Naiki, H., and Gejyo, F. (1999). Kinetic analysis of amyloid fibril formation. *Methods Enzymol,* Vol. 309, pp. 305-318, ISSN 0076-6879

Naiki, H., and Nakakuki, K. (1996). First-order kinetic model of Alzheimer's beta-amyloid fibril extension in vitro. *Lab Invest,* Vol. 74, pp. 374-383, ISSN 0023-6837

Nakabeppu, Y. (2007). Oxidative damage in nucleic acids and Parkinson's disease. *J Neurosci Res,* Vol. 85, pp. 919-934, ISSN 0360-4012

Nakamura, K. (2008). Optical reporters for the conformation of alpha-synuclein reveal a specific interaction with mitochondria. *J Neurosci,* Vol. 28, pp. 12305-12317, ISSN 1529-2401

Nikoulina, S.E. (2002). Inhibition of glycogen synthase kinase 3 improves insulin action and glucose metabolism in human skeletal muscle. *Diabetes,* Vol. 51, pp. 2190-2198, ISSN 0012-1797

Nishikawa, K. (2003). Alterations of structure and hydrolase activity of parkinsonism-associated human ubiquitin carboxyl-terminal hydrolase L1 variants. *Biochem Biophys Res Commun,* Vol. 304, pp. 176-183, ISSN 0006-291X

Obeso, J.A. (2010). Missing pieces in the Parkinson's disease puzzle. *Nat Med,* Vol. 16, pp. 653-661, ISSN 1546-170X (Electronic)

Okada, S. (2005). No associations between Parkinson's disease and polymorphisms of the quinone oxidoreductase (NQO1, NQO2) genes. *Neurosci Lett,* Vol. 375, pp. 178-180, ISSN 0304-3940

Olanow, C.W. (2009). The scientific and clinical basis for the treatment of Parkinson disease (2009). *Neurology,* Vol. 72, pp. S1-136, ISSN 1526-632X (Electronic)

Ono, K. (2006). Anti-amyloidogenic effects of antioxidants: implications for the prevention and therapeutics of Alzheimer's disease. *Biochim Biophys Acta,* Vol. 1762, pp. 575-586, ISSN 0006-3002

Paisan-Ruiz, C. (2004). Cloning of the gene containing mutations that cause PARK8-linked Parkinson's disease. *Neuron,* Vol. 44, pp. 595-600, ISSN 0896-6273

Palacino, J.J. (2004). Mitochondrial dysfunction and oxidative damage in parkin-deficient mice. *J Biol Chem,* Vol. 279, pp. 18614-18622, ISSN 0021-9258

Park, J. (2006). Mitochondrial dysfunction in Drosophila PINK1 mutants is complemented by parkin. *Nature,* Vol. 441, pp. 1157-1161, ISSN 1476-4687 (Electronic)

Parker, W.D., Jr. (1989). Abnormalities of the electron transport chain in idiopathic Parkinson's disease. *Ann Neurol,* Vol. 26, pp. 719-723, ISSN 0364-5134

Pasinetti, G.M. (2001). Cyclooxygenase and Alzheimer's disease: implications for preventive initiatives to slow the progression of clinical dementia. *Arch Gerontol Geriatr,* Vol. 33, pp. 13-28

Patton, R.L. (2006). Amyloid-{beta} peptide remnants in AN-1792-immunized Alzheimer's disease patients: a biochemical analysis. *Am J Pathol,* Vol. 169, pp. 1048-1063, ISSN

Perl, D.P. (2010). Neuropathology of Alzheimer's disease. *The Mount Sinai journal of medicine, New York,* Vol. 77, pp. 32-42, ISSN 1931-7581 (Electronic)

Perry, G. (1985). Paired helical filaments from Alzheimer disease patients contain cytoskeletal components. *Proceedings of the National Academy of Sciences of the United States of America,* Vol. 82, pp. 3916-3920, ISSN 0027-8424

Perry, G. (1999). Activation of neuronal extracellular receptor kinase (ERK) in Alzheimer disease links oxidative stress to abnormal phosphorylation. *Neuroreport,* Vol. 10, pp. 2411-2415, ISSN 0959-4965

Pitschke, M. (1998). Detection of single amyloid beta-protein aggregates in the cerebrospinal fluid of Alzheimer's patients by fluorescence correlation spectroscopy. *Nat Med,* Vol. 4, pp. 832-834, ISSN 1078-8956

Poorkaj, P. (1998). Tau is a candidate gene for chromosome 17 frontotemporal dementia. *Annals of neurology,* Vol. 43, pp. 815-825, ISSN 0364-5134

Przedborski, S. (2004). MPTP as a mitochondrial neurotoxic model of Parkinson's disease. *J Bioenerg Biomembr,* Vol. 36, pp. 375-379, ISSN 0145-479X

Qian, L. (2010). Neuroinflammation is a key player in Parkinson's disease and a prime target for therapy. *J Neural Transm,* Vol. 117, pp. 971-979, ISSN 1435-1463 (Electronic)

Qu, W. (2009). Kaempferol derivatives prevent oxidative stress-induced cell death in a DJ-1-dependent manner. *J Pharmacol Sci,* Vol. 110, pp. 191-200, ISSN 1347-8613

Rabinovic, A.D. (2000). Role of oxidative changes in the degeneration of dopamine terminals after injection of neurotoxic levels of dopamine. *Neuroscience,* Vol. 101, pp. 67-76, ISSN 0306-4522

Reddy, P.H. (2011). Abnormal tau, mitochondrial dysfunction, impaired axonal transport of mitochondria, and synaptic deprivation in Alzheimer's disease. *Brain research,* Vol. 1415, pp. 136-148, ISSN 1872-6240 (Electronic)

Reed, M.N. (2009). Cognitive effects of cell-derived and synthetically derived Abeta oligomers. *Neurobiol Aging,* Vol. 1558-1497 (Electronic)

Rogers, S.L. (1998). Donepezil improves cognition and global function in Alzheimer disease: a 15-week, double-blind, placebo-controlled study. Donepezil Study Group. *Arch Intern Med,* Vol. 158, pp. 1021-1031, ISSN 0003-9926

Roher, A.E. (1996). Morphology and toxicity of A beta-(1-42) dimer derived from neuritic and vascular amyloid deposits of Alzheimer's disease. *J Biol Chem,* Vol. 271, pp. 20631-20635,

Sairam, K. (2003). Non-steroidal anti-inflammatory drug sodium salicylate, but not diclofenac or celecoxib, protects against 1-methyl-4-phenyl pyridinium-induced dopaminergic neurotoxicity in rats. *Brain Res,* Vol. 966, pp. 245-252, ISSN 0006-8993

Santa-Maria, I. (2007). Tramiprosate, a drug of potential interest for the treatment of Alzheimer's disease, promotes an abnormal aggregation of tau. *Mol Neurodegener,* Vol. 2, pp. 17, ISSN 1750-1326

Satake, W. (2009). Genome-wide association study identifies common variants at four loci as genetic risk factors for Parkinson's disease. *Nat Genet,* Vol. 41, pp. 1303-1307, ISSN 1546-1718

Sawamura, N. (2001). Site-specific phosphorylation of tau accompanied by activation of mitogen-activated protein kinase (MAPK) in brains of Niemann-Pick type C mice. *The Journal of biological chemistry,* Vol. 276, pp. 10314-10319, ISSN 0021-9258

Schapira, A.H., and Gegg, M. (2011). Mitochondrial contribution to Parkinson's disease pathogenesis. *Parkinsons Dis,* Vol. 2011, pp. 159160, ISSN 2042-0080 (Electronic)

Schapira, A.H., and Jenner, P. (2011). Etiology and pathogenesis of Parkinson's disease. *Mov Disord,* Vol. 26, pp. 1049-1055, ISSN 1531-8257 (Electronic)

Schenk, D. (1999). Immunization with amyloid-beta attenuates Alzheimer-disease-like pathology in the PDAPP mouse. *Nature,* Vol. 400, pp. 173-177, ISSN 0028-0836

Schmechel, A. (2003). Alzheimer beta-amyloid homodimers facilitate A beta fibrillization and the generation of conformational antibodies. *J Biol Chem,* Vol. 278, pp. 35317-35324, ISSN 0021-9258

Schonbeck, U. (1998). Generation of biologically active IL-1 beta by matrix metalloproteinases: a novel caspase-1-independent pathway of IL-1 beta processing. *J Immunol,* Vol. 161, pp. 3340-3346, ISSN 0022-1767

Schoneich, C. (2003). Free radical reactions of methionine in peptides: Mechanisms relevant to beta-amyloid oxidation and Alzheimer's disease. *Journal of the American Chemical Society,* Vol. 125, pp. 13700-13713, ISSN

Selkoe, D.J., and Schenk, D. (2003). Alzheimer's disease: molecular understanding predicts amyloid-based therapeutics. *Annu Rev Pharmacol Toxicol,* Vol. 43, pp. 545-584, ISSN 0362-1642

Semchuk, K.M. (1992). Parkinson's disease and exposure to agricultural work and pesticide chemicals. *Neurology,* Vol. 42, pp. 1328-1335, ISSN 0028-3878

Shelton, S.B., and Johnson, G.V. (2004). Cyclin-dependent kinase-5 in neurodegeneration. *Journal of neurochemistry,* Vol. 88, pp. 1313-1326, ISSN 0022-3042

Shoji, M. (2000). Age-related amyloid beta protein accumulation induces cellular death and macrophage activation in transgenic mice. *J Pathol,* Vol. 191, pp. 93-101, ISSN

Siebert, A. (2009). Nrf2 activators provide neuroprotection against 6-hydroxydopamine toxicity in rat organotypic nigrostriatal cocultures. *J Neurosci Res,* Vol. 87, pp. 1659-1669, ISSN 1097-4547 (Electronic)

Siegel, D. (1997). The reduction of alpha-tocopherolquinone by human NAD(P)H: quinone oxidoreductase: the role of alpha-tocopherolhydroquinone as a cellular antioxidant. *Mol Pharmacol,* Vol. 52, pp. 300-305, ISSN 0026-895X

Simon-Sanchez, J. (2009). Genome-wide association study reveals genetic risk underlying Parkinson's disease. *Nat Genet,* Vol. 41, pp. 1308-1312, ISSN 1546-1718

Skovronsky, D.M. (2000). In vivo detection of amyloid plaques in a mouse model of Alzheimer's disease. *Proc Natl Acad Sci U S A,* Vol. 97, pp. 7609-7614, ISSN 0027-8424

Smith, M.A. (1997). Iron accumulation in Alzheimer disease is a source of redox-generated free radicals. *Proc Natl Acad Sci U S A,* Vol. 94, pp. 9866-9868, ISSN 0027-8424

Snow, A.D. (1995). Differential binding of vascular cell-derived proteoglycans (perlecan, biglycan, decorin, and versican) to the beta-amyloid protein of Alzheimer's disease. *Arch Biochem Biophys,* Vol. 320, pp. 84-95, ISSN 0003-9861

Snow, A.D. (1994). Heparan sulfate proteoglycan in diffuse plaques of hippocampus but not of cerebellum in Alzheimer's disease brain. *Am J Pathol,* Vol. 144, pp. 337-347, ISSN 0002-9440

Son, H.J. (2011). A novel compound PTIQ protects the nigral dopaminergic neurons in MPTP-induced animal model of Parkinson's disease. *Br J Pharmacol,* Vol. 1476-5381

Spencer, J.P. (1998). Conjugates of catecholamines with cysteine and GSH in Parkinson's disease: possible mechanisms of formation involving reactive oxygen species. *J Neurochem,* Vol. 71, pp. 2112-2122, ISSN 0022-3042

Spillantini, M.G. (1998). Mutation in the tau gene in familial multiple system tauopathy with presenile dementia. *Proceedings of the National Academy of Sciences of the United States of America,* Vol. 95, pp. 7737-7741, ISSN 0027-8424

Spillantini, M.G. (1997). Alpha-synuclein in Lewy bodies. *Nature,* Vol. 388, pp. 839-840, ISSN 0028-0836

Spittaels, K. (2000). Glycogen synthase kinase-3beta phosphorylates protein tau and rescues the axonopathy in the central nervous system of human four-repeat tau transgenic mice. *The Journal of biological chemistry,* Vol. 275, pp. 41340-41349, ISSN 0021-9258

Stewart, W.F. (1997). Risk of Alzheimer's disease and duration of NSAID use. *Neurology,* Vol. 48, pp. 626-632, ISSN 0028-3878

Stine, W.B., Jr. (2003). In vitro characterization of conditions for amyloid-beta peptide oligomerization and fibrillogenesis. *J Biol Chem,* Vol. 278, pp. 11612-11622, ISSN 0021-9258

Strauss, K.M. (2005). Loss of function mutations in the gene encoding Omi/HtrA2 in Parkinson's disease. *Hum Mol Genet,* Vol. 14, pp. 2099-2111, ISSN 0964-6906

Stringer, J.L. (2004). Presence and induction of the enzyme NAD(P)H: quinone oxidoreductase 1 in the central nervous system. *J Comp Neurol,* Vol. 471, pp. 289-297, ISSN 0021-9967

Su, J.H. (1992). Localization of heparan sulfate glycosaminoglycan and proteoglycan core protein in aged brain and Alzheimer's disease. *Neuroscience,* Vol. 51, pp. 801-813, ISSN 0306-4522

Sullivan, M. (2007). Tramiprosate falls short in phase III Alzheimer's trial. *Clin Psychiatry News,* Vol. 35, pp. 27, ISSN

Suo, Z. (2002). Participation of protease-activated receptor-1 in thrombin-induced microglial activation. *J Neurochem,* Vol. 80, pp. 655-666, ISSN 0022-3042

T. Yamada, E.G.M., R.L. Schelper (1993). Histological and biochemical pathology in a family with autosomal dominant Parkinsonism and dementia. *Neurol Psychiatry Brain Res,* Vol. 26–35

Tabner, B.J. (2001). Production of reactive oxygen species from aggregating proteins implicated in Alzheimer's disease, Parkinson's disease and other neurodegenerative diseases. *Curr Top Med Chem,* Vol. 1, pp. 507-517, ISSN 1568-0266

Tanner, C.M. (2009). Occupation and risk of parkinsonism: a multicenter case-control study. *Arch Neurol,* Vol. 66, pp. 1106-1113, ISSN 1538-3687 (Electronic)

Tikka, T. (2001). Minocycline, a tetracycline derivative, is neuroprotective against excitotoxicity by inhibiting activation and proliferation of microglia. *J Neurosci,* Vol. 21, pp. 2580-2588, ISSN 1529-2401 (Electronic)

Tseng, H.C. (2002). A survey of Cdk5 activator p35 and p25 levels in Alzheimer's disease brains. *FEBS letters,* Vol. 523, pp. 58-62, ISSN 0014-5793

Van Laar, V.S. (2009). Proteomic identification of dopamine-conjugated proteins from isolated rat brain mitochondria and SH-SY5Y cells. *Neurobiol Dis,* Vol. 34, pp. 487-500, ISSN 1095-953X (Electronic) van Muiswinkel, F.L. (2004). Expression of NAD(P)H:quinone oxidoreductase in the normal and Parkinsonian substantia nigra. *Neurobiol Aging,* Vol. 25, pp. 1253-1262, ISSN 0197-4580

Verbeek, M.M. (1997). Differences between the pathogenesis of senile plaques and congophilic angiopathy in Alzheimer disease. *J Neuropathol Exp Neurol,* Vol. 56, pp. 751-761, ISSN 0022-3069

Vu, T.K. (1991). Molecular cloning of a functional thrombin receptor reveals a novel proteolytic mechanism of receptor activation. *Cell,* Vol. 64, pp. 1057-1068, ISSN 0092-8674

Warner, T.T., and Schapira, A.H. (2003). Genetic and environmental factors in the cause of Parkinson's disease. *Ann Neurol,* Vol. 53 Suppl 3, pp. S16-23; discussion S23-15, ISSN 0364-5134

Wilcock, G.K. (2000). Efficacy and safety of galantamine in patients with mild to moderate Alzheimer's disease: multicentre randomised controlled trial. Galantamine International-1 Study Group. *Br Med J,* Vol. 321, pp. 1445-1449, ISSN 0959-8138

Wilhelmus, M.M. (2007). Heat shock proteins and amateur chaperones in amyloid-Beta accumulation and clearance in Alzheimer's disease. *Mol Neurobiol,* Vol. 35, pp. 203-216, ISSN 0893-7648

Wilms, H. (2003). Activation of microglia by human neuromelanin is NF-kappaB dependent and involves p38 mitogen-activated protein kinase: implications for Parkinson's disease. *FASEB J,* Vol. 17, pp. 500-502, ISSN 1530-6860 (Electronic)

Wischik, C.M. (1989). Cell biology of the Alzheimer tangle. *Current opinion in cell biology,* Vol. 1, pp. 115-122, ISSN 0955-0674

Woo, M.S. (2008). Inhibition of MMP-3 or -9 suppresses lipopolysaccharide-induced expression of proinflammatory cytokines and iNOS in microglia. *J Neurochem,* Vol. 106, pp. 770-780, ISSN 1471-4159 (Electronic)

Wright, T.M. (2006). Tramiprosate. *Drugs Today (Barc),* Vol. 42, pp. 291-298, ISSN 1699-3993

Wu, D.C. (2002). Blockade of microglial activation is neuroprotective in the 1-methyl-4-phenyl-1,2,3,6-tetrahydropyridine mouse model of Parkinson disease. *J Neurosci,* Vol. 22, pp. 1763-1771, ISSN 1529-2401 (Electronic)

Xu, Y. (2005). Conformational transition of amyloid beta-peptide. *Proc Natl Acad Sci U S A,* Vol. 102, pp. 5403-5407, ISSN 0027-8424

Zafar, K.S. (2007). A comparative study of proteasomal inhibition and apoptosis induced in N27 mesencephalic cells by dopamine and MG132. *J Neurochem,* Vol. 102, pp. 913-921, ISSN 0022-3042

Zafar, K.S. (2006). Overexpression of NQO1 protects human SK-N-MC neuroblastoma cells against dopamine-induced cell death. *Toxicol Lett,* Vol. 166, pp. 261-267, ISSN 0378-4274

Zafar, K.S. (2006). A potential role for cyclized quinones derived from dopamine, DOPA, and 3,4-dihydroxyphenylacetic acid in proteasomal inhibition. *Mol Pharmacol,* Vol. 70, pp. 1079-1086, ISSN 0026-895X

Zecca, L. (2008). Human neuromelanin induces neuroinflammation and neurodegeneration in the rat substantia nigra: implications for Parkinson's disease. *Acta Neuropathol,* Vol. 116, pp. 47-55, ISSN 0001-6322

Zecca, L. (2003). The neuromelanin of human substantia nigra: structure, synthesis and molecular behaviour. *J Neural Transm Suppl,* Vol. 145-155, ISSN 0303-6995

Zeevalk, G.D. (2008). Glutathione and Parkinson's disease: is this the elephant in the room? *Biomed Pharmacother,* Vol. 62, pp. 236-249, ISSN 0753-3322

Zhang, W. (2005). Aggregated alpha-synuclein activates microglia: a process leading to disease progression in Parkinson's disease. *FASEB J,* Vol. 19, pp. 533-542, ISSN 1530-6860

Zhang, Y. (2000). Parkin functions as an E2-dependent ubiquitin- protein ligase and promotes the degradation of the synaptic vesicle-associated protein, CDCrel-1. *Proc Natl Acad Sci U S A,* Vol. 97, pp. 13354-13359, ISSN 0027-8424

Zimprich, A. (2004). Mutations in LRRK2 cause autosomal-dominant parkinsonism with pleomorphic pathology. *Neuron,* Vol. 44, pp. 601-607, ISSN 0896-6273

6

Nitrooxidative Stress and Neurodegeneration

Michal Fiedorowicz and Pawel Grieb
Mossakowski Medical Research Centre, Polish Academy of Sciences, Warsaw Poland

1. Introduction

Stress is the force on unit areas within a material that develops as a result of the externally applied force (Enciclopedia Britannica, 2011).

When I wrote the first paper on the stress syndrome in 1936, I tried to demonstrate that stress (…) is clearly a definable biological and medical phenomenon whose mechanisms can be objectively identified and with which we can cope much better once we know how to handle it (…) Stress is the nonspecific response of the body to any demand, whether is caused by, or results in, pleasant or unpleasant conditions (Selye, 1985).

Oxidative stress is defined as a persistent imbalance between antioxidants and pro-oxidants in favor of the latter, resulting in (often) irreversible cellular damages (Probiox, 2011).

Nitrosative Stress: A condition that occurs when the production of highly reactive nitrogen-containing chemicals, such as nitrous oxide, exceed the ability of the (...) body to neutralize and eliminate them. Nitrosative stress can lead to reactions that alter protein structure thus interfering with normal body functions (Oxford Dictionary of Sports Science & Medicine, 2007).

The four quotations collected above illustrate confusion with the notion of stress. In physics, in Hooke's law, 'stress' means a force acting on an elastic material and producing a proportional amount of deformation, or strain. However, according to Selye, who introduced the notion of 'stress' into (bio)medicine, it is not a kind of force acting on an organism (such force is called 'stressor'), but a response of an organism to such a force. In fact, Selye's definition of 'stress' is more similar to the notion of 'strain' in Hooke's law. Contemporary uses of the term 'stress' in biomedical scientific literature are very diverse; the last two examples define stress as an imbalance which occurs inside a body and leads to its damage. These definitions are very different from Selye's definition of stress.

Several distinguished authors wrote reviews about oxidative and nitrosative stress, but many either did not define these terms at all, or defined them vaguely and indirectly. For example, in a recent review one of the most prominent biochemists working in the field of redox and free radicals biochemistry professor Barry Halliwell only listed reasons why tissue injury causes oxidative stress and what oxidative stress means in the context of human disease (Halliwell, 2009); it seems that he implicitly defined oxidative stress as a result of tissue injury (or, perhaps, response to it) rather than its cause. However most authors, indeed, use terms 'oxidative stress' and 'nitrosative stress' to describe situations of persistent imbalance between production and removal of oxidising free radicals leading to their increased level and resulting in harmful effects on biological molecules, cells and tissues. For example professor Helmut Sies defined 'oxidative stress' as a condition occurring when the generation of reactive oxygen species (ROS) in a system exceeds the system's ability to neutralize and eliminate them. This imbalance can result from a lack of antioxidant capacity caused by disturbance in production, distribution, or by an overabundance of ROS from endogenous sources or environmental stressors (Brenneisen et al., 2005; Sies, 1997). Shouldn't we conclude that oxidative stress is always linked to the damage of biological macromolecules and the disruption of cellular homeostasis? However, the title of the other paper from Sies's laboratory includes the phrase "Peroxynitrite signalling: (...) activation of stress-responsive pathways" (Klotz et al., 2002), which is suggestive of that cells not only receive harm from nitrooxidative stress but also can respond to in an orderly manner, which depends on circumstances and may be either positive or detrimental.

Concise and amazingly fitting definition of the term 'stress' we found in the English-Polish dictionary (Stanislawski, 1999). This definition, translated back to English, reads the following: 'stress is the pressure of circumstances'. In the case of oxidative and nitrosative stress the said circumstances are disturbances in the balance between production and removal of reactive forms of oxygen and nitrogen, most of which are free radicals. The amount of literature on this subject is so large, that its comprehensive review would require a multi-thousand-page book. In the present chapter we will concentrate on the following specific subjects: (1) why nitrooxidative stress is considered harmful, (2) cellular metabolism of reactive oxygen and nitrogen species, and (3) how nitrooxidative stress can contribute to some major neurodegenerative diseases.

2. Free radicals

The recent version of the International Union of Pure and Applied Chemistry (IUPAC) *Recommendations on Nomenclature of Inorganic Chemistry* (IUPAC, 2005), known as *the Red Book*, defines a **radical** as an atom or molecule with one or more unpaired electrons. An unpaired electron may be indicated in a formula by a superscript dot. A radical may have positive, negative or zero charge. Metals and their ions or complexes often possess unpaired electrons but, by convention, they are not considered to be radicals. The terms 'radical' and 'free radical' are frequently used interchangeably, although more correctly radicals may be called 'free' only when they can freely diffuse in their environment.

The aforementioned definition is also strictly applicable to organic radicals, i.e. radicals containing carbon. However, we shall bear in mind that not long time ago such a view was difficult to accept. This was because, after many futile attempts to isolate carbon-containing radicals, XIX-century chemists concluded that carbon must always be tetravalent (i.e. form four bonds) and organic radicals cannot exist. Although the first organic free radical, the trityl (triphenylmethyl) radical (fig. 1), was discovered by Gomberg in 1900, for many years this discovery was viewed only as a curiosity (Henderson, 2000). Besides, trityl radical does not contain oxygen.

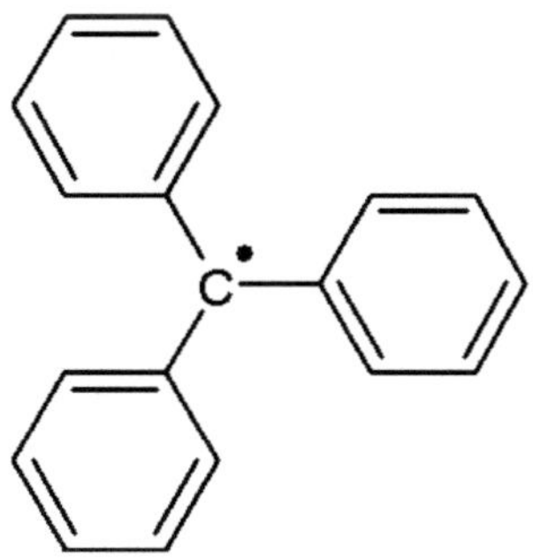

Fig. 1. Trityl (triphenylmethyl) radical.

The concept of oxygen free radicals toxicity as the major contributor to various pathologies has been developed in the middle of XX century, at the intersection of studies on mechanisms of oxygen toxicity and on toxic effects of ionizing radiation. On one hand, it was already very well known that eukaryotic organisms cannot survive without oxygen, yet at the same time oxygen is toxic. This Janus-faced property of oxygen is sometimes called the 'paradox of aerobic life', or the 'oxygen paradox' (Fridovich, 1975). Toxic effects of exposure to oxygen at increased partial pressure, particularly evident in human central nervous system and lungs, have been described in the late XIX century, but after more than 50 years their mechanism remained unknown (Donald, 1947). On the other hand, harmful effects on living organisms of ionizing radiation, which become known shortly after its discovery (Inkret et al., 1995), were already explained, mostly by the intracellular radiolysis of water molecules into H^+ and OH^- radicals. These radicals either by itself cause oxidative damage to the cells, or further recombine to nascent toxic radicals such as superoxide.

In 1954 the presence of free radicals in biological materials not subjected to ionizing radiation was discovered (Commoner et al., 1954). Almost at the same time Gershman, Gilbert and collaborators put forward a hypothesis that the majority of harmful effects of both oxygen and ionizing radiation could be attributed to the same mechanism, namely the formation of oxygen radicals (Gerschman et al., 1954). This hypothesis was later developed into the theory that oxygen radicals are continuously generated in all living cells, starting point of their cellular metabolism being the formation of superoxide radical anion (Fridovich, 1983). Halliwell and Gutteridge (1984) called this concept 'the superoxide theory of oxygen toxicity'. Currently it is generally accepted that oxygen free radicals are ubiquitous in the living matter; they are continuously produced by a variety of reactions (enzymatic and nonenzymatic), and at the same time continuously removed by the other variety of reactions. Indeed, the generation of oxygen radicals in living cells is not a pathology, but the fundamental physiological phenomenon.

Moreover, molecular oxygen (O_2) by itself is a double radical (a biradical), having two unpaired electrons with parallel spin states. This arangement is quite fortunate, as it makes O_2 a stable radical and prevents spontaneous ignition of carbon-based materials in the oxygen atmosphere. On the other hand, as a consequence, oxidation by molecular oxygen can easily occur only by the transfer of single electrons. However, organic molecules which are substrates for biological oxidations do not contain unpaired electrons. Therefore molecular oxygen could accept a pair of electrons from an organic substrate only when one of the electrons of oxygen or one of the electrons from the donating substrate inverts its spin. This can happen, but would require a substantial activation energy.

The solution utilised by living cells to decrease activation energy for oxidations relies on conducting two oxidations stepwise, by a close sequence of two single-electron transfers (Miles, 2003). This arrangement works nicely, but its side effect is a relatively high probability that products of the first one-electron reduction of oxygen, i.e. oxygen radicals, will not engage in the second one-electron reduction step but enter the intracellular (or extracellular) milieu instead.

As mentioned already, oxygen free radicals have potential to react with (that is, to oxidize) practically any organic molecule they come in contact with. These reactions may inflict damage to cellular constituents including macromolecules (proteins, nucleic acids), aminoacids, sugars, lipids (polyunsaturated fatty acids in particular) etc. However, under normal metabolic conditions the actual concentration of free radicals in biological matter (i.e. living cells and extracellular material) is pretty small. Chance et al. (1979) estimated that in rat liver equilibrium concentration of superoxide anion radical is in the order of 10^{-12} to 10^{-11} M and that of hydrogen peroxide is only 3 orders of magnitude greater. Only if equilibrium is disturbed, which may be called nitrooxidative stress, oxygen free radicals and products of their metabolism which are strong oxidants, all called collectively reactive oxygen and nitrogen species (ROS and RNS), do have potential for inflicting damage to vital constituents of the living cells (McCord, 2000).

3. Cellular metabolism of reactive oxygen and nitrogen species

Reactions of ROS and RNS which occur in living cells are irreversible and may be presented as a cascade (fig. 2) that starts with generation of **superoxide radical** ($O_2^{\bullet -}$). This free radical appears mainly in mitochondria; some authors estimate that 2-4% of oxygen metabolized by mitochondrial respiratory chain leaves it as superoxide (Turrens, 2003). $O_2^{\bullet -}$ is also a product of certain enzymatic reactions localized outside mitochondria, in particular NADH oxidation conducted by non-mitochondrial NADH oxidases called NOX (Sorce & Krause, 2009). Some NOX isoenzymes are end parts of 'plasma respiratory chains' called also 'plasma membrane oxidoreductases' (PMOR) present in many cell types including neurons (Wright & Kuhn, 2002). ECTO-NOX present on cell surface are supposed to release $O_2^{\bullet -}$ into the extracellular milieu, while other isoforms of NOX produce superoxide radical intracellularly.

An additional source of superoxide radical is **singlet oxygen** ($^1O_2$), generated in photosensitization reaction which takes place *in vivo* upon exposure of cells to light, e.g. in the retina. Although not a free radical, $^1O_2$ is a highly reactive molecule, thus it belongs to ROS. Some authors claim that singlet oxygen by itself can damage membranes and other cell components (Winkler et al., 1999). Importantly, singlet oxygen cannot be removed enzymatically but only in reactions with non-enzymatic antioxidants. Singlet oxygen can be also reduced to $O_2^{\bullet -}$.

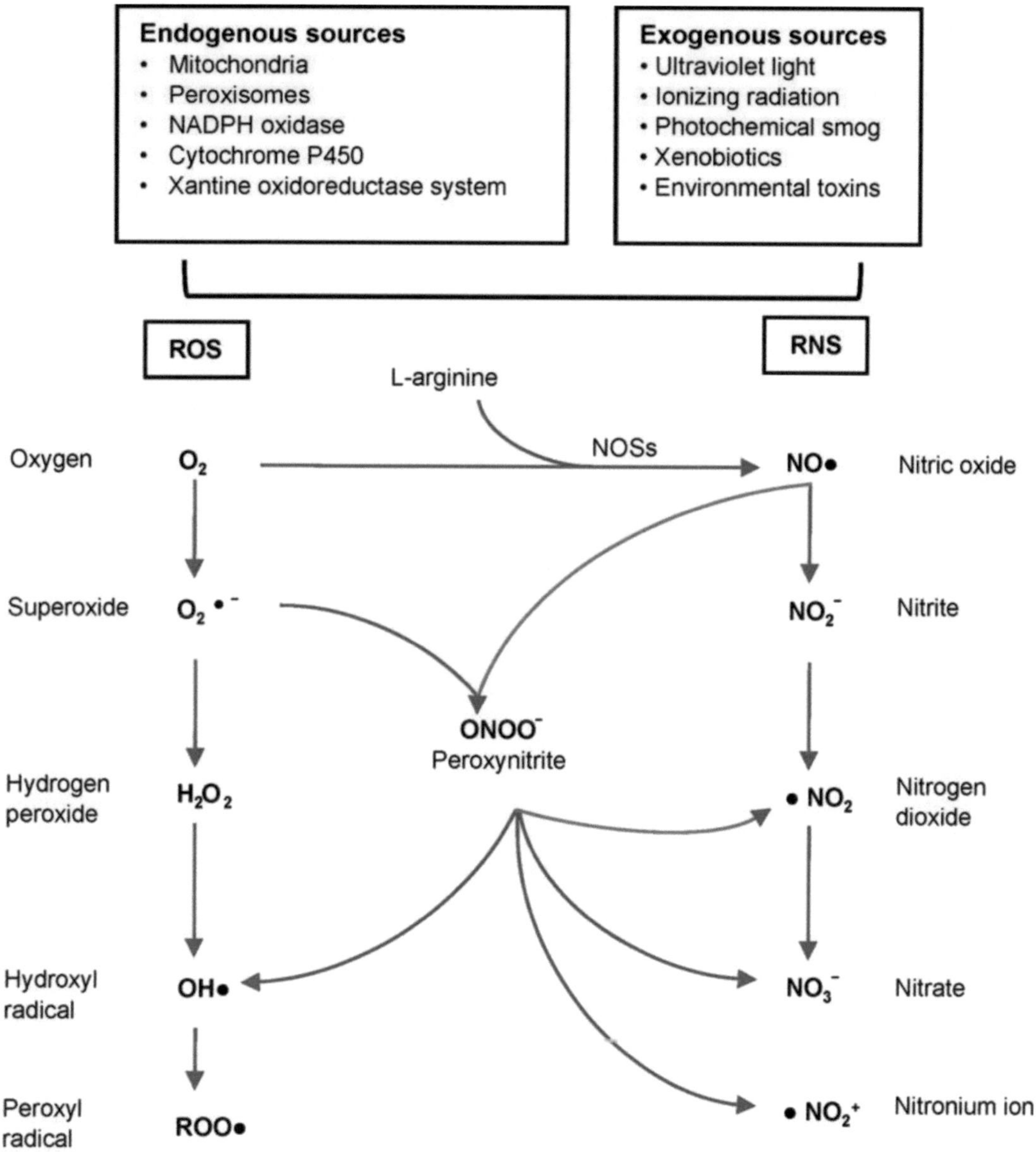

Fig. 2. Cascade of radical reactions in the cell and the most important reactive oxygen and nitrogen species. Main sources of ROS and RNS are listed in the upper part of the figure. Reproduced from Mangialasche et al. (2009). © Elsevier, with permission.

Cells can be damaged directly by superoxide radical (Benov, 2001), or by its metabolites, hydroxyl radical and peroxynitrites. Compared to other radicals superoxide is not very reactive chemically; moreover it may react only either with itself (dismutation), with another radical such as nitric oxide, or with a a metal. Hovewer, although dismutation of $O_2^{\bullet -}$ occurs spontaneously, it is a second order reaction with respect to substrate concentration, ineffective in removing it at low concentrations. Since even in subnanomolar concentrations superoxide is toxic, in particular to some mitochondrial enzymes (e.g. aconitase), all cells are equipped with enzymes superoxide dismutases (SOD), which very efficiently convert superoxide to hydrogen peroxide (see below).

Of all ROS, **hydrogen peroxide** is a molecule with the longest half-life, and it may achieve the highest intracellular concentration. Moreover, it has the ability to diffuse across biological membranes. Hydrogen peroxide by itself is not particularly toxic or dangerous to the cells, but in reaction catalyzed by iron ions (Fe^{2+}) it is converted to hydroxyl radical ($OH^{\bullet}$) (Buonocore et al., 2010). This reaction, known as the Haber-Weiss reaction, generates hydroxyl radicals from H_2O_2 and superoxide. It can occur in cells, being responsible for oxidative stress. It is a two-step catalytic cycle. The first step involves reduction of ferric ion to ferrous:

$$Fe^{3+} + O_2^{\bullet -} \rightarrow Fe^{2+} + O_2$$

The second step, known as the Fenton reaction, regenerates ferric ion:

$$Fe^{2+} + H_2O_2 \rightarrow Fe^{3+} + OH^- + OH^{\bullet}$$

Hydroxyl radical is regarded the most cell-damaging oxidant (Cheng et al., 2002). Its half life is extremely short (10^{-6} s, 3 orders of magnitude shorter than $O_2^{\bullet -}$) and it acts locally, very close to site of its generation. It reacts mainly with alkyl groups or with polyunsaturated fatty acids, initiating chain peroxidation (see below).

Peroxynitrite ($ONOO^-$), the most important RNS, is a product of reaction of superoxide radical with nitric oxide. It is not a radical but is a potent oxidant and nitrating agent. It can nitrate tyrosine residues of proteins (generating nitrotyrosine) - this protein modification can affect enzyme activities and increase susceptibility of proteins to proteolysis (Abello et al., 2009). It also oxidizes fatty acids and induces DNA strand breaks (Ascenzi et al., 2010).

ROS and RNS react with many important biomolecules. **Lipid chain peroxidation** is particularly important since it affects functioning of biological membranes: their fluidity, permeability, ion transportation and inhibits metabolic processes. Peroxidation of mitochondrial membrane lipids (e.g. cardiolipin) may induce apoptosis (Kagan et al., 2009). Lipids containing polyunsaturated faty acids (PUFA) are particularly vulnerable to peroxidation. Lipid chain peroxidation consists of three phases: initiation, propagation and termination (fig. 3). Initiation phase includes hydrogen atom abstraction in reaction with diiferent radicals (e.g. $OH^{\bullet}$) and produces a lipid radical ($L^{\bullet}$). $L^{\bullet}$ reacts with oxygen to produce lipid peroxyl radical ($LOO^{\bullet}$) that can abstract hydrogen atoms from another lipids to produce lipid hydroxyperoxide (LOOH) and another radical (propagation). This reaction can repeated many times - one hydroxyl radical can damage thousands of PUFA chains. The 'chain peroxidation' terminates when two radicals react together forming non-radical species (Catala, 2010).

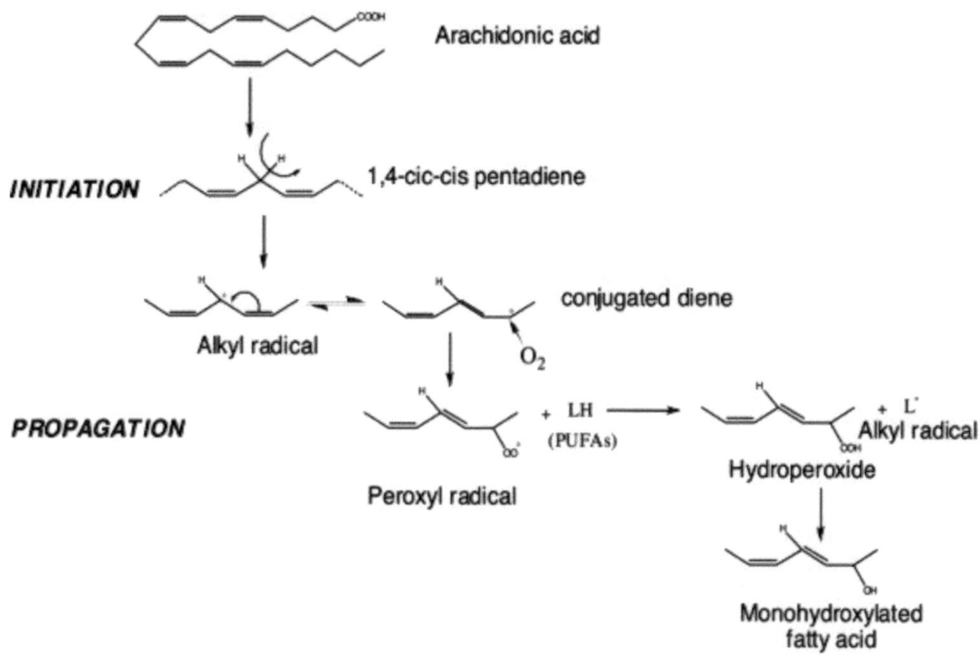

Fig. 3. Lipid peroxidation mechanism. Arachidonic acid was used as an example. Reproduced from Catala (2010). © Elsevier, with permission.

Cells possess various mechanisms responsible for minimizing free radical hazard – 'low-weight' non-catalytic antioxidants and antioxidant enzymes. Superoxide dismutases can be regarded as 'first line of defense' against ROS. This group of enzymes catalyze reaction of superoxide radical dismutation (i.e. conversion of $O_2^{\bullet-}$ to H_2O_2). Although this reaction occurs spontaneously, lack of catalyst would increase $O_2^{\bullet-}$ concentration, potentiate chain lipid peroxidation and lead to more intensive generation of RNS. Mammals possess three isoforms of superoxide dismutases: 'cytoplasmic' (CuZn-SOD, SOD1), 'mitochondrial' (Mn-SOD, SOD2) and 'extracellular' (EC-SOD, SOD3). Most of cellular dismutase activity (50-80%) is attributed to SOD1 (Faraci & Didion, 2004) but it is SOD2 that is thought to be crucial for cell functioning. SOD2 gene knockout was lethal in mice (Huang et al., 2001) and decrease in SOD2 activity ($Sod2^{+/-}$) led to neuronal loss and cancer progression (Van Remmen et al., 2003).

It should be also stressed that recently ROS and RNS are regarded not only as toxic byproducts of metabolism but also as **important signaling molecules**. Two important and thoroughly examined ones are hydrogen peroxide and nitric oxide. Hydrogen peroxide has relatively long half-life and can penetrate biological membrane. Concentration of H_2O_2 in the cell is also relatively high. It is believed to be involved in various processes including immune cell activation, remodeling of vessels, cell growth and many others (see reviews by Veal et al. (2007) or by Giorgio et al. (2007)). Hydrogen peroxide level is precisely regulated by growth factors. It inhibits phosphatases that are involved in propagation of signal induced by growth factors. It also induces tyrosine phosphorylation by activation of MAP kinases.

Observation that at least some of ROS and RNS are important signaling molecules and their levels are precisely regulated in the cell leads to the idea of 'redox homeostasis'. It is hypothesized that ROS/RNS are especially involved in regulation of proliferation and cell death of cells (Clement & Pervaiz, 1999). Reducing environment and low levels of ROS/RNS would suppress proliferation and is characteristic for 'resting' cells (see also fig. 7). Higher level of oxidants would promote proliferation and a bit higher apoptosis. However, above some range apoptosis would be suppressed due to oxidation of caspases (Hampton & Orrenius, 1998).

4. Nitrooxidative stress – Contribution to the pathomechanisms of neurodegenerative disorders

Neurodegenerative diseases - innate or acquired disorders of nervous system - can be defined by degeneration and death of neuronal cells. There is a regional or even cell-type-specific selectivity of neuronal failure and loss in different diseases. For example in Alzheimer's disease loss of cholinergic neurons occur mainly in the forebrain, in Parkinson's disease dopaminergic neurons in substiantia nigra are selectively injured and in glaucoma retinal ganglion cells are degenerating. Neuronal tissue seems to be vulnerable to damage caused by reactive forms of oxygen and nitrogen: oxygen metabolism is high and neurons contain high amounts of PUFA. Also oxidative/nitrosative damage to the neuronal tissue seems to be an early hallmark of degeneration in different pathologies. Thus, despite region-specific sensitivity, damage resulting from processes including ROS and RNS may be proposed as unifying mechanism for neurodegeneration (Ischiropoulos & Beckman, 2003). Common mechanisms involved in neurodegenerative disease leading to oxidative stress could include the inhibition of mitochondrial metabolism, neuronal excitotoxicity, and neuroinflammation (Golden & Patel, 2009). Examples further in this chapter show that nitrooxidative stress can be a key player in pathomechanisms of diverse neurodegenerative diseases.

4.1 Nitrooxidative stress and Alzheimer's disease

Alzheimer's disease (AD) is the most common type of dementia and in fact the most common neurodegenerative disorder. Most of the cases are sporadic but 5-10% of cases are familial and associated with mutations in genes of proteins involved in amyloid-β (Aβ) metabolism. The disease is characterized by progressive cognitive decline and neuropathological alterations: senile plaques built up by Aβ peptide and neurofibrillary tangles composed of hyperphosphorylated tau protein. Gross brain atrophy prominent in AD is caused by massive loss of neurons mostly in the temporal lobe and parietal lobe, and parts of the frontal cortex and cingulate gyrus. Possibilities of therapeutic interventions are currently modest.

Numerous reports demonstrate both oxidative and nitrosative damage in the brains of AD patients (reviewed by Mangialasche et al. (2009)). This damage concerns lipids since numerous markers of lipid peroxidation (*inter alia* malondialdehyde, acrolein, 4-hydroxy-2-nonenal and F2-isoprostanes) were found to be upregulated in brains of AD patients. Also markers of nucleic acid damage (like 8-hydroxydeoxyguanosine) or protein modification (like 3-nitrotyrosine (3-NT) or protein carbonyls) were upregulated.

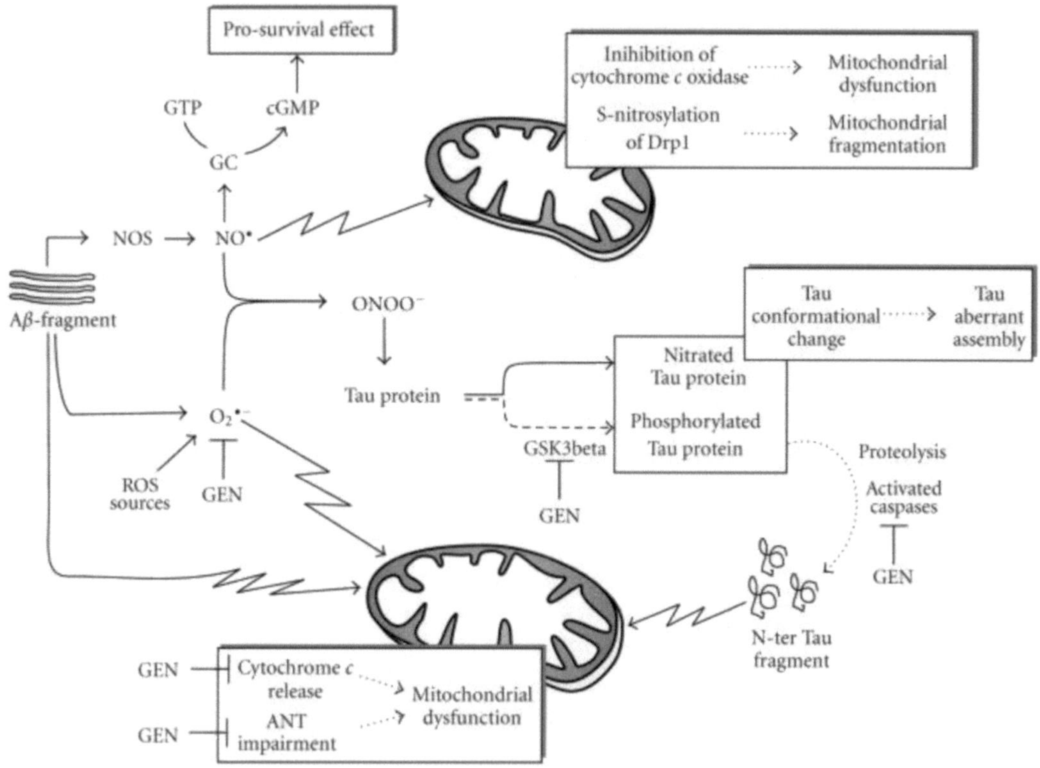

Fig. 4. Overview of the interplay between Aβ, Tau, oxidative/nitrosative stress, and mitochondria. Reproduced from Bobba et al. (2010). © Antonella Bobba et al., open access article.

Importantly, increased oxidative damage seems to be an early event in AD pathology since it is observed already in mildly cognitively impaired patients (Keller et al., 2005). This observations led to an idea of using various markers of oxidative/nitrosative damage as an early marker of AD pathology allowing to start therapeutical intervention in an early stage of the disease (see review by Galasko & Montine (2010)). Currently, F_2-isoprostane, a lipid peroxidation product, seems to be the most promising biomarker (de Leon et al., 2007; Pratico et al., 2002). Unfortunately while distinguishing AD and non-AD patients with markers measured in the cerebrospinal fluid seems to be pretty reliable there are some problems with applying these measures to plasma or urine samples.

Results obtained in different animal models of AD are consistent with those observed in patients. Oxidative lipid damage seem to be an early event in transgenic mouse models of AD amyloidosis and in fact precede Aβ plaque formation (Pratico et al., 2001).

One simple explanation of increased nitrooxidative stress in AD is Aβ toxicity. This is in concert with Aβ hypothesis that is currently the most popular one and assumes that formation of Aβ plaques is a central event in AD patophysiology. Aβ is thought to be capable of forming of free radicals by generation of hydrogen peroxide (Jomova et al., 2010). This potential of Aβ to generate free radicals was confirmed by *in vitro* studies (Ill-Raga et al., 2010) and is connected with its affinity to redox metals (eg. copper and iron). From the other side in experimental models nitrooxidative stress precedes Aβ plaques formation. There is also data showing that oxidative stress can actually alter metabolism of Aβ precursor protein and tau and thus promote formation of plaques and tangles (Li et al., 2004; Lovell et al., 2004; Ohyagi et al., 2000).

An apparent hallmark of AD is decreased brain energy metabolism. Even when corrected for decreased number of neurons brain glucose metabolism is markedly decreased in AD patients (Heiss et al., 1991; Ogawa et al., 1996). This altered energetics may be attributed to mitochondrial dysfunction and promote production of ROS and RNS. Recent reports showed that it could be Aβ that affects mitochondria and alters their functioning. Aβ can access the mitochondrial matrix and accumulate in the mitochondria affecting activity of mitochondrial enzymes and potentiate release of ROS (Chen & Yan, 2006).

Last but not least inflammatory processes seem to be a part of AD pathology - microglia are present in the Aβ plaques and in their surroundings (Rozemuller et al., 2005; Schwab & McGeer, 2008). Also Aβ can *in vitro* activate microglia (Jekabsone et al., 2006). Activation of microglia is associated with production of ROS and potentially leads to damage of neighbouring neurons (Block et al., 2007).

4.2 Nitrooxidative stress and Parkinson's disease

Parkinson's disease (PD) is the second most common neurodegenerative disease. Disease progression starts with motor deficiencies – rigidity, shaking, slowness of movement and as progresses difficulties with gait and walking arise. In the advanced stages of the disease symptoms also include cognitive decline and behavioural changes. Pathologic hallmarks of PD are degeneration and death of dopaminergic neurons in substantia nigra and presence of Lewy bodies – intracellular aggregates of protein α-synuclein. Treatment includes stimulation of dopamine signalling, e.g. by supplementation with dopamine precursor – L-DOPA or by administration of dopamine agonists (Lew, 2007).

Nitrooxidative stress is evident in the brains of PD patients. Increased levels of lipid peroxidation products: 4-hydroxy-2-nonenal and thiobarbituric acid reactive substances were found in substantia nigra of PD patients (Yoritaka et al., 1996). Also markers of oxidative damage to DNA and RNA like 8-hydroxyguanosine were found to be upregulated in this region (Zhang et al., 1999). Protein oxidation was found to be increased in PD, eg. levels of protein carbonyls were higher than in age-matched controls (Alam et al., 1997).

Also data obtained from animal models of PD imply increased nitrooxidative stress. PINK1 and DJ-1 null mice had increased levels of oxidative stress markers (Andres-Mateos et al., 2007; Gautier et al., 2008). Toxicity of overexpressed α-synuclein in mice is also thought to be associated with free radicals (Masliah et al., 2000).

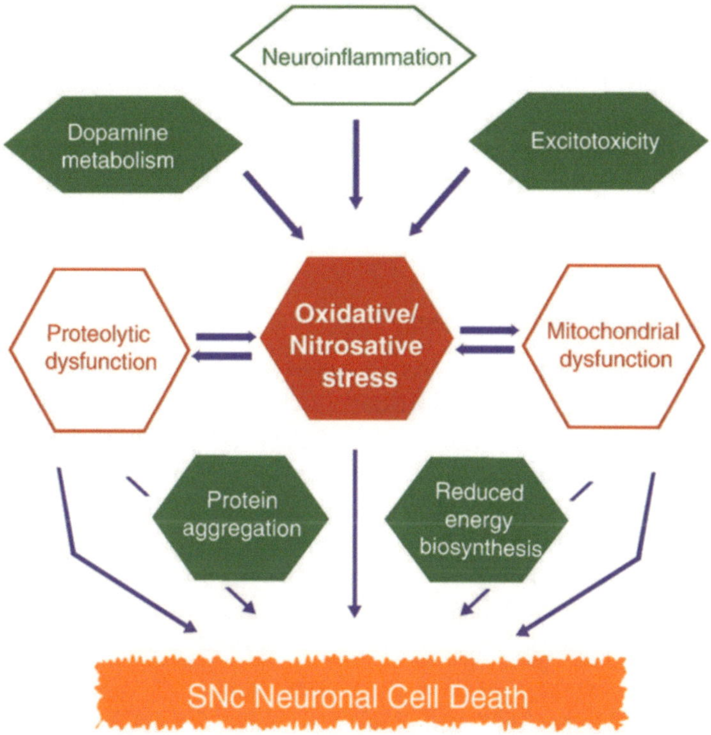

Fig. 5. Oxidative and nitrosative stress as a central event in PD pathology. SNc - substantia nigra compacta. Reproduced from Tsang & Chung (2009). © Elsevier, with permission.

This upregulation of oxidative/nitrosative stress might be related to mitochondrial dysregulation observed in PD patients (see fig. 5). There is direct evidence showing decreased activity of mitochondrial complex I isolated from substantia nigra and frontal cortex of PD patients (Parker, Jr. et al., 2008; Schapira et al., 1990). Also increased oxidation of this protein complex has been shown in PD patients (Keeney et al., 2006). It seems that abnormalities in functioning of complex I lead to increased generation of ROS. Importantly, administration of several complex I inhibitors lead to PD symptoms: motor deficiencies and death of dopaminergic neurons. Accidental exposure to 1-methyl-4-phenyl-1,2,3,6-tetrahydropyridine (MPTP, impurity in illegally synthesized recreational drug 1-methyl-4-phenyl-4-propionoxypiperidine, MPPP) that is precursor of neurotoxic 1-methyl-4-phenylpyridinium (MPP^+) leads to a rapid development of irreversible parkinsonian symptoms (Langston et al., 1983). Due to its selectivity, MPTP administration to laboratory animals is widely used as a model of PD. On the other hand ROS and RNS might be involved in decrease of complex I activity especially by involvement of $ONOO^-$ (Navarro & Boveris, 2009).

Overstimulation of N-methyl-D-aspartate receptor (i.e. excitotoxicity) can be also involved in PD pathology. Resulting Ca^{2+} influx leads to activation of NO synthase and overproduction of NO that can react with $O_2^{\bullet -}$ (overproduced due to mitochondrial dysregulation) and generate highly toxic $ONOO^-$. This mechanism seems to work in mice treated with MPTP since various NO synthase knockout mice were resistant to MPTP toxicity (Liberatore et al., 1999; Przedborski et al., 1996).

Activation of microglia is also present in PD pathology. Such activation was observed in PD patients *in vivo* by PET imaging (Gerhard et al., 2006). It was also noted in the brains of MPTP-intoxicated patients (Langston et al., 1999) and in animals that received MPTP in order to induce PD symptoms (Czlonkowska et al., 1996; Kohutnicka et al., 1998). One link between this persistent activation of microglia and pathology is increased production of ROS/RNS.

4.3 Nitrooxidative stress and glaucoma

Glaucoma - neurodegenerative disease of the retina - is the most common cause of irreversible blindness worldwide (Resnikoff et al., 2004). Progression of glaucoma is associated with gradual narrowing of visual field, typically starting from the periphery. It is sometimes called 'a sneaky theft of sight' since progression of the disease may remain unnoticed for many years. Pathological changes in glaucoma concern retinal ganglion cells and its axons that build optic nerve (Foster et al., 2002). Some recent data point that glaucoma is not limited to retina and optic nerve but also affect upstream components of the visual pathway (Gupta & Yucel, 2007). Current treatment strategies concentrate on lowering intraocular pressure (IOP), a condition observed in most but not all of the cases of glaucoma.

Measuring nitrooxidative damage biomarkers is a bit easier in case of glaucoma as aqueous humor and vitreous humor are pretty easily accessible. MDA level was two times higher in aqueous humor obtained from patients with open angle glaucoma than from healthy controls (Ghanem et al., 2010; Yildirim et al., 2005). Also open angle glaucoma patients had higher level of oxidative DNA damages in cells of trabecular meshwork (structure engaged in control of IOP). Importantly these alterations correlated well with IOP and narrowing of visual field (Izzotti et al., 2003; Sacca et al., 2005). Glutathione, ascorbic acid and tyrosine - low molecular antioxidants were downregulated in glaucoma patients (Ferreira et al., 2004), whereas SOD activity was diminished.

Also in animal models of glaucoma markers of oxidative/nitrosative stress were upregulated. MDA was upregulated in a model of high-pressure glaucoma (Moreno et al., 2004). Also carbonyl groups in retinas from these animals were upregulated. SOD activity in a model of high-pressure glaucoma was diminished (Moreno et al., 2004).

Signs of mitochondrial dysregulation were also noted in glaucoma patients. Abu-Amero et al. (2006) revealed association between primary open-angle glaucoma and changes in mitochondrial DNA. They also found that mitochndrial respiratory activity was significantly decreased in these patients. In normal tension glaucoma mutations in genes coding mitochondrial proteins were found (Mabuchi et al., 2007; Wolf et al., 2009).

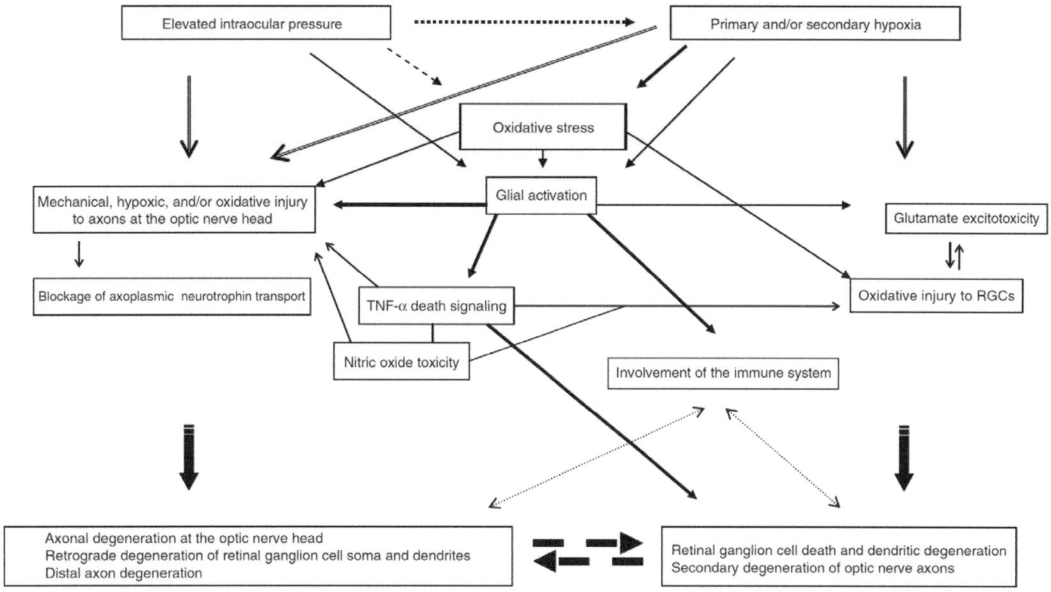

Fig. 6. Multiple proposed pathogenic mechanisms in glaucoma seem to related to oxidative stress as a common pathway. Reproduced from Tezel (2006). © Elsevier, with permission.

It is well known that glutamate administered into vitreous humor is toxic for retinal ganglion cells (Lucas & Newhouse, 1957; Quigley, 1999). Also N-methyl-D-aspartate intravitreous administration causes massive retinal ganglion cell loss (Nakazawa et al., 2005). The ability of glial cells to buffer extracellular glutamate might be impaired (Martin et al., 2002; Moreno et al., 2005). Although, some earlier reports demonstrated elevated glutamate in glaucoma patients and in some glaucoma models (Brooks et al., 1997; Dkhissi et al., 1999; Dreyer et al., 1996), other groups did not observe glutamate elevation in similar settings (Carter-Dawson et al., 2002; Honkanen et al., 2003).

Immune component is also present in glaucoma (Tezel, 2011). Upregulation of different components of immune system was found in glaucoma patients (Kuehn et al., 2006; Wax et al., 1998; Yang, 2004). Also in various animal models immune response was upregulated (Johnson et al., 2007; Steele et al., 2006). So called 'para-inflammation' – weak but persistent activation of immune system seem to be the case in glaucoma. Oxidized macromolecules stimulate resident immune cells including microglia and seem to stimulate para-inflammation (Xu et al., 2009).

5. Antioxidant therapies in neurodegenerative diseases: Rationales and precautions

As shown above, ROS and RNS could be regarded as 'key players' in pathologies of various neurodegenerative diseases. This leads to idea that antioxidant supplementation can be a reasonable therapeutic strategy in neurodegenerative disorders. One can imagine two major strategies to reduce nitrooxidative stress in these pathologic conditions (Uttara et al., 2009):

- 'upstream' to nitroxidative stress
- 'downstream' to nitrooxidative stress

'Upstream' antioxidant therapies would lead to reduction of ROS/RNS production. This could be achieved by chelating metals that catalyze generation of free radicals (like hydroxyl radical), inhibition of enzymatic reactions leading to generation of ROS/RNS or its precursors (e.g. hydrogen peroxide or nitric oxide). 'Downstream' antioxidant therapies would include agents reducing or preventing inflammation but also direct antioxidants, i.e. 'antioxidants' in traditional and narrow meaning. Some examples of antioxidants are listed in table 1.

	Mechanism of action	Examples
Upstream antioxidants	Preventing formation of free radicals	- Chelators - Inhibitors of oxidases - Inhibitors of nitric oxide synthase - Antagonists of glutamate receptors - Calcium antagonists - Anti-inflammatory drugs
Downstream antioxidants	Scavenging free radicals (direct antioxidants)	- Tocopherols - Flavonoids - Selenium-containigs compounds (e.g. ebselen) - Polyenes (carotene, lycopene, retinol)
	Catalizing decomposition of free radicals	- Mimetics of superoxide dismutase and/or catalase (e.g. tempol)
	Preventing secondary burden by ROS/RNS	- Creatine - Carnitine - Lipoic acid - Nicotinamide - N-butyl-α-phenylnitrone

Table 1. Examples of upstream and downstream antioxidants.

Many of the known antioxidants were tested in various animal models of neurodegenerative diseases and some of them were also tested in clinical trials (see reviews by (Moosmann & Behl, 2002; Tan et al., 2003; Uttara et al., 2009)). It is hard to summarize this data but one has to admit that outcomes are somehow disappointing. Theoretically, the best we can expect in case of antioxidant therapy in neurodegenerative diseases is cessation of degenerative processes. This means that we can count on stopping the process that is normally already pretty advanced, in many diseases the first symptoms appear only when 40-50% of cells are lost.

Another lesson from these numerous studies concerns features which should characterize an antioxidant that could be potentially protective in neurodegenerative diseases. Ability to cross the brain-blood barrier (BBB) seems to be the crucial one (Gilgun-Sherki et al., 2001).

Many of the known antioxidants have poor ability to cross BBB. The way the molecule crosses BBB can be also of importance, e.g. vitamin C is transported as its oxidised form, dehydroascorbic acid, by glucose transporter and then reduced back to ascorbic acid. However, reducing dehydroascorbic acid consumes glutathione. This means that vitamin C supplementation would not lead to increase in the net cerebral antioxidant capacity (Tan et al., 2003).

There are some issues and controversies concerning antioxidant therapies *per se*. For years antioxidants used to be shown unequivocally as safe and widely applicable drugs. However, recent clinical trials suggest more careful approach to antioxidant application. In some cases they can even potentiate the damage (Halliwell, 2000; Salganik, 2001). One of the many possible reasons is that ROS and RNS are not only damaging agents but as mentioned before also play a vital signalling role in the cell. Cells and organisms maintain redox homeostasis and too low levels of ROS and RNS can also be detrimental. Potential side-effects of antioxidants are summarised in fig. 7.

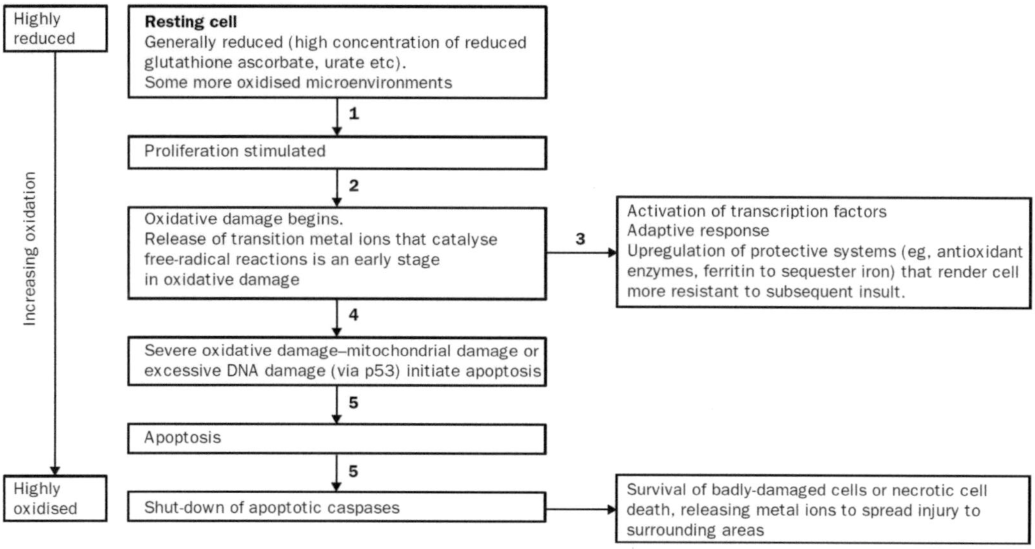

Fig. 7. Potential side-effects of antioxidants. Antioxidants might: (1) inhibit cell proliferation by preventing transient oxidations that stimulate protein phosphorylation and transcription factors; (2) protect against oxidative damage by scavenging excess ROS/RNS; (3) prevent adaptation to oxidative damage by decreasing transcription-factor activation; (4) accelerate oxidative damage by reducing transition-metal ions into their lower oxidation states that are better promoters of free-radical damage; and (5) inhibit free-radical-induced apoptosis, either beneficial to the organism or deleterious. Reproduced from Halliwell (2000). © Elsevier, with permission.

Good examples illustrating are mimetics of SOD, e.g. TEMPOL and other nitroxides, stable radicals that convert superoxide radical to hydrogen peroxide. Administration of substances that would help in eliminating superoxide radical seems to be a good therapeutic strategy and proved to be effective in many settings (Wilcox, 2010). On the other hand deleterious effects of SOD overexpression are well known, as they have been demonstrated in many settings including cell lines (Groner et al., 1986) and transgenic animals (Avraham et al., 1988; Ceballos-Picot et al., 1991). Increased oxidative stress in Down's syndrome seems to be associated with SOD-1 overexpression (Sinet, 1982). Dose-dependency curve for SOD and also its mimetics in different experimental settings is 'bell-shaped', i.e. after reaching maximum protective effect further increasing the dose leads to decreasing the protective effect (McCord, 2008).

6. Conclusions

Nitrooxidative stress seems to be not only a common phenomenon in various neurodegenerative disorders, but also a common mechanism of neurodegeneration. Obviously, there are 'disease-specific' factors that activate and inter-play with nitrooxidative stress but neurodegenerative diseases seem to share some factors that are 'key players' in their pathology: excitotoxicity, mitochondrial disruption and neuroinflammation.

Antioxidant supplementation seemed to be an excellent therapeutic and prophylactic strategy for various neurodegenerative disorders. Recently, antioxidant supplementation occurred not as safe as we previously thought. Also efficacy of these therapies is somehow controversial. Perhaps we need antioxidants that are precisely 'targeted' and evaluate accurate dosing of these substances.

7. References

Abello, N.; Kerstjens, H.A.; Postma, D.S. & Bischoff, R. (2009). Protein tyrosine nitration: selectivity, physicochemical and biological consequences, denitration, and proteomics methods for the identification of tyrosine-nitrated proteins. J Proteome Res , Vol. 8, No. 7, (2009), pp. 3222-3238, ISSN 1535-3893

Abu-Amero, K.K.; Morales, J. & Bosley, T.M. (2006). Mitochondrial abnormalities in patients with primary open-angle glaucoma. Invest Ophthalmol Vis Sci , Vol. 47, No. 6, (2006), pp. 2533-2541, ISSN 0146-0404

Alam, Z.I.; Daniel, S.E.; Lees, A.J.; Marsden, D.C.; Jenner, P. & Halliwell, B. (1997). A generalised increase in protein carbonyls in the brain in Parkinson's but not incidental Lewy body disease. J Neurochem , Vol. 69, No. 3, (1997), pp. 1326-1329, ISSN 0022-3042

Andres-Mateos, E.; Perier, C.; Zhang, L.; Blanchard-Fillion, B.; Greco, T.M.; Thomas, B.; Ko, H.S.; Sasaki, M.; Ischiropoulos, H.; Przedborski, S.; Dawson, T.M. & Dawson, V.L. (2007). DJ-1 gene deletion reveals that DJ-1 is an atypical peroxiredoxin-like peroxidase. Proc Natl Acad Sci U S A , Vol. 104, No. 37, (2007), pp. 14807-14812, ISSN 0027-8424

Ascenzi, P.; di, M.A.; Sciorati, C. & Clementi, E. (2010). Peroxynitrite-An ugly biofactor? Biofactors , Vol. 36, No. 4, (2010), pp. 264-273, ISSN 0951-6433

Avraham, K.B.; Schickler, M.; Sapoznikov, D.; Yarom, R. & Groner, Y. (1988). Down's syndrome: abnormal neuromuscular junction in tongue of transgenic mice with elevated levels of human Cu/Zn-superoxide dismutase. Cell , Vol. 54, No. 6, (1988), pp. 823-829, ISSN 0092-8674

Benov, L. (2001). How superoxide radical damages the cell. Protoplasma , Vol. 217, No. 1-3, (2001), pp. 33-36, ISSN 0033-183X

Block, M.L.; Zecca, L. & Hong, J.S. (2007). Microglia-mediated neurotoxicity: uncovering the molecular mechanisms. Nat Rev Neurosci , Vol. 8, No. 1, (2007), pp. 57-69, ISSN 1471-003X

Bobba, A.; Petragallo, V.A.; Marra, E. & Atlante, A. (2010). Alzheimer's proteins, oxidative stress, and mitochondrial dysfunction interplay in a neuronal model of Alzheimer's disease. Int J Alzheimers Dis , Vol. 2010. pii: 621870., No. (2010), pp. 621870-, ISSN 2090-0252

Brenneisen, P.; Steinbrenner, H. & Sies, H. (2005). Selenium, oxidative stress, and health aspects. Mol Aspects Med , Vol. 26, No. 4-5, (2005), pp. 256-267, ISSN 0098-2997

Brooks, D.E.; Garcia, G.A.; Dreyer, E.B.; Zurakowski, D. & Franco-Bourland, R.E. (1997). Vitreous body glutamate concentration in dogs with glaucoma. Am J Vet Res , Vol. 58, No. 8, (1997), pp. 864-867, ISSN

Buonocore, G.; Perrone, S. & Tataranno, M.L. (2010). Oxygen toxicity: chemistry and biology of reactive oxygen species. Semin Fetal Neonatal Med , Vol. 15, No. 4, (2010), pp. 186-190, ISSN 1744-165X

Carter-Dawson, L.; Crawford, M.L.; Harwerth, R.S.; Smith, E.L., III; Feldman, R.; Shen, F.F.; Mitchell, C.K. & Whitetree, A. (2002). Vitreal glutamate concentration in monkeys with experimental glaucoma. Invest Ophthalmol Vis Sci , Vol. 43, No. 8, (2002), pp. 2633-2637, ISSN

Catala, A. (2010). A synopsis of the process of lipid peroxidation since the discovery of the essential fatty acids. Biochem Biophys Res Commun , Vol. 399, No. 3, (2010), pp. 318-323, ISSN 0006-291X

Ceballos-Picot, I.; Nicole, A.; Briand, P.; Grimber, G.; Delacourte, A.; Defossez, A.; Javoy-Agid, F.; Lafon, M.; Blouin, J.L. & Sinet, P.M. (1991). Neuronal-specific expression of human copper-zinc superoxide dismutase gene in transgenic mice: animal model of gene dosage effects in Down's syndrome. Brain Res , Vol. 552, No. 2, (1991), pp. 198-214, ISSN 0006-8993

Chance, B.; Sies, H. & Boveris, A. (1979). Hydroperoxide metabolism in mammalian organs. Physiol Rev , Vol. 59, No. 3, (1979), pp. 527-605, ISSN 0031-9333

Chen, X. & Yan, S.D. (2006). Mitochondrial Abeta: a potential cause of metabolic dysfunction in Alzheimer's disease. IUBMB Life , Vol. 58, No. 12, (2006), pp. 686-694, ISSN 1521-6543

Cheng, F.C.; Jen, J.F. & Tsai, T.H. (2002). Hydroxyl radical in living systems and its separation methods. J Chromatogr B Analyt Technol Biomed Life Sci , Vol. 781, No. 1-2, (2002), pp. 481-496, ISSN 1570-0232

Clement, M.V. & Pervaiz, S. (1999). Reactive oxygen intermediates regulate cellular response to apoptotic stimuli: an hypothesis. Free Radic Res , Vol. 30, No. 4, (1999), pp. 247-252, ISSN 1071-5762

Commoner, B.; Townsend, J. & Pake, G.E. (1954). Free radicals in biological materials. Nature , Vol. 174, No. 4432, (1954), pp. 689-691, ISSN 0028-0836

Czlonkowska, A.; Kohutnicka, M.; Kurkowska-Jastrzebska, I. & Czlonkowski, A. (1996). Microglial reaction in MPTP (1-methyl-4-phenyl-1,2,3,6-tetrahydropyridine) induced Parkinson's disease mice model. Neurodegeneration , Vol. 5, No. 2, (1996), pp. 137-143, ISSN 1055-8330

de Leon, M.J.; Mosconi, L.; Li, J.; De, S.S.; Yao, Y.; Tsui, W.H.; Pirraglia, E.; Rich, K.; Javier, E.; Brys, M.; Glodzik, L.; Switalski, R.; Saint Louis, L.A. & Pratico, D. (2007).

Longitudinal CSF isoprostane and MRI atrophy in the progression to AD. J Neurol , Vol. 254, No. 12, (2007), pp. 1666-1675, ISSN 0340-5354

Dkhissi, O.; Chanut, E.; Wasowicz, M.; Savoldelli, M.; Nguyen-Legros, J.; Minvielle, F. & Versaux-Botteri, C. (1999). Retinal TUNEL-positive cells and high glutamate levels in vitreous humor of mutant quail with a glaucoma-like disorder. Invest Ophthalmol Vis Sci , Vol. 40, No. 5, (1999), pp. 990-995, ISSN

Donald, K.W. (1947). Oxygen poisoning in man; signs and symptoms of oxygen poisoning. Br Med J , Vol. 1, No. 4507, (1947), pp. 712-717, ISSN 0007-1447

Dreyer, E.B.; Zurakowski, D.; Schumer, R.A.; Podos, S.M. & Lipton, S.A. (1996). Elevated glutamate levels in the vitreous body of humans and monkeys with glaucoma. Arch Ophthalmol , Vol. 114, No. 3, (1996), pp. 299-305, ISSN 0003-9950

Enciclopedia Britannica (2011). Hooke's law, 01.10.2011, Available from http://www.britannica.com/EBchecked/topic/271336/Hookes-law

Faraci, F.M. & Didion, S.P. (2004). Vascular protection: superoxide dismutase isoforms in the vessel wall. Arterioscler Thromb Vasc Biol , Vol. 24, No. 8, (2004), pp. 1367-1373, ISSN 1079-5642

Ferreira, S.M.; Lerner, S.F.; Brunzini, R.; Evelson, P.A. & Llesuy, S.F. (2004). Oxidative stress markers in aqueous humor of glaucoma patients. Am J Ophthalmol , Vol. 137, No. 1, (2004), pp. 62-69, ISSN 0002-9394

Foster, P.J.; Buhrmann, R.; Quigley, H.A. & Johnson, G.J. (2002). The definition and classification of glaucoma in prevalence surveys. Br J Ophthalmol , Vol. 86, No. 2, (2002), pp. 238-242, ISSN 0007-1161

Fridovich, I. (1975). Oxygen: boon and bane. Am Sci , Vol. 63, No. 1, (1975), pp. 54-59, ISSN 0003-0996

Fridovich, I. (1983). Superoxide radical: an endogenous toxicant. Annu Rev Pharmacol Toxicol , Vol. 23, No. (1983), pp. 239-257, ISSN 0362-1642

Galasko, D. & Montine, T.J. (2010). Biomarkers of oxidative damage and inflammation in Alzheimer's disease. Biomark Med , Vol. 4, No. 1, (2010), pp. 27-36, ISSN 1752-0363

Gautier, C.A.; Kitada, T. & Shen, J. (2008). Loss of PINK1 causes mitochondrial functional defects and increased sensitivity to oxidative stress. Proc Natl Acad Sci U S A , Vol. 105, No. 32, (2008), pp. 11364-11369, ISSN 0027-8424

Gerhard, A.; Pavese, N.; Hotton, G.; Turkheimer, F.; Es, M.; Hammers, A.; Eggert, K.; Oertel, W.; Banati, R.B. & Brooks, D.J. (2006). In vivo imaging of microglial activation with [11C](R)-PK11195 PET in idiopathic Parkinson's disease. Neurobiol Dis , Vol. 21, No. 2, (2006), pp. 404-412, ISSN 0969-9961

Gerschman, R.; Gilbert, D.L.; Nye, S.W.; Dwyer, P. & Fenn, W.O. (1954). Oxygen poisoning and x-irradiation: a mechanism in common. Science , Vol. 119, No. 3097, (1954), pp. 623-626, ISSN 0036-8075

Ghanem, A.A.; Arafa, L.F. & El Baz, A. (2010). Oxidative stress markers in patients with primary open-angle glaucoma. Curr Eye Res , Vol. 35, No. 4, (2010), pp. 295-301, ISSN 0271-3683

Gilgun-Sherki, Y.; Melamed, E. & Offen, D. (2001). Oxidative stress induced-neurodegenerative diseases: the need for antioxidants that penetrate the blood brain barrier. Neuropharmacology , Vol. 40, No. 8, (2001), pp. 959-975, ISSN 0028-3908

Giorgio, M.; Trinei, M.; Migliaccio, E. & Pelicci, P.G. (2007). Hydrogen peroxide: a metabolic by-product or a common mediator of ageing signals? Nat Rev Mol Cell Biol , Vol. 8, No. 9, (2007), pp. 722-728, ISSN 1471-0072

Golden, T.R. & Patel, M. (2009). Catalytic antioxidants and neurodegeneration. Antioxid Redox Signal , Vol. 11, No. 3, (2009), pp. 555-570, ISSN 1523-0864

Groner, Y.; Elroy-Stein, O.; Bernstein, Y.; Dafni, N.; Levanon, D.; Danciger, E. & Neer, A. (1986). Molecular genetics of Down's syndrome: overexpression of transfected human Cu/Zn-superoxide dismutase gene and the consequent physiological changes. Cold Spring Harb Symp Quant Biol , Vol. 51 Pt 1:381-93., No. (1986), pp. 381-393, ISSN 0091-7451

Gupta, N. & Yucel, Y.H. (2007). What changes can we expect in the brain of glaucoma patients? Surv Ophthalmol , Vol. 52 Suppl 2:S122-6., No. (2007), pp. S122-S126, ISSN 0039-6257

Halliwell, B. (2000). The antioxidant paradox. Lancet , Vol. 355, No. 9210, (2000), pp. 1179-1180, ISSN 0140-6736

Halliwell, B. (2009). The wanderings of a free radical. Free Radic Biol Med , Vol. 46, No. 5, (2009), pp. 531-542, ISSN 0891-5849

Halliwell, B. & Gutteridge, J.M. (1984). Oxygen toxicity, oxygen radicals, transition metals and disease. Biochem J , Vol. 219, No. 1, (1984), pp. 1-14, ISSN 0264-6021

Hampton, M.B. & Orrenius, S. (1998). Redox regulation of apoptotic cell death. Biofactors , Vol. 8, No. 1-2, (1998), pp. 1-5, ISSN 0951-6433

Heiss, W.D.; Szelies, B.; Kessler, J. & Herholz, K. (1991). Abnormalities of energy metabolism in Alzheimer's disease studied with PET. Ann N Y Acad Sci , Vol. 640:65-71., No. (1991), pp. 65-71, ISSN 0077-8923

Henderson, N. (2000). The Discovery of Organic Free Radicals by Moses Gomberg, 24.10.2011, Available from http://portal.acs.org/portal/acs/corg/content?_nfpb=true&_pageLabel=PP_ARTICLEMAIN&node_id=924&content_id=WPCP_007609&use_sec=true&sec_url_var=region1&__uuid=2010c927-eb9f-41c8-89b1-ff0c459381c7

Honkanen, R.A.; Baruah, S.; Zimmerman, M.B.; Khanna, C.L.; Weaver, Y.K.; Narkiewicz, J.; Waziri, R.; Gehrs, K.M.; Weingeist, T.A.; Boldt, H.C.; Folk, J.C.; Russell, S.R. & Kwon, Y.H. (2003). Vitreous amino acid concentrations in patients with glaucoma undergoing vitrectomy. Arch Ophthalmol , Vol. 121, No. 2, (2003), pp. 183-188, ISSN 0003-9950

Huang, T.T., Carlson, E.J., Kozy, H.M., Mantha, S., Goodman, S.I., Ursell, P.C. & Epstein, C.J. (2001). Genetic modification of prenatal lethality and dilated cardiomyopathy in Mn superoxide dismutase mutant mice. Free Radic Biol Med , Vol. 31, No. 9, (2001), pp. 1101-1110, ISSN 0891-5849

Ill-Raga, G.; Ramos-Fernandez, E.; Guix, F.X.; Tajes, M.; Bosch-Morato, M.; Palomer, E.; Godoy, J.; Belmar, S.; Cerpa, W.; Simpkins, J.W.; Inestrosa And NC & Munoz, F.J. (2010). Amyloid-beta peptide fibrils induce nitro-oxidative stress in neuronal cells. J Alzheimers Dis , Vol. 22, No. 2, (2010), pp. 641-652, ISSN 1387-2877

Inkret, W.C.; Meinhold, C.B. & Taschner, J.C. (1995). A brief history of radiation protection standards. Los Alamos Science , Vol. 23, No. (1995), pp. 116-123, ISSN 0273-7116

Ischiropoulos, H. & Beckman, J.S. (2003). Oxidative stress and nitration in neurodegeneration: cause, effect, or association? J Clin Invest , Vol. 111, No. 2, (2003), pp. 163-169, ISSN 0021-9738

IUPAC (2005). *Nomenclature of Inorganic Chemistry. IUPAC Recommendations 2005.* RSC Publishing - IUPAC, ISBN 0-85404-438-8, Cambridge

Izzotti, A.; Sacca, S.C.; Cartiglia, C. & De Flora, S. (2003). Oxidative deoxyribonucleic acid damage in the eyes of glaucoma patients. Am J Med , Vol. 114, No. 8, (2003), pp. 638-646, ISSN 0002-9343

Jekabsone, A.; Mander, P.K.; Tickler, A.; Sharpe, M. & Brown, G.C. (2006). Fibrillar beta-amyloid peptide Abeta1-40 activates microglial proliferation via stimulating TNF-alpha release and H2O2 derived from NADPH oxidase: a cell culture study. J Neuroinflammation , Vol. 3:24., No. (2006), pp. 24-, ISSN 1742-2094

Johnson, E.C.; Jia, L.; Cepurna, W.O.; Doser, T.A. & Morrison, J.C. (2007). Global changes in optic nerve head gene expression after exposure to elevated intraocular pressure in a rat glaucoma model. Invest Ophthalmol Vis Sci , Vol. 48, No. 7, (2007), pp. 3161-3177, ISSN 0146-0404

Jomova, K.; Vondrakova, D.; Lawson, M. & Valko, M. (2010). Metals, oxidative stress and neurodegenerative disorders. Mol Cell Biochem , Vol. 345, No. 1-2, (2010), pp. 91-104, ISSN 0300-8177

Kagan, V.E.; Bayir, H.A.; Belikova, N.A.; Kapralov, O.; Tyurina, Y.Y.; Tyurin, V.A.; Jiang, J.; Stoyanovsky, D.A.; Wipf, P.; Kochanek, P.M.; Greenberger, J.S.; Pitt, B.; Shvedova, A.A. & Borisenko, G. (2009). Cytochrome c/cardiolipin relations in mitochondria: a kiss of death. Free Radic Biol Med , Vol. 46, No. 11, (2009), pp. 1439-1453, ISSN 0891-5849

Keeney, P.M.; Xie, J.; Capaldi, R.A. & Bennett, J.P., Jr. (2006). Parkinson's disease brain mitochondrial complex I has oxidatively damaged subunits and is functionally impaired and misassembled. J Neurosci , Vol. 26, No. 19, (2006), pp. 5256-5264, ISSN

Keller, J.N.; Schmitt, F.A.; Scheff, S.W.; Ding, Q.; Chen, Q.; Butterfield, D.A. & Markesbery, W.R. (2005). Evidence of increased oxidative damage in subjects with mild cognitive impairment. Neurology , Vol. 64, No. 7, (2005), pp. 1152-1156, ISSN 0028-3878

Klotz, L.O.; Schroeder, P. & Sies, H. (2002). Peroxynitrite signaling: receptor tyrosine kinases and activation of stress-responsive pathways. Free Radic Biol Med , Vol. 33, No. 6, (2002), pp. 737-743, ISSN 0891-5849

Kohutnicka, M.; Lewandowska, E.; Kurkowska-Jastrzebska, I.; Czlonkowski, A. & Czlonkowska, A. (1998). Microglial and astrocytic involvement in a murine model of Parkinson's disease induced by 1-methyl-4-phenyl-1,2,3,6-tetrahydropyridine (MPTP). Immunopharmacology , Vol. 39, No. 3, (1998), pp. 167-180, ISSN 0162-3109

Kuehn, M.H.; Kim, C.Y.; Ostojic, J.; Bellin, M.; Alward, W.L.; Stone, E.M.; Sakaguchi, D.S.; Grozdanic, S.D. & Kwon, Y.H. (2006). Retinal synthesis and deposition of complement components induced by ocular hypertension. Exp Eye Res , Vol. 83, No. 3, (2006), pp. 620-628, ISSN 0014-4835

Langston, J.W.; Ballard, P.; Tetrud, J.W. & Irwin, I. (1983). Chronic Parkinsonism in humans due to a product of meperidine-analog synthesis. Science , Vol. 219, No. 4587, (1983), pp. 979-980, ISSN 0036-8075

Langston, J.W.; Forno, L.S.; Tetrud, J.; Reeves, A.G.; Kaplan, J.A. & Karluk, D. (1999). Evidence of active nerve cell degeneration in the substantia nigra of humans years after 1-methyl-4-phenyl-1,2,3,6-tetrahydropyridine exposure. Ann Neurol , Vol. 46, No. 4, (1999), pp. 598-605, ISSN 0364-5134

Lew, M. (2007). Overview of Parkinson's disease. Pharmacotherapy , Vol. 27, No. 12 Pt 2, (2007), pp. 155S-160S, ISSN 0277-0008

Li, F.; Calingasan, N.Y.; Yu, F.; Mauck, W.M.; Toidze, M.; Almeida, C.G.; Takahashi, R.H.; Carlson, G.A.; Flint, B.M.; Lin, M.T. & Gouras, G.K. (2004). Increased plaque burden in brains of APP mutant MnSOD heterozygous knockout mice. J Neurochem , Vol. 89, No. 5, (2004), pp. 1308-1312, ISSN 0022-3042

Liberatore, G.T.; Jackson-Lewis, V.; Vukosavic, S.; Mandir, A.S.; Vila, M.; McAuliffe, W.G.; Dawson, V.L.; Dawson, T.M. & Przedborski, S. (1999). Inducible nitric oxide synthase stimulates dopaminergic neurodegeneration in the MPTP model of Parkinson disease. Nat Med , Vol. 5, No. 12, (1999), pp. 1403-1409, ISSN 1078-8956

Lovell, M.A.; Xiong, S.; Xie, C.; Davies, P. & Markesbery, W.R. (2004). Induction of hyperphosphorylated tau in primary rat cortical neuron cultures mediated by oxidative stress and glycogen synthase kinase-3. J Alzheimers Dis , Vol. 6, No. 6, (2004), pp. 659-671, ISSN 1387-2877

Lucas, D.R. & Newhouse, J.P. (1957). The toxic effect of sodium L-glutamate on the inner layers of the retina. AMA Arch Ophthalmol , Vol. 58, No. 2, (1957), pp. 193-201, ISSN

Mabuchi, F.; Tang, S.; Kashiwagi, K.; Yamagata, Z.; Iijima, H. & Tsukahara, S. (2007). The OPA1 gene polymorphism is associated with normal tension and high tension glaucoma. Am J Ophthalmol , Vol. 143, No. 1, (2007), pp. 125-130, ISSN 0002-9394

Mangialasche, F.; Polidori, M.C.; Monastero, R.; Ercolani, S.; Camarda, C.; Cecchetti, R. & Mecocci, P. (2009). Biomarkers of oxidative and nitrosative damage in Alzheimer's disease and mild cognitive impairment. Ageing Res Rev , Vol. 8, No. 4, (2009), pp. 285-305, ISSN 1568-1637

Martin, K.R.; Levkovitch-Verbin, H.; Valenta, D.; Baumrind, L.; Pease, M.E. & Quigley, H.A. (2002). Retinal glutamate transporter changes in experimental glaucoma and after optic nerve transection in the rat. Invest Ophthalmol Vis Sci , Vol. 43, No. 7, (2002), pp. 2236-2243, ISSN 0146-0404

Masliah, E.; Rockenstein, E.; Veinbergs, I.; Mallory, M.; Hashimoto, M.; Takeda, A.; Sagara, Y.; Sisk, A. & Mucke, L. (2000). Dopaminergic loss and inclusion body formation in alpha-synuclein mice: implications for neurodegenerative disorders. Science , Vol. 287, No. 5456, (2000), pp. 1265-1269, ISSN 0036-8075

McCord, J.M. (2000). The evolution of free radicals and oxidative stress. Am J Med , Vol. 108, No. 8, (2000), pp. 652-659, ISSN 0002-9343

McCord, J.M. (2008). Superoxide dismutase, lipid peroxidation, and bell-shaped dose response curves. Dose Response , Vol. 6, No. 3, (2008), pp. 223-238, ISSN 1559-3258

Miles, B. (2003). Oxygen metabolism and oxygen toxicity, 06.05.2011, Available from http://www.tamu.edu/classes/bmiles/lectures/Oxygen%20Metabolism%20and%20Oxygen%20Toxicity.pdf

Moosmann, B. & Behl, C. (2002). Antioxidants as treatment for neurodegenerative disorders. Expert Opin Investig Drugs , Vol. 11, No. 10, (2002), pp. 1407-1435, ISSN 1354-3784

Moreno, M.C.; Campanelli, J.; Sande, P.; Sanez, D.A.; Keller Sarmiento, M.I. & Rosenstein, R.E. (2004). Retinal oxidative stress induced by high intraocular pressure. Free Radic Biol Med , Vol. 37, No. 6, (2004), pp. 803-812, ISSN 0891-5849

Moreno, M.C.; Sande, P.; Marcos, H.A.; de, Z.N.; Keller Sarmiento, M.I. & Rosenstein, R.E. (2005). Effect of glaucoma on the retinal glutamate/glutamine cycle activity. FASEB J , Vol. 19, No. 9, (2005), pp. 1161-1162, ISSN 0892-6638

Nakazawa, T.; Shimura, M.; Endo, S.; Takahashi, H.; Mori, N. & Tamai, M. (2005). N-Methyl-D-Aspartic acid suppresses Akt activity through protein phosphatase in retinal ganglion cells. Mol Vis , Vol. 11:1173-82., No. (2005), pp. 1173-1182, ISSN 1090-0535

Navarro, A. & Boveris, A. (2009). Brain mitochondrial dysfunction and oxidative damage in Parkinson's disease. J Bioenerg Biomembr , Vol. 41, No. 6, (2009), pp. 517-521, ISSN 0145-479X

Ogawa, M.; Fukuyama, H.; Ouchi, Y.; Yamauchi, H. & Kimura, J. (1996). Altered energy metabolism in Alzheimer's disease. J Neurol Sci , Vol. 139, No. 1, (1996), pp. 78-82, ISSN 0022-510X

Ohyagi, Y.; Yamada, T.; Nishioka, K.; Clarke, N.J.; Tomlinson, A.J.; Naylor, S.; Nakabeppu, Y.; Kira, J. & Younkin, S.G. (2000). Selective increase in cellular A beta 42 is related to apoptosis but not necrosis. Neuroreport , Vol. 11, No. 1, (2000), pp. 167-171, ISSN 0959-4965

Oxford Dictionary of Sports Science & Medicine (2007). Nitrosative stress, 25.09.2011, Available from
http://www.answers.com/topic/nitrosative-stress#ixzz1Yz0Phmmz

Parker, W.D., Jr.; Parks, J.K. & Swerdlow, R.H. (2008). Complex I deficiency in Parkinson's disease frontal cortex. Brain Res , Vol. 1189:215-8. Epub@2007 Nov 1., No. (2008), pp. 215-218, ISSN 0006-8993

Pratico, D.; Clark, C.M.; Liun, F.; Rokach, J.; Lee, V.Y. & Trojanowski, J.Q. (2002). Increase of brain oxidative stress in mild cognitive impairment: a possible predictor of Alzheimer disease. Arch Neurol , Vol. 59, No. 6, (2002), pp. 972-976, ISSN 0003-9942

Pratico, D.; Uryu, K.; Leight, S.; Trojanoswki, J.Q. & Lee, V.M. (2001). Increased lipid peroxidation precedes amyloid plaque formation in an animal model of Alzheimer amyloidosis. J Neurosci , Vol. 21, No. 12, (2001), pp. 4183-4187, ISSN 0270-6474

Probiox (2011). What is Oxidative Stress?, 29.08.2011, Available from
http://www.probiox.com/uk/pages/oxidative_def.html

Przedborski, S.; Jackson-Lewis, V.; Yokoyama, R.; Shibata, T.; Dawson, V.L. & Dawson, T.M. (1996). Role of neuronal nitric oxide in 1-methyl-4-phenyl-1,2,3,6-tetrahydropyridine (MPTP)-induced dopaminergic neurotoxicity. Proc Natl Acad Sci U S A , Vol. 93, No. 10, (1996), pp. 4565-4571, ISSN 0027-8424

Quigley, H.A. (1999). Neuronal death in glaucoma. Prog Retin Eye Res , Vol. 18, No. 1, (1999), pp. 39-57, ISSN 1350-9462

Resnikoff, S.; Pascolini, D.; Etya'ale, D.; Kocur, I.; Pararajasegaram, R.; Pokharel, G.P. & Mariotti, S.P. (2004). Global data on visual impairment in the year 2002. Bull World Health Organ , Vol. 82, No. 11, (2004), pp. 844-851, ISSN 0042-9686

Rozemuller, A.J.; van Gool, W.A. & Eikelenboom, P. (2005). The neuroinflammatory response in plaques and amyloid angiopathy in Alzheimer's disease: therapeutic implications. Curr Drug Targets CNS Neurol Disord , Vol. 4, No. 3, (2005), pp. 223-233, ISSN 1568-007X

Sacca, S.C.; Pascotto, A.; Camicione, P.; Capris, P. & Izzotti, A. (2005). Oxidative DNA damage in the human trabecular meshwork: clinical correlation in patients with primary open-angle glaucoma. Arch Ophthalmol , Vol. 123, No. 4, (2005), pp. 458-463, ISSN 0003-9950

Salganik, R.I. (2001). The benefits and hazards of antioxidants: controlling apoptosis and other protective mechanisms in cancer patients and the human population. J Am Coll Nutr , Vol. 20, No. 5 Suppl, (2001), pp. 464S-472S, ISSN 0731-5724

Schapira, A.H.; Cooper, J.M.; Dexter, D.; Clark, J.B.; Jenner, P. & Marsden, C.D. (1990). Mitochondrial complex I deficiency in Parkinson's disease. J Neurochem , Vol. 54, No. 3, (1990), pp. 823-827, ISSN 0022-3042

Schwab, C. & McGeer, P.L. (2008). Inflammatory aspects of Alzheimer disease and other neurodegenerative disorders. J Alzheimers Dis , Vol. 13, No. 4, (2008), pp. 359-369, ISSN 1387-2877

Selye, H. (1985). The nature of stress, 01.10.2011, Available from http://www.icnr.com/articles/the-nature-of-stress.html

Sies, H. (1997). Oxidative stress: oxidants and antioxidants. Exp Physiol , Vol. 82, No. 2, (1997), pp. 291-295, ISSN 0958-0670

Sinet, P.M. (1982). Metabolism of oxygen derivatives in down's syndrome. Ann N Y Acad Sci , Vol. 396, No. (1982), pp. 83-94, ISSN 0077-8923

Sorce, S. & Krause, K.H. (2009). NOX enzymes in the central nervous system: from signaling to disease. Antioxid Redox Signal , Vol. 11, No. 10, (2009), pp. 2481-2504, ISSN 1523-0864

Stanislawski, J. (1999). *The Great English-Polish Dictionary.* Philip Wilson, ISBN 83-7236-048-0, Warsaw

Steele, M.R.; Inman, D.M.; Calkins, D.J.; Horner, P.J. & Vetter, M.L. (2006). Microarray analysis of retinal gene expression in the DBA/2J model of glaucoma. Invest Ophthalmol Vis Sci , Vol. 47, No. 3, (2006), pp. 977-985, ISSN 0146-0404

Tan, D.X.; Manchester, L.C.; Sainz, R.; Mayo, J.C.; Alvares, F.L. & Reiter, R.J. (2003). Antioxidant strategies in treatment against neurodegenerative disorders. Expert Opin Ther Patents , Vol. 13, No. 10, (2003), pp. 1513-1543, ISSN 1354-3776

Tezel, G. (2006). Oxidative stress in glaucomatous neurodegeneration: mechanisms and consequences. Prog Retin Eye Res , Vol. 25, No. 5, (2006), pp. 490-513, ISSN 1350-9462

Tezel, G. (2011). The immune response in glaucoma: a perspective on the roles of oxidative stress. Exp Eye Res , Vol. 93, No. 2, (2011), pp. 178-186, ISSN

Tsang, A.H. & Chung, K.K. (2009). Oxidative and nitrosative stress in Parkinson's disease. Biochim Biophys Acta , Vol. 1792, No. 7, (2009), pp. 643-650, ISSN 0006-3002

Turrens, J.F. (2003). Mitochondrial formation of reactive oxygen species. J Physiol , Vol. 552, No. Pt 2, (2003), pp. 335-344, ISSN 0022-3751

Uttara, B.; Singh, A.V.; Zamboni, P. & Mahajan, R.T. (2009). Oxidative stress and neurodegenerative diseases: a review of upstream and downstream antioxidant therapeutic options. Curr Neuropharmacol , Vol. 7, No. 1, (2009), pp. 65-74, ISSN 1570-159X

Van Remmen, H.; Ikeno, Y.; Hamilton, M.; Pahlavani, M.; Wolf, N.; Thorpe, S.R.; Alderson, N.L.; Baynes, J.W.; Epstein, C.J.; Huang, T.T.; Nelson, J.; Strong, R. & Richardson, A. (2003). Life-long reduction in MnSOD activity results in increased DNA damage and higher incidence of cancer but does not accelerate aging. Physiol Genomics , Vol. 16, No. 1, (2003), pp. 29-37, ISSN 1094-8341

Veal, E.A.; Day, A.M. & Morgan, B.A. (2007). Hydrogen peroxide sensing and signaling. Mol Cell , Vol. 26, No. 1, (2007), pp. 1-14, ISSN 1097-2765

Wax, M.B.; Tezel, G. & Edward, P.D. (1998). Clinical and ocular histopathological findings in a patient with normal-pressure glaucoma. Arch Ophthalmol , Vol. 116, No. 8, (1998), pp. 993-1001, ISSN 0003-9950

Wilcox, C.S. (2010). Effects of tempol and redox-cycling nitroxides in models of oxidative stress. Pharmacol Ther , Vol. 126, No. 2, (2010), pp. 119-145, ISSN

Winkler, B.S.; Boulton, M.E.; Gottsch, J.D. & Sternberg, P. (1999). Oxidative damage and age-related macular degeneration. Mol Vis , Vol. 5, No. (1999), pp. 32-42, ISSN 1090-0535

Wolf, C.; Gramer, E.; Muller-Myhsok, B.; Pasutto, F.; Reinthal, E.; Wissinger, B. & Weisschuh, N. (2009). Evaluation of nine candidate genes in patients with normal tension glaucoma: a case control study. BMC Med Genet , Vol. 10:91., No. (2009), pp. 91-, ISSN 1471-2350

Wright, M.V. & Kuhn, T.B. (2002). CNS neurons express two distinct plasma membrane electron transport systems implicated in neuronal viability. J Neurochem , Vol. 83, No. 3, (2002), pp. 655-664, ISSN 0022-3042

Xu, H.; Chen, M. & Forrester, J.V. (2009). Para-inflammation in the aging retina. Prog Retin Eye Res , Vol. 28, No. 5, (2009), pp. 348-368, ISSN 1350-9462

Yang, X.L. (2004). Characterization of receptors for glutamate and GABA in retinal neurons. Prog Neurobiol , Vol. 73, No. 2, (2004), pp. 127-150, ISSN 0002-9394

Yildirim, O.; Ates, N.A.; Ercan, B.; Muslu, N.; Unlu, A.; Tamer, L.; Atik, U. & Kanik, A. (2005). Role of oxidative stress enzymes in open-angle glaucoma. Eye (Lond) , Vol. 19, No. 5, (2005), pp. 580-583, ISSN 0950-222X

Yoritaka, A.; Hattori, N.; Uchida, K.; Tanaka, M.; Stadtman, E.R. & Mizuno, Y. (1996). Immunohistochemical detection of 4-hydroxynonenal protein adducts in Parkinson disease. Proc Natl Acad Sci U S A , Vol. 93, No. 7, (1996), pp. 2696-2701, ISSN 0027-8424

Zhang, J.; Perry, G.; Smith, M.A.; Robertson, D.; Olson, S.J.; Graham, D.G. & Montine, T.J. (1999). Parkinson's disease is associated with oxidative damage to cytoplasmic DNA and RNA in substantia nigra neurons. Am J Pathol , Vol. 154, No. 5, (1999), pp. 1423-1429, ISSN 0002-9440

7

Molecular Mechanisms of Acute Brain Injury and Ensuing Neurodegeneration

Francisco J. Ortega, Jose M. Vidal-Taboada,
Nicole Mahy and Manuel J. Rodríguez
*Unitat de Bioquímica i Biologia Molecular, Facultat de Medicina,
Institut d'Investigacions Biomèdiques August Pi i Sunyer (IDIBAPS),
Universitat de Barcelona and Centro de Investigación Biomédica en Red sobre
Enfermedades Neurodegenerativas (CIBERNED), Barcelona
Spain*

1. Introduction

Injury to the central nervous system (CNS), including stroke, traumatic brain injury and spinal cord injury, cause devastating and irreversible damage and loss of function. For example, stroke affects very large patient populations, results in major suffering for the patients and their relatives, and involves a significant cost to society. CNS damage implies disruption of the intricate internal circuits involved in cognition, the sensory-motor functions, and other important functions. There are currently no treatments available to properly restore such lost functions. New therapeutic proposals will emerge from an understanding of the interdependence of molecular and cellular responses to CNS injury, in particular the inhibitory mechanisms that block regeneration and those that enhance neuronal plasticity.

In this chapter we explore the hypothesis that different CNS insults induce similar molecular and cellular processes that lead to neuronal death and the ensuing neurodegeneration. Thus, acute CNS injury is characterized by immediate, massive neuronal death and marked tissue injury that arise from interdependent mechanisms such as glutamate-mediated excitotoxicity, failure of energy production, acidosis, generation of reactive oxygen species (ROS), and a potent inflammatory reaction. Acute brain injury can also activate a neurodegenerative process whose effects are time-dependent and related to the initial severity of the primary insult. In addition to misfolded protein aggregation, the same common molecular and cellular processes, including chronic excitotoxicity, calcium homeostasis dysregulation, energy failure and chronic inflammation, underlie the pathology of neurodegenerative diseases.

2. Acute CNS disorders have common molecular mechanisms

Acute CNS injury is characterized by immediate, massive neuronal death and marked tissue injury as a result of uncontrolled local necrosis. This primary injury expands in the surrounding tissue for weeks through interdependent mechanisms such as glutamate receptor over-stimulation, failure of cellular energetics, acidosis, the generation of ROS, and a potent inflammatory response, all of which further cell death and tissue destruction (Figure 1).

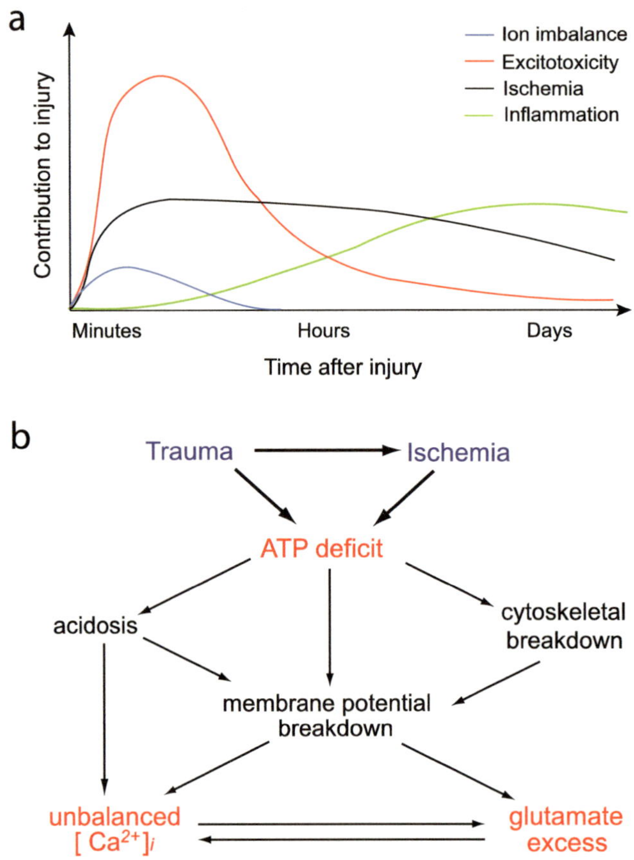

Fig. 1. Pathophysiology of traumatic brain injury and ischemia. a) Kinetics of the main events taking place in the lesioned CNS after an acute injury. b) ATP availability, intracellular calcium and extracellular glutamate determine the cascade of the interdependent molecular processes leading to neuronal death

2.1 Molecular mechanisms of excitotoxicity after acute CNS injury

Glutamate accounts for most of the excitatory synaptic activity in the CNS through three groups of receptors: two ionotropic receptors (N-Methyl-D-aspartate (NMDA) and α-amino-3-hydroxy-5-methyl-4-isoxazole propionic acid (AMPA)-kainate receptors); and one group of metabotropic receptors, which are coupled to G proteins. Although non-NMDA receptors are not initially permeable to calcium, glutamate release in the synaptic cleft increases post-synaptic and glial membrane permeability, which leads to a transient increase in intracellular calcium concentration ($[Ca^{2+}]_i$) (Obrenovitch et al., 2000). Excessive activation of glutamate receptors can directly trigger neuronal death through a process characterized by chronic glutamate release and the consequent $[Ca^{2+}]_i$ dys-homeostasis in neurons and astrocytes (Lau

& Tymianski, 2010) with the formation of intracellular calcium precipitates (Rodríguez et al., 2001). This process, defined as excitotoxicity, also involves cellular influxes of Na^+ and Cl^- and efflux of K^+, and the resulting cell swelling (Chen et al., 1998, Katayama et al., 1995).

The link between excitotoxicity, excessive $[Ca^{2+}]_i$ increase, and neuronal death (Figure 1) has been established from data obtained from neuronal cultures and rodent models of hypoxia-ischemia and of cerebral lesions (Lau & Tymianski, 2010, Verkhratsky, 2007). In these studies, the induced neuronal death can be blocked with intracellular calcium chelators (Tymianski et al., 1993) or voltage-operated calcium channel antagonists, extracellular calcium removal, or emptying of the cellular calcium stores (Verkhratsky, 2007). In addition, an increase in $[Ca^{2+}]_i$ plays a direct role in the neuronal damage observed during cerebral ischemia and epileptic seizures (Verkhratsky, 2007).

Therefore, control of the cellular calcium homeostasis is a key element in ensuring an adequate cellular response at any moment. When intracellular calcium movements overload this homeostatic balance, the extrusion systems are activated and Ca^{2+}/Na^+ antiporters and mitochondrial Ca^{2+} uniporter lead to a reduction in intracytosolic calcium (Lau & Tymianski, 2010). Once the first wave is stopped, calcium-binding proteins release calcium, which is extruded by the highly efficient plasma membrane calcium ATPases (Verkhratsky, 2007). A similar process takes place in mitochondria, in the nuclear envelope, the endoplasmic-reticulum network, and the secretory vesicles. All of these systems have a critical dependence on energy availability and the interplay between them decreases the cytoplasmatic calcium levels in a coordinated way (Beck et al., 2004). Any alteration of the cellular energy metabolism will alter calcium homeostasis and vice versa (Berridge, 1998).

The mechanisms by which calcium exerts its toxic actions remain controversial. It has been proposed that an increase in $[Ca^{2+}]_i$ may over-stimulate cellular processes that normally operate at low levels, or it may trigger certain cascades that are not usually functional (Tymianski & Tator, 1996). Some of the mechanisms directly activated by calcium or Ca^{2+}-calmodulin include energy depletion due to a loss of mitochondrial membrane potential, the production of ROS, membrane gap formation through an over-activation of phospholipase A2, calpain-induced cytoskeleton breakdown, and endonuclease mediated DNA degradation (Nicholls et al., 2003, Verkhratsky, 2007). Also, excessive calcium induces peroxidation of phospholipids and a release of arachidonic acid, which is metabolized to proinflammatory eicosanoids.

In addition to causing calcium dys-homeostasis, excitotoxicity also induces acidosis inside the cells and in the extracellular space. There are several mechanisms by which pH decreases with neuronal injury. Mitochondrial damage forces the cell to a shift from aerobic to anaerobic metabolism and as a result the glucose is oxidized to lactate with the formation of only two ATPs and the release of two protons (Chan et al., 2006). After trauma and ischemia, extracellular lactate increases dramatically and the pH decreases. To ensure neuronal viability during human hypoxia, oxygen is reserved for neurons and astroglial glycogen is oxidized to lactate, which is rapidly transported into neurons for its complete oxidation, to satisfy the high energy demand and prevent further damage (Sibson et al., 1998). Protons also appear during some chemical reactions such as phospholipid hydrolysis. In parallel, calcium influx causes a rapid cytoplasmic acidification (Werth & Thayer, 1994) through the membrane Na^+/H^+ exchanger that restores the Na^+ gradient and the Ca^{2+}-dependent displacement of protons bound to cytoplasmic anions (Tymianski & Tator, 1996).

Although the mechanisms by which acidosis produces neuronal damage remain unclear, some hypotheses have been proposed. Protons may reduce K^+ conductance and thus facilitate action potentials. Moreover, reinforced by energetic depletion, a pH decrease inhibits the Na^+/Ca^{2+} exchange, thereby contributing to the breakdown of membrane potential and increasing the $[Ca^{2+}]_i$ again. Acidosis may also inhibit neurotransmitter re-uptake, enhance free radical production and accelerate DNA damage (Tymianski & Tator, 1996). However, a pH decrease also helps prevent further neuronal damage by NMDA receptor blockade and Ca^{2+} influx reduction into the cell (Kaku et al., 1993).

As a consequence of the excessive $[Ca^{2+}]_i$ and acidosis nucleation of calcium phosphate crystals (i.e. hydroxyapatite crystals) frequently occurs in the cytoplasm of injured neurons and astrocytes, leading to a process of tissue calcification. Cellular microcalcification has been observed in a variety of human pathologies, such as vascular dementia, Alzheimer's disease (AD), Parkinson's disease (PD), astrogliomas, and post-traumatic epilepsy, and also develops in rodent excitotoxic models of CNS injury in a common pattern. (Ramonet et al., 2006, Rodríguez et al., 2001). Excitotoxic paradigms in rat CNS lead to intracellular calcium precipitation similar to brain calcification in humans (Ramonet et al., 2002, 2006). These experiments demonstrate that calcium deposit formation does not depend on the glutamate receptor subtype initially stimulated, but rather on the cell type involved. Although the significance of cell calcification is unknown, some findings point to calcium precipitation as a mechanism to overcome excitotoxicity. The homogeneous morphology of these deposits in CNS areas and pathologies suggests common synaptic processes (Ramonet et al., 2006), where variability depends on cellular type (astrocyte or neuron), glutamatergic activity, and energy availability. Thus, hydroxyapatite formation brings about a reduction in free calcium ions with no energy expenditure, which may constitute an alternative homeostatic step in reducing excitotoxicity after CNS damage. (Ramonet et al., 2006, Rodriguez et al., 2000)

2.2 Energy availability determines cell survival or death

Ultimately, acute brain damage can be viewed as an energy crisis that results from either an impaired energy production, as in ischemia or hypoglycemia, or pathologically elevated energy demands, as in a sustained seizure (Sapolsky, 2001). Early energy depletion leads to ischemic cell death. Within a few minutes, the membrane potential is lost and thus the neuronal and glial cells become depolarized. This activates the presynaptic, voltage-dependent calcium channels and results in the release of excitatory amino acids into the extracellular space, thereby inducing further neuronal calcium overload, release of intracellular ROS and depletion of glutathione (Orrenius et al., 2003). This primary injury then expands through an excitotoxic spiral, which involves ever-increasing mitochondrial dysfunction, an increase in $[Ca^{2+}]_i$, the release of glutamate, membrane depolarization, ROS production, acidosis, and NMDA receptor desensitization (Figure 2). If the homeostatic threshold is exceeded, the activation of proteases would further accelerates this cycle, which finally results in excitotoxic cell death (Mattson, 2006, Orrenius et al., 2003).

Neuronal demise resulting from excitotoxicity was classically believed to lack the regulated series of events involved in a death program and was therefore considered to be invariably necrotic. However, key regulators of apoptosis, such as p53, Bcl-2 and caspases, are also involved in excitotoxicity and ischemic CNS injury, and a wide continuous spectrum of situations between apoptosis and necrosis has finally been redefined (Nicotera et al., 1999).

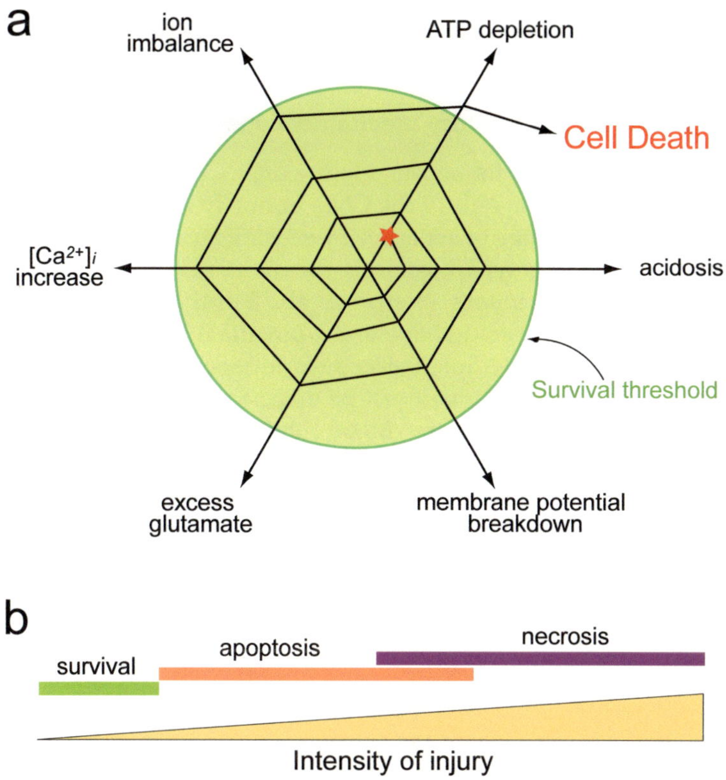

Fig. 2. Accelerating loops of excitotoxicity and cell death. a) An initial insult causes a limited disturbance of cellular homeostasis; the starting point (red star) being for example the ATP depletion due to a discrete localized hypoxia. Looping mechanisms cause an ever increasing mitochondrial dysfunction and acidosis, an increase in $[Ca^{2+}]_i$ and in glutamate release, with membrane depolarization and ion imbalance. Beyond a certain threshold, the activation of cell death program would further accelerate the cycles leading to neuronal death. b) Under mild injury, the initial aggression would be compensated by cellular defense mechanisms; with a more severe damage, neurons would die by apoptosis, necrosis or a mixed program (adapted from Nicotera et al., 1999).

After a stroke, collateral vessels maintain sufficient blood flow to allow the potential survival of cells in areas adjacent to the core of the infarct. Cells in this penumbra area have impaired function but remain viable for a period of time (Vosler et al., 2009). In the area where oxygen depletion is only moderate, cells can activate their own apoptotic program, which requires ATP to be executed. The mitochondria play a role in either necrotic or apoptotic cell death, depending on the severity of the initial insult (Beal, 2000). Apoptosis is favored after mild insults when ATP production of the cell is relatively well preserved, whereas necrosis occurs in response to a severe insult, such as severe ischemia. Cells then die rapidly due to cell swelling, activation of proteases, and cell membrane breakdown. Thus, for each cell type, the factors that determine the pattern of cell death at any moment are the intensity of the lesion, the $[Ca^{2+}]_i$ and the cellular energy production. The cell then prevents the uncontrolled release of intracellular compounds (e.g. glutamate) and the subsequent inflammatory response of tissue. As ATP decreases, the necrotic process starts presenting a hybrid pattern involving both cell death types (Figure 2).

2.3 Neuroinflammation as a retaliatory mechanism against CNS damage

Inflammatory cells participate in tissue remodeling after CNS injury. Microglia, which are generally considered the immune cells of the CNS, normally monitor the brain environment and respond to the functional state of synapses by sensing and eliminating defunct synapses (Wake et al., 2009), controlling synaptogenesis (Bessis et al., 2007) and clearing newborn adult hippocampal neuroprogenitors (Sierra et al., 2010). After CNS injury, microglia become reactive, adopt an amoeboid shape and upregulate a variety of surface molecules and the release of cytokines. In addition, marked recruitment, proliferation and activation of microglial cell precursors from the blood can be detected in damaged regions of the brain (Soulet & Rivest, 2008), and when the blood brain barrier (BBB) integrity has been compromised by the insult, a variety of inflammatory cells, such as activated leukocytes, rapidly penetrate the brain (Frijns & Kappelle, 2002). These inflammatory cells have a dual role in the early and late stages of stroke. For instance, regardless of the cellular origin, MMP-9 is initially detrimental but promotes brain regeneration and neurovascular remodeling in the later repair phase (Amantea et al., 2009), and therefore may be involved in further brain damage or repair.

In addition to microglia, astrocytes and endothelial cells are also involved in the intracerebral immune response to CNS injury. All of these cell types act, in part, by secreting cytokines, chemokines, neurotrophic or neurotoxic factors (Bailey et al., 2006). For example, activated microglial cells migrate towards dying neurons in response to neuroinflammation and can exacerbate local cell damage (Streit, 2005). Microglia also respond to interferon (IFN)γ and tumor necrosis factor (TNF)-α by expressing class I and II major histocompatibility complex molecules (MHC-I and -II, respectively) as well as co-stimulatory molecules, which allows them to function as antigen-presenting cells (Kettenmann et al., 2011). Astrocytes that also express MHC molecules, but lack co-stimulatory molecules, can present antigen to primed memory T cells but not to naive T cells (Neumann et al., 1996). Furthermore, astrocytes respond by releasing other complement proteins and acute-phase proteins, such as α1-antichymotrypsin and α2-macroglobulin, as well as neuronal growth factors and cytokines (Kettenmann et al., 2011). As a hallmark, microglia are normally the first cells in the brain to react to acute injury and recruit astrocytes by secreting acute-phase proteins, particularly those belonging to the complement system, and also by releasing cytokines, such as interleukin (IL)-1β and TNF-α, and ROS species (Kettenmann et al., 2011). Unlike their role in phagocytosis, activated microglia are classified as antigen-presenting cells, as they upregulate MHC-II, and under certain conditions following brain inflammation or injury, activated microglia aid in brain repair, providing a potent neuroprotection (Carson et al., 2006) or acting as a proneurogenic influence that supports the different steps of neurogenesis (Ekdahl et al., 2009).

Microglia do not constitute a unique cell population, but rather, show a range of phenotypes (Schwartz et al., 2006) that are closely related to the evolution of the lesion process (Graeber & Streit, 2010). In a dynamic equilibrium with the lesion microenvironment, these phenotypes range from the well-known proinflammatory activation state (classically activated or M1) to a neurotrophic one that is involved in cell repair and extracellular matrix remodeling (alternatively activated or M2) (Dirscherl et al., 2010). Thus, microglia differentiate into cells that exacerbate tissue injury or promote CNS repair when they receive signals from the close surroundings. M1 microglia/macrophages, activated via toll-like receptors and IFNγ, produce proinflammatory cytokines and oxidative metabolites that facilitate their role as indiscriminate killers of infectious agents and tumor cells (Mantovani et al., 2004), with collateral damage to healthy cells and tissue. Conversely, M2 microglia/macrophages form in the presence of IL-4 or IL-13, downregulate inflammation, and facilitate wound healing, with the induction of scavenger receptors and matrix-degrading enzymes that enhance phagocytosis and promote tissue repair, i.e., by promoting angiogenesis and matrix remodeling (Mantovani et al., 2004, Sica et al., 2006). Furthermore, the crosstalk between elements of the neuroinflammatory response and those that interact with neural stem cells might activate endogenous neurogenesis and facilitate brain repair (Rolls et al., 2007).

3. Acute brain injury can trigger neurodegeneration

Acute brain injury can also activate a neurodegenerative process whose effects are time-dependent and related to the initial severity of insult. For example, acute neurological injury and chronic brain damage have been linked in boxers, with a correlation between the prevalence of subdural hematoma and dementia pugilistica (Miele et al., 2006). Also, cerebrovascular diseases and processes initiated by ischemia reperfusion may be central in the pathogenesis of AD (Zlokovic, 2005), including abnormal protein aggregation processes.

Neurodegenerative disorders are characterized by distinct clinical features that result from a discrete progressive neuronal loss, leading to specific structural alterations in the brain and various forms of cerebral dysfunction over periods of years. However, common molecular and cellular processes, such as excitotoxicity, $[Ca^{2+}]_i$ increase, energy failure and chronic inflammation may also underlie different neurodegenerative diseases (Lau & Tymianski, 2010). In these situations, as described for acute CNS injury, a link between the over-activation of excitatory amino acid receptors, an increase in $[Ca^{2+}]_i$, energy failure, and neuronal death has also been established (Bano et al., 2005, Randall & Thayer, 1992).

3.1 Chronic excitotoxicity as part of neurodegenerative processes

Glutamate excitotoxicity has been inextricably linked to ischemic CNS injury and secondary injuries that occur following traumatic brain injury, whereas the chronic glutamate-mediated over-excitation of neurons is a newer concept that has linked excitotoxicity to neurodegenerative processes in amyotrophic lateral sclerosis (ALS), Huntington's disease, AD and PD (Lau & Tymianski, 2010). Such a chronic excitotoxic process can be triggered by a dysfunction of glutamate synapses, due to an anomaly at the pre-synaptic, post-synaptic, or astroglial level (Rodriguez et al., 2009b). For example, loss of ionotropic receptor selectivity and deficiencies in glial glutamate re-uptake are present in ALS (Obrenovitch et al., 2000). These dysfunctions also help to explain phenomena such as the aging-related hypoactivity of NMDA receptors observed in AD (Olney et al., 1997) and the AMPA-receptor increase detected in the hippocampus of aged-impaired rats (Le Jeune et al., 1996).

The contribution of excitotoxicity to the neurodegenerative process can be reproduced by the microinjection of low doses of glutamate agonist into the rodent brain. Due to the high affinity of ionotropic glutamate receptors for their specific agonists, NMDA, AMPA or kainate injected in non-saturable conditions can trigger calcium-mediated excitotoxicity in several rat brain areas and induce an ongoing neurodegenerative process (Bernal et al., 2000, Petegnief et al., 2004, Rodriguez et al., 2000, Rodriguez et al., 2004). For example, any microinjection of glutamate agonist in the rat medial septum triggers a persistent process that leads to a progressive septal atrophy with a cholinergic and GABAergic neuronal loss and a concomitant neuroinflammation that does not parallel the lesion (Rodriguez et al., 2009a). These paradigms also mimic the alterations of other neurotransmitter systems and neuromodulators found in human neurodegeneration. Thus, long-term ibotenic-induced lesion in the rat basal forebrain leads to a loss of cholinergic afferents and decreased extracellular noradrenaline, glutamate, and taurine. At a functional level, excitotoxic disruption of the septohippocampal pathway also consistently reproduces some of AD memory impairments (Waite et al., 1994).

CNS damage caused by an acute injury directly depends on the initial severity and the time elapsed after injury. But each variable activates different mechanisms. Comparison of the rat medial septum response to the insult caused by graded concentrations of AMPA with the time-course effects of a low dose of AMPA showed evidence of marked differences in the lesion dynamism (Rodriguez et al., 2009a). Thus, the medium dose of AMPA increased calcification and the degree of microglia reaction in the GABAergic region of the septal area, whereas atrophy and neuronal loss only reached a plateau with the higher AMPA doses. Results of a six-month study with a low AMPA-dose evidenced a progressive increase in neuronal death and septal atrophy with astrogliosis and microgliosis during the first month, and a total absence of calcium precipitates. Septal damage does not then increase with the intensity of an excitotoxic insult, but rather it progresses with time, meaning different mechanisms are involved in each situation.

3.2 Uncoupling of retaliatory systems and energy availability

Given the toxic effects of glutamate-mediated over-stimulation, adaptations that act to decrease synaptic accumulation of glutamate have the potential to be protective. Within these protective mechanisms, some are conducted to inhibit glutamate release during insults and some others involve retrograde signaling of inhibitory neurotransmitters and neuromodulators. Thus, the release of GABA, taurine and adenosine presents a retaliatory activity that has shown neuroprotective properties during glutamate-mediated neuronal insults (see Sapolsky, 2001 for a review). All of the processes mediated by these neuromodulators are interdependent and the coordination between the effects of GABA, taurine and adenosine helps avoid excessive synaptic glutamate and control neuronal damage.

Control of synaptic glutamate levels, when not coupled to energy production, renders neurons susceptible to death. Under controlled conditions, the stoichiometric coupling of glutamatergic activity and glucose metabolism accounts for 80% of total cerebral glucose (Sibson et al., 1998). Part of this energy is needed for glutamate recycling in a coordinated process involving astrocytes and neurons, with 15% of brain oxidative metabolism contributed by astroglia (Lebon et al., 2002). A reduction in energy availability and the consequent altered glutamate activity may then play a role in apoptotic or necrotic neuronal death (Ramonet et al., 2004).

However, the balance between retaliatory system actions and energy metabolism can be disrupted by glutamate-mediated neuronal injury and then play a role in the evoked neurodegenerative process. For example, AMPA microinjection in the medial septum induces a progressive neuronal loss associated with a long-term decline of the hippocampal functions and decreased GABAergic and glutamatergic activities (Rodriguez et al., 2005). By contrast, this same hippocampal lesion increases adenosine and taurine transmissions, glutamate recycling and glucose metabolism (Ramonet et al., 2004, Rodriguez et al., 2005). Over time, adenosine replaces GABA in the control of glutamate neurotransmission to avoid further excitotoxic damage when cholinergic and GABAergic processes are compromised. This same lesion paradigm induces apoptotic neuronal loss in the hippocampus with enhancement of neuronal glycolysis and a glutamate/glutamine cycle displacement towards glutamine production that decreases glutamate concentration (Ramonet et al., 2004). In addition, glutamine is removed from the synapses, probably through vessels, where it inhibits NO synthesis, exhibiting a clear vasodilatory effect. In this scenario, the hippocampal increase in neuronal energy metabolism, which is associated with a decreased glutamate neurotransmission and neuronal apoptotic death, reflects a neurodegenerative process with unfulfilled coordination of the retaliatory systems and a chronic energy requirement to execute the apoptotic program.

3.3 Neurodegeneration results from dysregulation of calcium homeostasis

As mentioned above, the over-activation of glutamate receptors results in a massive increase in the cytoplasm calcium levels, which requires considerable energy expenditure to restore $[Ca^{2+}]_i$ to its physiological basal level. Dysregulation of calcium homeostasis alters the rapid and coherent activation of neurons and is therefore ultimately responsible for many common aspects of brain dysfunction in neurodegenerative diseases. For example, calcium-mediated apoptosis may underlie the etiology of chronic neurodegenerative disorders such as AD and PD.

In AD pathogenesis, multiple cellular and molecular alterations involve alterations in synaptic calcium handling and perturbed cellular calcium homeostasis. With ageing neurons encounter increased oxidative stress and impaired energy metabolism, which compromise the control of membrane excitability and $[Ca^{2+}]_i$ dynamics (Camandola & Mattson, 2011). Also in AD, elevated intracellular calcium levels contribute to the enhanced amyloidogenic processing of the amyloid-beta precursor protein (APP) (Liang et al., 2010) and mediates its cytotoxic effects. The cytotoxic actions of amyloid beta (Aβ) involve calcium as a central mediator of pathological actions through two mechanisms. First, when aggregating at the cell surface Aβ generates ROS, which results in membrane lipid peroxidation (Mark et al., 1997) that ultimately impairs glucose and glutamate transporters thereby promoting excitotoxicity (Keller et al., 1997, Mark et al., 1997). As a second mechanism, Aβ oligomers may form calcium-permeable pores in the plasma membrane. Also, glutamate receptor-mediated calcium elevations cause changes in tau protein similar to those seen in neurofibrillary tangles (Mattson, 1990). Other studies report that preseniline-1 mutations perturb calcium dynamics at the glutamatergic and cholinergic synapses, suggesting a pivotal role for aberrant neuronal calcium regulation in AD.

Since alterations in calcium homeostasis have also been reported in other neurodegenerative disorders associated with an accumulation of misfolded protein aggregates, including PD, Huntington's disease, ALS, and transmissible spongiform encephalopathies (TSEs) (Camandola & Mattson, 2011), these alterations are considered a common pathophysiological factor linked to neuronal degeneration. Thus, neurodegenerative diseases that exhibit diverse clinical and neuropathological phenotypes share the common features of glutamate-mediated over-excitation and calcium dyshomeostasis. Together with misfolded protein aggregation, these features participate in the pathogenic process that progressively reduces cell function and survival within the nervous system, leading to neurological disability and often death. Therefore, the different CNS aggressions of genetic, infectious, environmental or other origins can induce the same neurodegenerative injury. This convergence is due to the multi-directional interactions between the neurons, glial cells, extracellular matrix, endothelia and host immune cells that regulate tissue homeostasis and orchestrate the tissue response to the insult.

3.4 Molecular mechanisms of misfolded protein aggregation

Nearly all neurodegenerative disorders, such as AD, PD, Huntington's disease, TSEs, Tauopathies, ALS, and frontotemporal lobar degeneration with ubiquitin-positive inclusions, share common neuropathology (Forman et al., 2004). Thus, since they primarily feature the presence of abnormal protein inclusions containing specific misfolded proteins, these disorders are also classified as misfolded protein diseases (MPD). Some of these misfolding proteins are polyglutamine, protease-resistant prion protein, Aβ, Tau, α-synuclein, SOD1, TDP-43 or FUS, and share no common sequence or structural identity (Morales et al., 2010; Soto et al., 2006). Protein aggregation defines neurodegenerative diseases broadly, but with significant differences between the affected areas of CNS and the damaged neuronal type. For example, cholinergic neurons are preferentially affected in AD, dopaminergic neurons in PD, and motor neurons in ALS.

Correct folding requires proteins to assume one particular structure and failure to adopt its proper structure is a major threat to cell function and viability. Consequently, elaborated systems have evolved to protect cells from misfolded proteins, including the molecular chaperones that promote proper protein folding and the ubiquitin-proteasome system that degrades the newly translated proteins that failed to fold correctly (Gitler & Shorter 2011). In this system, the misfolded protein accumulation often reflects the cellular response to an imbalanced protein homeostasis, and relates to a perturbation of cellular function and aging. As mentioned above, all of the protective systems need abundant concomitant cellular energy production, and the frequent hypoxic or hypoglycemic incidents associated with hypercholesterolemia, diabetes and hypertension reduce energy availability and participate in the pathogenesis of neurodegenerative diseases (Forman et al., 2004, Haces et al., 2010). Consequently, these misfolded proteins develop insidiously in patients over their lifetime, and manifest clinically until middle or late life, as a MPD.

The common pathogenic mechanism of MPD represents the initial aggregation and CNS deposition of one type of misfolded protein in the nucleus or cytosol of specific neurons and/or well-located extracellular space (Gadad et al., 2011). In fact, the amyloid formation follows a crystallization-like process, known as seeding-nucleation, which, through a slow interaction between misfolded protein monomers, initially forms an oligomeric nucleus, or seed, around which a second, faster phase of elongation takes place. The nuclei formation is a slow process and represents the limiting step, and the extent of amyloidosis depends on the number of seeds produced (Carulla et al., 2010). In time, the progressive aggregation of fibrillar structures, with short stretches of β-pleated sheet stabilized by intermolecular interactions and oriented perpendicular to the fibril axis, leads to abundant extended insoluble amyloidogenic proteins, with deleterious effects (Sanchez et al., 2011). The formation of different oligomeric aggregates also occurs, and the exposure of their hydrophobic amino acid residues on their external surface changes their solubility and interactions with their cellular targets. For example, in AD, a soluble 4 kDa peptide is initially produced and the amyloidogenic Aβ, which is identified as the main component of AD oligomers and senile plaques, readily interacts with other Aβ molecules to progressively form a wide range of oligomers and soluble aggregates (Carulla et al., 2005). This continued amyloidogenesis gives rise to the high molecular weight and insoluble amyloid fibrils that are highly abundant in senile plaques. Aβ plays a recurring role in protein phosphorylation, signal transduction mechanisms, cytoskeletal organization, multiprotein complex formation, and synaptotoxicity, and when analyzing its pathogenic aggregation, the oligomers present the higher neurotoxicity.

All Aβ aggregation states and actions are also influenced by the abnormal activity of transition metal ions. Trapped in fibrils, they completely alter their structure, are electrochemically active, and can generate ROS in the presence of hydrogen peroxide and reducing agents. The biometal age-related dyshomeostasis causes a variation of their activity, especially in metalloproteins like SOD1 or the prion protein. In fact, the variety of binding affinities and binding sites reported for copper to Aβ, α-synuclein, SOD1 and the prion protein indicate that, through these numerous possible interactions, the copper level may directly drive the diversity of the states and functions of these proteins (Drew et al., 2010).

TSEs are considered unique among MPD in that they are transmissible; besides many amyloid pathological aggregates also have the ability to do so, and epidemiological data show that they are not infectious. However, several intriguing experimental results argue for a general infectious principle in protein misfolding and aggregation diseases in the pioneering studies of Westermark (1985) and Higuchi (1983), on systemic amyloidosis associated with the deposition of Amyloid-A and apolipoprotein AII. In PD, the infectious protein would be SNCA, whose abnormal conversion of native from to β-sheet is triggered or supported by various drivers, such as hereditary factors, aging, oxidative stress, or environmental toxins (Taylor et al., 2002). Nevertheless, disease propagation by different protein infectious agents remains to be proven in most neurodegenerative diseases.

3.5 Amyloid beta deposition after acute brain injury

Aβ is a physiological peptide that has a constant turnover in the brain (Saido & Iwata, 2006), and the potential causes for its deposition is the determinant of three main factors: 1) increased expression of APP, 2) aberrant enzymatic cleavage of APP by β- and γ-secretase, and 3) disruption of Aβ clearance from the CNS through the BBB. Therefore, rats subjected to chronic hypoperfusion or cerebral ischemia (Koistinaho & Koistinaho, 2005, Pluta, 2004) may show transient up-regulation and accumulation of APP and Aβ in the cortex boundary and white matter with decreased blood flow, which suggests an interplay between cerebrovascular and amyloid pathology. Therefore, stroke and hypoperfusion are important risk factors for amyloidosis (De La Torre, 2008). In this regard, studies of brain imaging in humans (Johnson et al., 2005, Rombouts & Scheltens, 2005), and animal models of cerebral hypoperfusion and of impaired clearance of Aβ across the BBB by the receptor for advanced glycation end products (RAGE) (Deane et al., 2004), denote that cerebrovascular dysfunction may precede cognitive decline and the onset of neurodegenerative changes in AD (Drzezga et al., 2003). Both increased and impaired brain-to-blood transport of Aβ across the BBB have been observed in AD (Deane et al., 2003). In AD patients, and particularly after ischemia (Fukuda et al., 2004), matrix metalloproteinase machinery is also overexpressed in the cerebral vessels, which can degrade basement membranes and extracellular matrix proteins, and subsequently compromise the BBB integrity. As reviewed in detail elsewhere (Saido & Iwata, 2006), endothelial cells can also directly degrade Aβ-expressing enzymes such as insulin-degrading enzyme and neprilysin. Therefore, if the integrity of the endothelium is compromised by all of these mechanisms, an imbalance of the degradation and clearance of Aβ should be expected.

In addition to the RAGE, low-density lipoprotein receptor related protein 1 is expressed in the vascular-CNS barrier, and both are critical for the regulation of Aβ receptors at the BBB. Their impaired activity may also contribute to the Aβ accumulation resulting in neuroinflammation, disconnection between the cerebral blood flow and metabolism, altered synaptic transmission, neuronal injury, and amyloid deposition into parenchymal and neurovascular lesions (Deane et al., 2004), therefore both receptors are critical for regulation of Aβ homeostasis in the CNS. Indeed, Aβ-RAGE suppression of cerebral blood flow is mediated by endothelial cells secretion of Endothelin-1 (Deane et al., 2003), leading to hypoperfusion and negatively affecting the synthesis of proteins required for memory and learning, and eventually causing neuritic injury and neuronal death.

Axonal injury is one of the most common and important pathological features of brain trauma and ischemia. In these situations, APP is a marker of axonal injury and accumulates due to the disruption of fast anterograde axonal transport (Smith et al., 2003). In particular, lysis of the terminal swollen bulb of disconnected axons may serve as a vehicle for the release of potentially toxic proteins, peptides, and their aggregates into the brain parenchyma. One of these potential toxins is the Aβ peptide, which causes neurodegeneration, acute necrotic damage and long-lasting degenerative processes, that in turn will activate an inflammatory response.

Reactive microglia are closely associated with senile plaques in AD patients, and microglia can contain intracellular deposits of Aβ, which indicates a role for these cells in the clearance and/or processing of Aβ (Mandrekar et al., 2009, Weldon et al., 1998). Heat sock proteins (HSP), which exhibit chaperone activity and are overexpressed following many injuries including AD and stroke (Turturici et al., 2011), induced microglial phagocytosis of Aβ peptides, probably mediated through NF-κB and p38 MAPK pathways and TLR4. Certainly, a possible explanation for phagocytosis activation by microglia is that HSP70–associated peptides are more immunogenic for both MHC class I- and II-dependent systems than peptides alone (Mycko et al., 2004). On the other hand, senile plaque-associated microglia expressed significantly more MHC-II, IL-1, the receptor for macrophage-colony stimulating factor-1, myeloid cell-specific calcium-binding protein MRP14 and CD40, all of which are associated with mononuclear phagocyte activation and inflammation. In addition, CCR3 and CCR5 have also been found in microglia associated with AD plaques, whereas CXCR2 and CXCR3 have been associated with neuritic plaques (Hickman et al., 2008). The CX3CL1/CX3CR1 pathway plays a part in microglia neurotoxicity in vivo, but also participates in microglial phagocytosis of Aβ and activation of the astroglial response (Lee et al., 2010). Interestingly, early microglial recruitment in AD promotes Aβ clearance and is neuroprotective, whereas chronic proinflammatory cytokine production in response to Aβ deposition downregulates genes involved in Aβ clearance, promotes its accumulation, and contributes to neurodegeneration (Hickman et al., 2008). It is noteworthy that in AD patients the classic inflammatory response (immunoglobulin and leucocyte infiltration) is absent (Eikelenboom & Veerhuis, 1996).

The generation of Aβ is initiated by β-secretase cleavage of APP (also called β-site APP-cleaving enzyme, BACE1), which is mostly present in neurons (Vassar et al., 1999). Ischemia strengthens the expression and activity of BACE1 (Wen et al., 2004), and notably, the early post-hypoxic upregulation of BACE1 depends on the production of ROS mediated by the sudden interruption of the mitochondrial electron transport chain, while the later expression of BACE1 is caused by activation of hypoxia inducible factor 1-α (Guglielmotto et al., 2009). After stroke, the activation of caspase-3 induces the ubiquitin-dependent stabilization of BACE1 (Tesco et al., 2007), thereby seeding the formation of oligomeric and fibrillar amyloid structures.

On the other hand, the intramembrane proteases presenilin 1 (PS1) and preselinin 2 (PS2) are part of the γ-secretase catalytic site, which in conjunction with BACE1, processes APP to generate Aβ. After an ischemic event, the γ-secretase activity is increased at the boundary of the infarct (Arumugam et al., 2006). Mutations in the genes encoding PS1 and PS2 cause early-onset familial AD (Thinakaran & Parent, 2004). In addition, mutant PS-expressing and PS-conditional knock out mice have shown aberrant neuroinflammatory response, which suggests a link between PS function and CNS innate immune response regulation (Beglopoulos et al., 2004). In this regard, TNF-α and IFNγ production upregulates BACE1 (Yamamoto et al., 2007) and stimulates γ-secretase-mediated cleavage of APP (Liao et al., 2004). Thus, proinflammatory cytokines would also contribute to AD-like pathology by promoting Aβ generation. Nonetheless, PS expression in microglial cells shows compensatory regulation where PS1 knockdown leads to increased PS2 and vice versa. But only PS2 depletion correlates with decreased γ-secretase function (Jayadev et al., 2010), and only PS2 might be implicated in Aβ phagocytosis by microglial cells (Farfara et al., 2011).

3.6 Chronic neuroinflammation

Neuroinflammation is a common characteristic of the pathological process in neurodegenerative diseases such as PD, AD, ALS, and multiple sclerosis (Graeber & Streit, 2010). Microgliosis is related to the molecular pathology of these diseases and has been associated with misfolded proteins, in the case of PD, ALS and Huntington's disease, where the misfolded proteins accumulate intracellularly, and with extracellular aggregates, as in the case of Aβ in AD. Activation of the microglia is also associated with the formation of calcium precipitates of hydroxyapatites, which are frequently observed in the specific CNS areas involved in neurodegenerative processes (Rodriguez et al., 2009b).

The benefits of such inflammation are substantial. For example, in the early stages of AD, reactive microglia phagocytose and degrade Aβ (Paresce et al., 1997), scavenges and eliminate the debris of dead or dying cells, and therefore protect the brain from its toxic effects (El Khoury et al., 2007) and the effects of other toxic agents released by dying cells (Figure 3). Furthermore, reactive astrocytes isolate neurons from senile plaques and release cytokines and growth factors that may help damaged neurons to survive and recover. However, when the disease progresses and a persistent proinflammatory cytokine production occurs, microglia release high amounts of TNF-α and IL-1β, and therefore lose their protective phenotype and their ability to phagocytose Aβ deposition. In these conditions, microglia become dysfunctional and fail to clear Aβ deposits (Hickman et al., 2008), hence promoting plaque formation (Bolmont et al., 2008). This chronic and uncontrolled inflammatory response can directly lead to the injury or death of neurons (Figure 3). In addition, activated microglia may also be directly involved in the generation of senile plaque pathology, either by the secretion of fibrilar and soluble Aβ (Chung et al., 1999) or by the release of biometals such as iron, which aggregates soluble Aβ fragments. For that reason, this innate immune response is currently considered a potential pathogenic factor for neurodegenerative diseases.

As explained above, microglia respond to tissue injury by adopting a diversity of phenotypes ranging from the deleterious M1 to the neuroprotective M2 (Halliday & Stevens, 2011, Henkel et al., 2009). This range of phenotypes is closely related to the evolution of the lesion process and their control will directly influence the outcome of the tissue. In addition, some microglial cells become increasingly dysfunctional with age and may play a direct role in the development of neurodegeneration (Block et al., 2007, Stoll et al., 2002). Whether microglia adopt a phenotype that mostly exacerbates tissue injury or one that promotes brain repair is likely to depend on the diversity of signals from the lesion environment and the response capacity of the aging cell.

In a complex crosstalk that is being progressively deciphered, astrocytes and inflammatory T-cell subsets influence the proinflammatory or anti-inflammatory responses of microglia, thus affecting their antigen-presenting cell properties and phagocytic capacity. Astrocytes generate local signals, such as glutamate, to communicate with neurons and these signals influence the outcome of the tissue during neurodegeneration (Allaman et al., 2011). They directly influence microglial behaviour by playing a critical role in the activation of microglia under infectious conditions (Ovanesov et al., 2008) and in multiple sclerosis, where MCP-1/CCL2 and IP-10/CXCL10 direct reactive gliosis (Tanuma et al., 2006). Some findings have implicated astrocytes in chronic microgliosis. For example, TNF-α secretion is crucial for rapid autocrine microglial activation with both neuroprotective and cytotoxic effects, a process that is also fed by TNF-α released by reactive astrocytes (Suzumura et al., 2006). These opposing TNF-α actions depend on the activation of two specific receptors: TNFR1, which has a low affinity and an intracellular death domain, and TNFR2, which has a high affinity and is mainly involved in neuroprotection (Fontaine et al., 2002). Therefore, at low concentrations, TNF-α only binds to TNFR2 and potentiates neuronal survival, whereas the subsequent TNF-α secretion by microglia and astrocytes activates TNFR1 in neurons and astrocytes and contributes to cell injury (Bernardino et al., 2008).

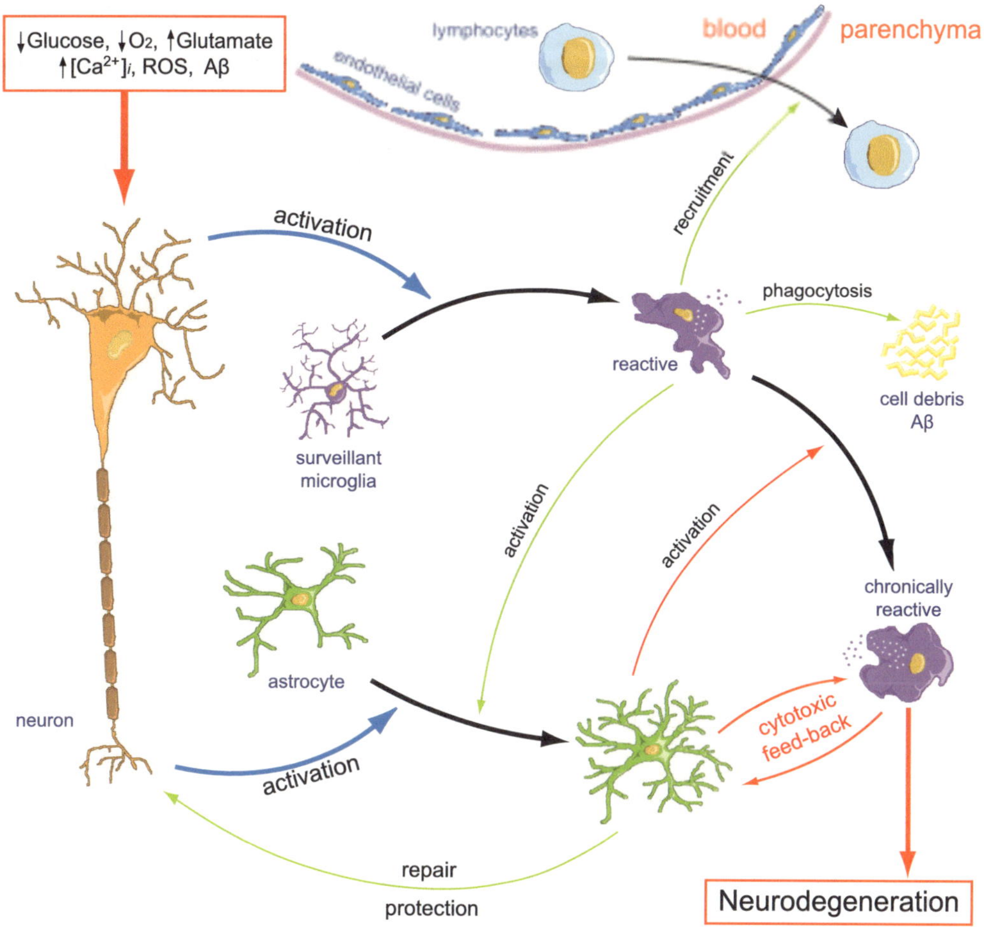

Fig. 3. Cellular processes involving chronic neuroinflammation after brain injury. Physiological modifications (molecules inside a red square) alter neurons, which in turn release activation signals to astrocytes and microglia. Reactive microglia mediate different pro-inflammatory and neuroprotective processes (green arrows) in coordination with reactive astrocytes. With increasing activation signals or reaction times, reactive microglia become increasingly dysfunctional and adopt a chronic reactive phenotype mostly cytotoxic that directly participates of neurodegeneration. Astrocytes may also promote this microglia cytotoxic activity by releasing activation signals (red arrows)

Thus, chronic microgliosis after CNS injury and during neurodegeneration involves a putative transition from an initial neuroprotective activity to a cytotoxic activity, and the interaction of astrocytes in the lesion site that promote the cytotoxic microglial phenotype through the secretion of TNF-α and other signals (Donato et al., 2009, Suzumura et al., 2006). In this scenario, the interplay between the trophic, neuroprotective, inflammatory and cytotoxic functions of microglia and astrocytes in acute and chronic CNS injury will determine the evolution of the neurodegenerative process. Control of this time-depending crosstalk requires a precise and dynamic analysis of the interactions so as to effectively develop approaches to neuroprotection and restoration of the injured tissue.

4. Conclusions

CNS injuries such as stroke, traumatic brain injury and spinal cord injury, are characterized by the appearance of common parameters that determine the outcome of the tissue and account for the ensuing neurodegenerative process underlied by glutamate-mediated excitotoxicity, calcium dyshomeostasis and neuroinflammation. At the tissue level, the pathogenesis of each disorder depends primarily on the availability of energy but also on the neuronal type involved, the synaptic density, the glial interactions, and the vicinity of vascularization. These parameters also underlie the ensuing neurodegenerative process that will determine the dynamics and progression of the disease but also the success of regenerative therapies.

The literature suggests that several treatment interventions can promote the regeneration of damaged tissue after an acute injury. The degree of such regeneration remains modest, but the diversity of mechanisms that may promote tissue recovery increases the options for developing new therapies. Therefore, future therapeutic approaches should include dealing with excitotoxicity and energy production, and controlling neuroinflammatory pathways, as complementary treatments to those addressed to overcome the inhibitory mechanisms that block regeneration and to enhance neuronal plasticity.

5. Acknowledgements

This research was supported by grants SAF2008-01902 and IPT-010000-2010-35 from the Ministerio de Ciencia e Innovación, and by grant 2009SGR1380 from the Generalitat de Catalunya, Spain.

6. References

Allaman, I., Belanger, M. & Magistretti, P.J. (2011). Astrocyte-neuron metabolic relationships: for better and for worse. *Trends Neurosci*, Vol. 34, No. 2, pp. 76-87, ISSN 1878-108X

Amantea, D., Nappi, G., Bernardi, G., Bagetta, G. & Corasaniti, M.T. (2009). Post-ischemic brain damage: pathophysiology and role of inflammatory mediators. *FEBS J*, Vol. 276, No. 1, pp. 13-26, ISSN 1742-4658

Arumugam, T.V., Chan, S.L., Jo, D.G., Yilmaz, G., Tang, S.C., Cheng, A., Gleichmann, M., Okun, E., Dixit, V.D., Chigurupati, S., Mughal, M.R., Ouyang, X., Miele, L., Magnus, T., Poosala, S., Granger, D.N. & Mattson, M.P. (2006). Gamma secretase-mediated Notch signaling worsens brain damage and functional outcome in ischemic stroke. *Nat Med*, Vol. 12, No. 6, pp. 621-3, ISSN 1078-8956

Bailey, S.L., Carpentier, P.A., Mcmahon, E.J., Begolka, W.S. & Miller, S.D. (2006). Innate and adaptive immune responses of the central nervous system. *Crit Rev Immunol*, Vol. 26, No. 2, pp. 149-88, ISSN 1040-8401

Bano, D., Young, K.W., Guerin, C.J., Lefeuvre, R., Rothwell, N.J., Naldini, L., Rizzuto, R., Carafoli, E. & Nicotera, P. (2005). Cleavage of the plasma membrane Na^+/Ca^{2+} exchanger in excitotoxicity. *Cell*, Vol. 120, No. 2, pp. 275-85, ISSN 0092-8674

Beal, M.F. (2000). Energetics in the pathogenesis of neurodegenerative diseases. *Trends Neurosci*, Vol. 23, No. 7, pp. 298-304, ISSN 0166-2236

Beck, A., Nieden, R.Z., Scheinder, H.P. & Deitmer, J.W. (2004). Calcium release from intracellular stores in rodent astrocytes and neurons in situ. *Cell Calcium*, Vol. 35 No. pp. 47-58, ISSN 0143-4160

Beglopoulos, V., Sun, X., Saura, C.A., Lemere, C.A., Kim, R.D. & Shen, J. (2004). Reduced beta-amyloid production and increased inflammatory responses in presenilin conditional knock-out mice. *J Biol Chem*, Vol. 279, No. 45, pp. 46907-14, ISSN 0021-9258

Bernal, F., Saura, J., Ojuel, J. & Mahy, N. (2000). Differential vulnerability of hippocampus, basal ganglia and prefrontal cortex to long-term NMDA excitotoxicity. *Exp Neurol*, Vol. 161, No. pp. 686-695, ISSN 0014-4886

Bernardino, L., Agasse, F., Silva, B., Ferreira, R., Grade, S. & Malva, J.O. (2008). Tumor necrosis factor-alpha modulates survival, proliferation, and neuronal differentiation in neonatal subventricular zone cell cultures. *Stem Cells*, Vol. 26, No. 9, pp. 2361-2371, ISSN 1066-5099

Berridge, M.J. (1998). Neuronal calcium signaling. *Neuron*, Vol. 21, No. pp. 13-26, ISSN 0896-6273

Bessis, A., Bechade, C., Bernard, D. & Roumier, A. (2007). Microglial control of neuronal death and synaptic properties. *Glia*, Vol. 55, No. 3, pp. 233-8, ISSN 0894-1491

Block, M.L., Zecca, L. & Hong, J.S. (2007). Microglia-mediated neurotoxicity: uncovering the molecular mechanisms. *Nat.Rev.Neurosci.*, Vol. 8, No. pp. 57-69, ISSN 1471-003X

Bolmont, T., Haiss, F., Eicke, D., Radde, R., Mathis, C.A., Klunk, W.E., Kohsaka, S., Jucker, M. & Calhoun, M.E. (2008). Dynamics of the microglial/amyloid interaction indicate a role in plaque maintenance. *J Neurosci*, Vol. 28, No. 16, pp. 4283-92, ISSN 1529-2401

Camandola S & Mattson MP. (2011) Aberrant subcellular neuronal calcium regulation in aging and Alzheimer's disease. Biochim Biophys Acta, Vol 1813, pp. 965-973, ISSN 0005-2728

Carson, M.J., Thrash, J.C. & Walter, B. (2006). The cellular response in neuroinflammation: The role of leukocytes, microglia and astrocytes in neuronal death and survival. *Clin Neurosci Res*, Vol. 6, No. 5, pp. 237-245, ISSN 1566-2772

Carulla, N., Caddy, G.L., Hall, D.R., Zurdo, J., Gairi, M., Feliz, M., Giralt, E., Robinson, C.V. & Dobson, C.M. (2005). Molecular recycling within amyloid fibrils. *Nature*, Vol. 436, No. 7050, pp. 554-8, ISSN 1476-4687

Carulla, N., Zhou, M., Giralt, E., Robinson, C.V. & Dobson, C.M. (2010). Structure and intermolecular dynamics of aggregates populated during amyloid fibril formation studied by hydrogen/deuterium exchange. *Acc Chem Res*, Vol. 43, No. 8, pp. 1072-9, ISSN 1520-4898

Chan, S.L., Liu, D., Kyriazis, G.A., Bagsiyao, P., Ouyang, X. & Mattson, M.P. (2006). Mitochondrial uncoupling protein-4 regulates calcium homeostasis and sensitivity to store-depletion-induced apoptosis in neural cells. *J Biol Chem*, Vol. 281 No. 49 pp.37391-37403, ISSN 0021-9258

Chen, Q., Olney, J.W., Lukasiewicz, P.D., Almli, T. & Romano, C. (1998). Ca^{2+}-independent excitotoxic neurodegeneration in isolated retina, an intact neural net: a role for Cl^- and inhibitory transmitters. *Mol Pharmacol*, Vol. 53, No. 3, pp. 564-572, ISSN 0026-895X

Chung, H., Brazil, M.I., Soe, T.T. & Maxfield, F.R. (1999). Uptake, degradation, and release of fibrillar and soluble forms of Alzheimer's amyloid beta-peptide by microglial cells. *J Biol Chem*, Vol. 274, No. 45, pp. 32301-8, ISSN 0021-9258

De La Torre, J.C. (2008). Alzheimer's disease prevalence can be lowered with non-invasive testing. *J Alzheimers Dis*, Vol. 14, No. 3, pp. 353-9, ISSN 1387-2877

Deane, R., Du Yan, S., Submamaryan, R.K., Larue, B., Jovanovic, S., Hogg, E., Welch, D., Manness, L., Lin, C., Yu, J., Zhu, H., Ghiso, J., Frangione, B., Stern, A., Schmidt, A.M., Armstrong, D.L., Arnold, B., Liliensiek, B., Nawroth, P., Hofman, F., Kindy, M., Stern, D. & Zlokovic, B. (2003). RAGE mediates amyloid-beta peptide transport across the blood-brain barrier and accumulation in brain. *Nat Med*, Vol. 9, No. 7, pp. 907-13, ISSN 1078-8956

Deane, R., Wu, Z. & Zlokovic, B.V. (2004). RAGE (yin) versus LRP (yang) balance regulates alzheimer amyloid beta-peptide clearance through transport across the blood-brain barrier. *Stroke*, Vol. 35, No. 11 Suppl 1, pp. 2628-31, ISSN 1524-4628

Dirscherl, K., Karlstetter, M., Ebert, S., Kraus, D., Hlawatsch, J., Walczak, Y., Moehle, C., Fuchshofer, R. & Langmann, T. (2010). Luteolin triggers global changes in the microglial transcriptome leading to a unique anti-inflammatory and neuroprotective phenotype. *J Neuroinflammation*, Vol. 7, No. 3, pp. 3, ISSN 1742-2094

Donato, R., Sorci, G., Riuzzi, F., Arcuri, C., Bianchi, R., Brozzi, F., Tubaro, C. & Giambanco, I. (2009). S100B's double life: intracellular regulator and extracellular signal. *Biochim Biophys Acta*, Vol. 1793, No. 6, pp. 1008-1022, ISSN 0304-4165

Drew, S.C., Masters, C.L. & Barnham, K.J. (2010). Alzheimer's Abeta peptides with disease-associated N-terminal modifications: influence of isomerisation, truncation and mutation on Cu2+ coordination. *PLoS One*, Vol. 5, No. 12, pp. e15875, ISSN 1932-6203

Drzezga, A., Lautenschlager, N., Siebner, H., Riemenschneider, M., Willoch, F., Minoshima, S., Schwaiger, M. & Kurz, A. (2003). Cerebral metabolic changes accompanying conversion of mild cognitive impairment into Alzheimer's disease: a PET follow-up study. *Eur J Nucl Med Mol Imaging*, Vol. 30, No. 8, pp. 1104-13, ISSN 1619-7070

Eikelenboom, P. & Veerhuis, R. (1996). The role of complement and activated microglia in the pathogenesis of Alzheimer's disease. *Neurobiol Aging*, Vol. 17, No. 5, pp. 673-80, ISSN 0197-4580

Ekdahl, C.T., Kokaia, Z. & Lindvall, O. (2009). Brain inflammation and adult neurogenesis: the dual role of microglia. *Neuroscience*, Vol. 158, No. 3, pp. 1021-1029, ISSN 0306-4522

El Khoury, J., Toft, M., Hickman, S.E., Means, T.K., Terada, K., Geula, C. & Luster, A.D. (2007). Ccr2 deficiency impairs microglial accumulation and accelerates progression of Alzheimer-like disease. *Nat Med*, Vol. 13, No. 4, pp. 432-8, ISSN 1078-8956

Farfara, D., Trudler, D., Segev-Amzaleg, N., Galron, R., Stein, R. & Frenkel, D. (2011). gamma-Secretase component presenilin is important for microglia beta-amyloid clearance. *Ann Neurol*, Vol. 69, No. 1, pp. 170-80, 1531-8249

Fontaine, V., Mohand-Said, S., Hanoteau, N., Fuchs, C., Pfizenmaier, K. & Eisel, U. (2002). Neurodegenerative and neuroprotective effects of tumor Necrosis factor (TNF) in retinal ischemia: opposite roles of TNF receptor 1 and TNF receptor 2. *J Neurosci*, Vol. 22, No. 7, pp. RC216, ISSN 1529-2401

Forman, M.S., Trojanowski, J.Q. & Lee, V.M. (2004). Neurodegenerative diseases: a decade of discoveries paves the way for therapeutic breakthroughs. *Nat Med*, Vol. 10, No. 10, pp. 1055-63, ISSN 1078-8956

Frijns, C.J. & Kappelle, L.J. (2002). Inflammatory cell adhesion molecules in ischemic cerebrovascular disease. *Stroke*, Vol. 33, No. 8, pp. 2115-22, ISSN 1524-4628

Fukuda, S., Fini, C.A., Mabuchi, T., Koziol, J.A., Eggleston, L.L., Jr. & Del Zoppo, G.J. (2004). Focal cerebral ischemia induces active proteases that degrade microvascular matrix. *Stroke*, Vol. 35, No. 4, pp. 998-1004, ISSN 1524-4628

Gadad, B.S., Britton, G.B. & Rao, K.S. (2011). Targeting oligomers in neurodegenerative disorders: lessons from alpha-synuclein, tau, and amyloid-beta peptide. *J Alzheimers Dis*, Vol. 24 Suppl 2, No. pp. 223-32, ISSN 1875-8908

Gitler, A.D., Shorter, J. (2011) RNA-binding proteins with prion-like domains in ALS and FTLD-U. *Prion*, Vol 1, No. 3, pp. 5 ISSN 1933-690X

Graeber, M.B. & Streit, W.J. (2010). Microglia: biology and pathology. *Acta Neuropathol*, Vol. 119, No. 1, pp. 89-105, ISSN 1432-0533

Guglielmotto, M., Aragno, M., Autelli, R., Giliberto, L., Novo, E., Colombatto, S., Danni, O., Parola, M., Smith, M.A., Perry, G., Tamagno, E. & Tabaton, M. (2009). The up-regulation of BACE1 mediated by hypoxia and ischemic injury: role of oxidative stress and HIF1alpha. *J Neurochem*, Vol. 108, No. 4, pp. 1045-56, ISSN 0022-3042

Haces, M.L., Montiel, T. & Massieu, L. (2010). Selective vulnerability of brain regions to oxidative stress in a non-coma model of insulin-induced hypoglycemia. *Neuroscience*, Vol. 165, No. 1, pp. 28-38, ISSN 0306-4522

Halliday, G.M. & Stevens, C.H. (2011). Glia: initiators and progressors of pathology in Parkinson's disease. *Mov Disord*, Vol. 26, No. 1, pp. 6-17, ISSN 0885-3185

Henkel, J.S., Beers, D.R., Zhao, W. & Appel, S.H. (2009). Microglia in ALS: the good, the bad, and the resting. *J Neuroimmune Pharmacol*, Vol. 4, No. 4, pp. 389-98, ISSN 1557-1904

Hickman, S.E., Allison, E.K. & El Khoury, J. (2008). Microglial dysfunction and defective beta-amyloid clearance pathways in aging Alzheimer's disease mice. *J Neurosci*, Vol. 28, No. 33, pp. 8354-60, ISSN 10270-6474

Higuchi, K., Matsumura, A., Honma, A., Takeshita, S., Hashimoto, K., Hosokawa, M., Yasuhira, K., Takeda, T. (1983) Systemic senile amyloid in senescence-accelerated mice. A unique fibril protein demonstrated in tissues from various organs by the unlabeled immunoperoxidase method. *Lab Invest*, Vol. 48 No. 2 pp. 231-240. ISSN 0023-6837

Jayadev, S., Case, A., Eastman, A.J., Nguyen, H., Pollak, J., Wiley, J.C., Moller, T., Morrison, R.S. & Garden, G.A. (2010). Presenilin 2 is the predominant gamma-secretase in microglia and modulates cytokine release. *PLoS One*, Vol. 5, No. 12, pp. e15743, ISSN 1932-6203

Johnson, N.A., Jahng, G.H., Weiner, M.W., Miller, B.L., Chui, H.C., Jagust, W.J., Gorno-Tempini, M.L. & Schuff, N. (2005). Pattern of cerebral hypoperfusion in Alzheimer disease and mild cognitive impairment measured with arterial spin-labeling MR imaging: initial experience. *Radiology*, Vol. 234, No. 3, pp. 851-9, ISSN 0033-8419

Kaku, D.A., Giffard, R.G. & Choi, D.W. (1993). Neuroprotective effects of glutamate antagonists and extracellular acidity. *Science*, Vol. 260, No. pp. 1516-1518,

Katayama, Y., Maeda, T., Koshinaga, M., Kawamata, T. & Tsubokawa, T. (1995). Role of excitatory amino acid-mediated ionic fluxes in traumatic brain injury. *Brain Pathol*, Vol. 5, No. pp. 427-435, ISSN 1750-3639

Keller, J.N., Pang, Z., Geddes, J.W., Begley, J.G., Germeyer, A., Waeg, G. & Mattson, M.P. (1997). Impairment of glucose and glutamate transport and induction of mitochondrial oxidative stress and dysfunction in synaptosomes by amyloid beta-peptide: role of the lipid peroxidation product 4-hydroxynonenal. *J Neurochem*, Vol. 69, No. 1, pp. 273-84, ISSN 0022-3042

Kettenmann, H., Hanisch, U.K., Noda, M. & Verkhratsky, A. (2011). Physiology of microglia. *Physiol Rev*, Vol. 91, No. 2, pp. 461-553, ISSN 1522-1210

Koistinaho, M. & Koistinaho, J. (2005). Interactions between Alzheimer's disease and cerebral ischemia-focus on inflammation. *Brain Res Brain Res Rev*, Vol. 48 No. pp. 240-250, ISSN 0165-0173

Lau, A. & Tymianski, M. (2010). Glutamate receptors, neurotoxicity and neurodegeneration. *Pflugers Arch*, Vol. 460, No. 2, pp. 525-42, ISSN 1432-2013

Le Jeune, H., Cçcyre, D., Rowe, W., Meaney, M.J. & Quirion, R. (1996). Ionotropic glutamate receptor subtypes in the aged memory-impaired and unimpaired Long-Evans rat. *Neuroscience*, Vol. 74, No. 2, pp. 349-363, ISSN 0306-4522

Lebon, V., Petersen, K.F., Cline, G.W., Shen, J., Mason, G.F., Dufour, S., Behar, K.L., Shulman, G.I. & Rothman, D.L. (2002). Astroglial contribution to brain energy metabolism in humans revealed by ^{13}C nuclear magnetic resonance spectroscopy: elucidation of the dominant pathway for neurotransmitter glutamate repletion and measurement of astrocytic oxidative metabolism. *J Neurosci*, Vol. 22, No. 5, pp. 1523-1531, ISSN 0270-6474

Lee, S., Varvel, N.H., Konerth, M.E., Xu, G., Cardona, A.E., Ransohoff, R.M. & Lamb, B.T. (2010). CX3CR1 deficiency alters microglial activation and reduces beta-amyloid deposition in two Alzheimer's disease mouse models. *Am J Pathol*, Vol. 177, No. 5, pp. 2549-62, ISSN 1525-2191

Liang, B., Duan, B.Y., Zhou, X.P., Gong, J.X. & Luo, Z.G. (2010). Calpain activation promotes BACE1 expression, amyloid precursor protein processing, and amyloid plaque formation in a transgenic mouse model of Alzheimer disease. *J Biol Chem*, Vol. 285, No. 36, pp. 27737-44, ISSN 1083-351X

Liao, Y.F., Wang, B.J., Cheng, H.T., Kuo, L.H. & Wolfe, M.S. (2004). Tumor necrosis factor-alpha, interleukin-1beta, and interferon-gamma stimulate gamma-secretase-mediated cleavage of amyloid precursor protein through a JNK-dependent MAPK pathway. *J Biol Chem*, Vol. 279, No. 47, pp. 49523-32, ISSN 0021-9258

Mandrekar, S., Jiang, Q., Lee, C.Y., Koenigsknecht-Talboo, J., Holtzman, D.M. & Landreth, G.E. (2009). Microglia mediate the clearance of soluble Abeta through fluid phase macropinocytosis. *J Neurosci*, Vol. 29, No. 13, pp. 4252-4262, ISSN 0270-6474

Mantovani, A., Sica, A., Sozzani, S., Allavena, P., Vecchi, A. & Locati, M. (2004). The chemokine system in diverse forms of macrophage activation and polarization. *Trends Immunol*, Vol. 25, No. 12, pp. 677-86, ISSN 1471-4906

Mark, R.J., Lovell, M.A., Markesbery, W.R., Uchida, K. & Mattson, M.P. (1997). A role for 4-hydroxynonenal, an aldehydic product of lipid peroxidation, in disruption of ion homeostasis and neuronal death induced by amyloid beta-peptide. *J Neurochem*, Vol. 68, No. 1, pp. 255-64, ISSN 0022-3042

Mattson, M.P. (1990). Antigenic changes similar to those seen in neurofibrillary tangles are elicited by glutamate and Ca^{2+} influx in cultured hippocampal neurons. *Neuron,* Vol. 2, No. pp. 105-117, ISSN 0896-6273

Mattson, M.P. (2006). Neuronal life-and-death signaling, apoptosis, and neurodegenerative disorders. *Antioxid Redox Signal.*, Vol. 8, No. 11-12, pp. 1997-2006, ISSN 1557-7716

Miele, V.J., Bailes, J.E., Cantu, R.C. & Rabb, C.H. (2006). Subdural hematomas in boxing: the spectrum of consequences. *Neurosurgery Focus*, Vol. 21 No. pp. E10, ISSN 1092-0684

Morales, R., Estrada, L.D., Diaz-Espinoza, R., Morales-Scheihing, D., Jara, M.C., Castilla, J. & Soto, C. (2010). Molecular cross talk between misfolded proteins in animal models of Alzheimer's and prion diseases. *J Neurosci*, Vol. 30, No. 13, pp. 4528-35, ISSN 1529-2401

Mycko, M.P., Cwiklinska, H., Szymanski, J., Szymanska, B., Kudla, G., Kilianek, L., Odyniec, A., Brosnan, C.F. & Selmaj, K.W. (2004). Inducible heat shock protein 70 promotes myelin autoantigen presentation by the HLA class II. *J Immunol*, Vol. 172, No. 1, pp. 202-13, ISSN 0022-1767

Neumann, H., Boucraut, J., Hahnel, C., Misgeld, T. & Wekerle, H. (1996). Neuronal control of MHC class II inducibility in rat astrocytes and microglia. *Eur J Neurosci*, Vol. 8, No. 12, pp. 2582-90, ISSN 0953-816X

Nicholls, D.G., Vesce, S., Kirk, L. & Chalmers, S. (2003). Interactions between mitochondrial bioenergetics and cytoplasmic calcium in cultured cerebellar granule cells. *Cell Calcium*, Vol. 34 No. pp. 407-424, ISSN 0143-4160

Nicotera, P., Leist, M. & Manzo, L. (1999). Neuronal cell death: a demise with different shapes. *Trends Pharmacol Sci*, Vol. 20, No. pp. 46-51, ISSN 0165-6147

Obrenovitch, T.P., Urenjak, J., Zilkha, E. & Jay, T.M. (2000). Excitotoxicity in neurological disorders--the glutamate paradox. *Int J Dev Neurosci*, Vol. 18, No. 2-3, pp. 281-287, ISSN 0736-5748

Olney, J.W., Wozniak, D.F. & Farber, N.B. (1997). Excitotoxic neurodegeneration in Alzheimer disease. *Arch Neurol*, Vol. 54, No. pp. 1234-1240, ISSN 0003-9942

Orrenius, S., Zhivotovsky, B. & Nicotera, P. (2003). Regulation of cell death: the calcium-apoptosis link. *Nat Rev Mol Cell Biol.*, Vol. 4, No. 7, pp. 552-565, ISSN 1471-0072

Ovanesov, M.V., Ayhan, Y., Wolbert, C., Moldovan, K., Sauder, C. & Pletnikov, M.V. (2008). Astrocytes play a key role in activation of microglia by persistent Borna disease virus infection. *J Neuroinflammation*, Vol. 5, No. pp. 50, ISSN 1742-2094

Paresce, D.M., Chung, H. & Maxfield, F.R. (1997). Slow degradation of aggregates of the Alzheimer's disease amyloid beta-protein by microglial cells. *J Biol Chem*, Vol. 272, No. 46, pp. 29390-7, ISSN 0021-9258

Petegnief, V., Ursu, G., Bernal, F. & Mahy, N. (2004). Nimodipine and TMB-8 potentiate the AMPA-induced lesion in the basal ganglia. *Neurochem Int*, Vol. 44 No. pp. 287-291, ISSN 0197-0186

Pluta, R. (2004). Alzheimer lesions after ischemia-reperfusion brain injury. *Folia Neuropathol*, Vol. 42 No. pp. 181-186, ISSN 0028-3894

Ramonet, D., De Yebra, L., Fredriksson, K., Bernal, F., Ribalta, T. & Mahy, N. (2006). Similar calcification process in acute and chronic human brain pathologies. *J Neurosci Res*, Vol. 83 No. pp. 147-156, ISSN 1097-4547

Ramonet, D., Pugliese, M., Rodríguez, M.J., De Yebra, L., Andrade, C., Adroer, R., Ribalta, T., Mascort, J. & Mahy, N. (2002). Calcium precipitation in acute and chronic brain diseases. *J Physiol-Paris*, Vol. 96, No. pp. 307-312, ISSN 0928-4257

Ramonet, D., Rodríguez, M.J., Fredriksson, K., Bernal, F. & Mahy, N. (2004). In vivo neuroprotective adaptation of the glutamate/glutamine cycle to neuronal death. *Hippocampus*, Vol. 14, No. 5, pp. 586-594, ISSN 1098-1063

Randall, R.D. & Thayer, S.A. (1992). Glutamate-induced calcium transient triggers delayed calcium overload and neurotoxicity in rat hippocampal neurons. *J Neurosci*, Vol. 12, No. 5, pp. 1882-95, ISSN 0270-6474

Rodriguez, M.J., Bernal, F., Andres, N., Malpesa, Y. & Mahy, N. (2000). Excitatory amino acids and neurodegeneration: a hypothetical role of calcium precipitation. *Int J Dev Neurosci*, Vol. 18, No. 2-3, pp. 299-307,

Rodriguez, M.J., Martinez-Sanchez, M., Bernal, F. & Mahy, N. (2004). Heterogeneity between hippocampal and septal astroglia as a contributing factor to differential in vivo AMPA excitotoxicity. *J Neurosci Res*, Vol. 77, No. 3, pp. 344-353, ISSN 0736-5748

Rodriguez, M.J., Prats, A., Malpesa, Y., Andres, N., Pugliese, M., Batlle, M. & Mahy, N. (2009a). Pattern of injury with a graded excitotoxic insult and ensuing chronic medial septal damage in the rat brain. *J Neurotrauma*, Vol. 26, No. 10, pp. 1823-34, ISSN 1557-9042

Rodriguez, M.J., Pugliese, M. & Mahy, N. (2009b). Drug abuse, brain calcification and glutamate-induced neurodegeneration. *Curr Drug Abuse Rev*, Vol. 2, No. 1, pp. 99-112, ISSN 1874-4745

Rodriguez, M.J., Robledo, P., Andrade, C. & Mahy, N. (2005). In vivo co-ordinated interactions between inhibitory systems to control glutamate-mediated hippocampal excitability. *J Neurochem*, Vol. 95, No. 3, pp. 651-661, ISSN 0022-3042

Rodríguez, M.J., Ursu, G., Bernal, F., Cusí, V. & Mahy, N. (2001). Perinatal human hypoxia-ischemia vulnerability correlates with brain calcification. *Neurobiol Dis*, Vol. 8, No. pp. 59-68, ISSN 0969-9961

Rolls, A., Shechter, R., London, A., Ziv, Y., Ronen, A., Levy, R. & Schwartz, M. (2007). Toll-like receptors modulate adult hippocampal neurogenesis. *Nat Cell Biol*, Vol. 9, No. 9, pp. 1081-8, ISSN 1465-7392

Rombouts, S. & Scheltens, P. (2005). Functional connectivity in elderly controls and AD patients using resting state fMRI: a pilot study. *Curr Alzheimer Res*, Vol. 2, No. 2, pp. 115-6, ISSN 1567-2050

Saido, T.C. & Iwata, N. (2006). Metabolism of amyloid beta peptide and pathogenesis of Alzheimer's disease. Towards presymptomatic diagnosis, prevention and therapy. *Neurosci Res*, Vol. 54, No. 4, pp. 235-53, ISSN 0168-0102

Sanchez, L., Madurga, S., Pukala, T., Vilaseca, M., Lopez-Iglesias, C., Robinson, C.V., Giralt, E. & Carulla, N. (2011). Abeta40 and Abeta42 amyloid fibrils exhibit distinct molecular recycling properties. *J Am Chem Soc*, Vol. 133, No. 17, pp. 6505-8, ISSN 1520-5126

Sapolsky, R.M. (2001). Cellular defenses against excitotoxic insults. *J Neurochem*, Vol. 76, No. pp. 1601-1611, ISSN 0022-3042

Schwartz, M., Butovsky, O., Bråck, W. & Hanisch, U.K. (2006). Microglial phenotype: is the commitment reversible? *Trends Neurosci*, Vol. 29 No. 2, pp. 68-74, ISSN 0166-2236

Sibson, N.R., Dhankhar, A., Mason, G.F., Rothman, D.L., Behar, K.L. & Shulman, R.G. (1998). Stoichiometric coupling of brain glucose metabolism and glutamatergic neuronal activity. *Proc Nat Acad Sci USA*, Vol. 95, No. pp. 316-321, ISSN 0027-8424

Sica, A., Schioppa, T., Mantovani, A. & Allavena, P. (2006). Tumour-associated macrophages are a distinct M2 polarised population promoting tumour progression: potential targets of anti-cancer therapy. *Eur J Cancer*, Vol. 42, No. 6, pp. 717-27, ISSN 0959-8049

Sierra, A., Encinas, J.M., Deudero, J.J., Chancey, J.H., Enikolopov, G., Overstreet-Wadiche, L.S., Tsirka, S.E. & Maletic-Savatic, M. (2010). Microglia shape adult hippocampal neurogenesis through apoptosis-coupled phagocytosis. *Cell Stem Cell*, Vol. 7, No. 4, pp. 483-95, ISSN 1875-9777

Smith, D.H., Chen, X.H., Iwata, A. & Graham, D.I. (2003). Amyloid beta accumulation in axons after traumatic brain injury in humans. *J Neurosurg*, Vol. 98, No. 5, pp. 1072-7, ISSN 0022-3085

Soto, C., Estrada, L. & Castilla, J. (2006). Amyloids, prions and the inherent infectious nature of misfolded protein aggregates. *Trends Biochem Sci*, Vol. 31, No. 3, pp. 150-5, ISSN 0968-0004

Soulet, D. & Rivest, S. (2008). Bone-marrow-derived microglia: myth or reality? *Curr Opin Pharmacol*, Vol. 8, No. 4, pp. 508-18, ISSN 1471-4892

Stoll, G., Jander, S. & Schroeter, M. (2002). Detrimental and beneficial effects of injury-induced inflammation and cytokine expression in the nervous system. *Adv Exp Med Biol*, Vol. 513, No. pp. 87-113, ISSN 0065-2598

Streit, W.J. (2005). Microglia and neuroprotection: implications for Alzheimer's disease. *Brain Res Brain Res Rev*, Vol. 48, No. 2, pp. 234-9, ISSN 0165-0173

Suzumura, A., Takeuchi, H., Zhang, G., Kuno, R. & Mizuno, T. (2006). Roles of glia-derived cytokines on neuronal degeneration and regeneration. *Ann N Y Acad Sci*, Vol. 1088, No. pp. 219-29, ISSN 0077-8923

Tanuma, N., Sakuma, H., Sasaki, A. & Matsumoto, Y. (2006). Chemokine expression by astrocytes plays a role in microglia/macrophage activation and subsequent neurodegeneration in secondary progressive multiple sclerosis. *Acta Neuropathol*, Vol. 112, No. 2, pp. 195-204, ISSN 0001-6322

Taylor, J.P., Hardy, J. & Fischbeck, K.H. (2002). Toxic proteins in neurodegenerative disease. *Science*, Vol. 296, No. 5575, pp. 1991-5, ISSN 1095-9203

Tesco, G., Koh, Y.H., Kang, E.L., Cameron, A.N., Das, S., Sena-Esteves, M., Hiltunen, M., Yang, S.H., Zhong, Z., Shen, Y., Simpkins, J.W. & Tanzi, R.E. (2007). Depletion of GGA3 stabilizes BACE and enhances beta-secretase activity. *Neuron*, Vol. 54, No. 5, pp. 721-37, ISSN 0896-6273

Thinakaran, G. & Parent, A.T. (2004). Identification of the role of presenilins beyond Alzheimer's disease. *Pharmacol Res*, Vol. 50, No. 4, pp. 411-8, ISSN 1043-6618

Turturici, G., Sconzo, G. & Geraci, F. (2011). Hsp70 and its molecular role in nervous system diseases. *Biochem Res Int*, Vol. 2011, No. pp. 618127, ISSN 2090-2255

Tymianski, M. & Tator, C.H. (1996). Normal and abnormal calcium homeostasis in neurons: a basis for the pathophysiology of traumatic and ischemic central nervous system injury. *Neurosurgery*, Vol. 38, No. 6, pp. 1176-1195, ISSN 0898-4921

Tymianski, M., Wallace, M.C., Spigelman, I., Uno, M., Carlen, P.L., Tator, C.H. & Charlton, M.P. (1993). Cell-permeant Ca^{2+} chelators reduce early excitotoxic and ischemic neuronal injury in vitro and in vivo. *Neuron*, Vol. 11, No. pp. 221-235, ISSN 0896-6273

Vassar, R., Bennett, B.D., Babu-Khan, S., Kahn, S., Mendiaz, E.A., Denis, P., Teplow, D.B., Ross, S., Amarante, P., Loeloff, R., Luo, Y., Fisher, S., Fuller, J., Edenson, S., Lile, J., Jarosinski, M.A., Biere, A.L., Curran, E., Burgess, T., Louis, J.C., Collins, F., Treanor, J., Rogers, G. & Citron, M. (1999). Beta-secretase cleavage of Alzheimer's amyloid precursor protein by the transmembrane aspartic protease BACE. *Science*, Vol. 286, No. 5440, pp. 735-741, ISSN 1095-9203

Verkhratsky, A. (2007). Calcium and cell death. *Subcell.Biochem.*, Vol. 45, No. pp. 465-480, ISSN 0306-0225

Vosler, P.S., Graham, S.H., Wechsler, L.R. & Chen, J. (2009). Mitochondrial targets for stroke: focusing basic science research toward development of clinically translatable therapeutics. *Stroke*, Vol. 40, No. 9, pp. 3149-55, ISSN 1524-4628

Waite, J., Chen, A., Wardlow, M. & Thal, L. (1994). Behavioural and biochemical consequences of combined lesions of the medial septum/diagonal band and nucleus basalis in the rat when ibotenic acid, quisqualic acid and AMPA are used. *Exp Neurol*, Vol. 30, No. pp. 214-229, ISSN 0014-4886

Wake, H., Moorhouse, A.J., Jinno, S., Kohsaka, S. & Nabekura, J. (2009). Resting microglia directly monitor the functional state of synapses in vivo and determine the fate of ischemic terminals. *J Neurosci*, Vol. 29, No. 13, pp. 3974-80, ISSN 1529-2401

Weldon, D.T., Rogers, S.D., Ghilardi, J.R., Finke, M.P., Cleary, J.P., O'hare, E., Esler, W.P., Maggio, J.E. & Mantyh, P.W. (1998). Fibrillar beta-amyloid induces microglial phagocytosis, expression of inducible nitric oxide synthase, and loss of a select population of neurons in the rat CNS in vivo. *J Neurosci*, Vol. 18, No. 6, pp. 2161-2173, ISSN 1529-2401

Wen, Y., Onyewuchi, O., Yang, S., Liu, R. & Simpkins, J.W. (2004). Increased beta-secretase activity and expression in rats following transient cerebral ischemia. *Brain Res*, Vol. 1009, No. 1-2, pp. 1-8, ISSN 0006-8993

Werth, J.L. & Thayer, S.A. (1994). Mitochondria buffer physiological calcium loads in cultured rat dorsal root ganglion neurons. *J Neurosci*, Vol. 14, No. pp. 348-356, ISSN 1529-2401

Westermark, P., Johnson, K.H., Pitkänen, P. (1985) Systemic amyloidosis: a review with emphasis on pathogenesis. *Appl Pathol*, Vol. 3 No. 1-2 pp. 55-68. ISSN 0252-1172

Yamamoto, M., Kiyota, T., Horiba, M., Buescher, J.L., Walsh, S.M., Gendelman, H.E. & Ikezu, T. (2007). Interferon-gamma and tumor necrosis factor-alpha regulate amyloid-beta plaque deposition and beta-secretase expression in Swedish mutant APP transgenic mice. *Am J Pathol*, Vol. 170, No. 2, pp. 680-92, ISSN 0002-9440

Zlokovic, B.V. (2005). Neurovascular mechanisms of Alzheimer's neurodegeneration. *Trend Neurosci*, Vol. 28 No. pp. 202-208, ISSN 0166-2236

8

Transmissible Spongiform Encephalopathies

Glaucia N. M. Hajj, Tiago G. Santos,
Michele C. Landemberger and Marilene H. Lopes
International Center for Research and Education,
A.C. Camargo Hospital, Antonio Prudente Foundation, São Paulo
Brazil

This chapter is dedicated to the loving memory of Prof. Ricardo Renzo Brentani, a brilliant scientist, a source of inspiration for younger generations and a wonderful man.

1. Introduction

1.1 Neurodegenerative disorders and transmissible spongiform encephalopathies

Neuronal death represents the primary pathology of neurodegenerative diseases such as Alzheimer's and Parkinson's disease and Amyotrophic Lateral Sclerosis. These diseases usually present with a slow onset and a chronic progression. Various regions of the brain, spinal cord, or peripheral nerves may be affected, leading to functional impairment and neuron loss. Neurodegenerative diseases are often categorized by symptoms that may include impairment in cognition, movement, strength, coordination, sensation, or autonomic control. However, the diagnosis of a specific neurodegenerative disease may be misleading, as there is both clinical and neuropathologic overlap among diseases and existing diagnostic tools are not always accurate. For most neurodegenerative diseases, neuronal dysfunction, such as synaptic loss, may occur long before neuronal death takes place (Soto, 2003;Shastry, 2003;Aguzzi and O'Connor, 2010).

A group of neurodegenerative diseases called protein conformational disorders includes relatively common diseases as well as some rare inherited disorders that involve the deposition of protein aggregates in the brain, leading to the selective loss of neurons in an age dependent manner. The protein conformational disorders include Alzheimer's disease (AD), Parkinson's disease (PD), Huntington's disease (HD), as well as polyglutamine disorders that include several forms of spinocerebellar ataxia, amyotrophic lateral sclerosis, and the transmissible spongiform encephalopathies (TSEs), also referred to as prion diseases (Table 1). These disorders affect a diverse neuronal population in discrete regions of the brain. Until recently, there were no molecular mechanisms known to be shared by all these diseases. However, accumulating evidence implicates protein misfolding and aggregation as a likely common underlying cause (Soto, 2003;Shastry, 2003;Aguzzi and O'Connor, 2010).

Correct cell maintenance depends upon the activity of proteins, whose function relies upon their three-dimensional structure. However, some proteins can also fold into stable alternative conformations that result in their aggregation and accumulation as fibrillar deposits. Although these deposits have similar morphological, structural, and staining/immunoreactivity characteristics, protein deposits found on different diseases may also have distinct biochemical or biological features. The precise causes of abnormal folding and accumulation of proteins are not understood. There is currently considerable debate regarding the toxic versus neuroprotective effect of aggregates, and whether small soluble oligomers of the same proteins, may represent the toxic entities (Aguzzi and O'Connor, 2010;Shastry, 2003;Soto, 2003).

The rarest, yet the most intriguing, of these protein conformational disorders are the TSEs or prion diseases. This group of diseases includes Creutzfeldt–Jakob disease (CJD), kuru, fatal familial insomnia (FFI), and Gerstmann–Straussler–Scheinker syndrome (GSS) in humans, scrapie in sheep, bovine spongiform encephalopathy (BSE) in cattle, and chronic wasting disease in cervids (Soto, 2003;Shastry, 2003;Aguzzi and O'Connor, 2010;Aguzzi et al., 2001;Aguzzi and Polymenidou, 2004;Gibbs, Jr. et al., 1968;Masters et al., 1981;Medori et al., 1992a;Medori et al., 1992b).

Diseases	Clinical Features	Structures affected	Likely cause
Alzheimer's disease	Progressive dementia	Hippocampus, cerebral cortex	Amyloid deposits
Amyotrophic lateral sclerosis	Movement disorder	Motor cortex, brainstem	Superoxide dismutase/ TDP-43 deposits
Charcot Marie Tooth	Muscular weakness	PNS	Axonal degeneration / demyelinization
Corticobasal degeneration	Impairment on cognition and movement	cerebral cortex and the basal ganglia	Unknown
Dementia with Lewy bodies	Impairment on cognition and movement	Cerebral cortex	Lewy bodies - deposits of synuclein and ubiquitin
Friedreich's ataxia	Coordination problems	Spinal cord and peripheral nerves	Mutation in Frataxin gene
Huntington's disease	Dementia, motor and psychiatric problems	Striatum, cerebral cortex	Huntingtin deposits
Multiple Sclerosis	sensory disturbance, visual loss, motor dysfunction	spinal cord and optic nerves	Demyelination
Parkinson's disease	Movement disorder	Substantia nigra, hypothalamus	Synuclein deposits
Pick's disease	behavior changes, speech difficulty, and impaired thinking	frontal lobes	Pick bodies, accumulation of Tau
Prion disorders	Dementia, ataxia, or psychiatric or insomnia problems	Various regions depending on the disease	Prion protein deposits
Progressive supranuclear palsy	Impairment on cognition and movement	most areas of the brain and in some parts of the spinal cord	unknown
Polyglutamine Diseases / Spinocerebellar ataxia	Coordination Problems	Cerebellum/ spinal cord	Accumulation of proteins (ataxins) presenting poly-Q repeats

Table 1. Brief list of well characterized neurodegenerative diseases (not inclusive, and diseases can present in ways in which they have not been listed). Protein conformational disorders are highlighted in bold. PNS = peripheral nervous system.

The most unique feature of the prion diseases is that they present both hereditary and transmissible forms and, as we will present further in this chapter, the identification of proteins as transmissible disease agents represents a breakthrough in the concepts of modern biology. Prion diseases are generally characterized by the aggregation of prions, also referred to PrP^{Sc}, into large plaques that are associated with the rapid loss of neurons in specific areas of the brain and corresponds to the onset of neurological and behavioral symptoms. The PrP^{Sc} protein is the abnormal isoform of the cellular prion protein (PrP^{C}) that is normally present in all tissues of the body and whose expression is particularly high in neurons. A change in the three-dimensional structure of PrP^{C} renders it into the highly insoluble PrP^{Sc}, which is resistant to degradation and proteinase digestion. The presence of PrP^{Sc} can alter the conformation of PrP^{C} in the cell, thus making it a productive infection. The unusual properties of prion propagation have presented challenges to researchers seeking to understand the pathogenic mechanisms of these diseases and have slowed the development of effective diagnostic tools and therapeutic strategies (Soto, 2003;Shastry, 2003;Aguzzi and O'Connor, 2010).

This chapter will focus on human prion disorders, their history, etiology, symptoms, and the therapeutic strategies tried so far. Instead of a comprehensive review of the abundant prion literature, our goal here is to present a general view of the mechanism of these diseases for the lay public, complemented by a list of references that will enable additional study for those who wish to further explore the mysteries of prions.

2. A historic overview

This section will present a historic view of the TSEs, from the early descriptions of scrapie, the prototypic prion disease that affects sheep and goats and which has been a concern since the 18th century, to kuru, an endemic form of human TSE that was transmitted via cannibalistic rituals among the aborigines of Papua New Guinea throughout the 1950s and 1960s. We will also discuss the transmission of prions via contaminated meat that resulted in patients who contracted a new variant of Creutzfeldt-Jakob disease and led to one of the largest catastrophes in the history of medicine.

2.1 From scrapie to kuru – The discovery of infectious prions

The disease named scrapie affects sheep and has been a matter of concern since the 18th century, mystifying farmers and negatively impacting local economies (Aguzzi, 2006). The name "scrapie" originates from the behavior of compulsive rubbing and scraping against fixed objects observed in affected sheep. Scrapie could be found in many countries of Europe, such as France, in which is called tremblante (trembling), Spain (Basqvilla disease), Germany (traberkrankheit - trotting disease), and Iceland (rida - tremor) amongst others, in addition to regions in Asia such as India and the Himalayas (Khujali or Mokoo) (Schneider et al., 2008;Prusiner, 1999).

Early descriptions of scrapie date back to the 17th century (Adams, 1975) or earlier, possibly including explicit references by agricultural writers at the time of the Romans (Schneider et al., 2008). The symptoms of scrapie are characterized by progressive ataxia, particularly in the hind limbs, and collapse. The disease typically affects sheep around four years of age and progresses rapidly, within weeks to months, to death of the animal (Adams, 1975). Naturally infected sheep may have an asymptomatic incubation period that varies from three to five years, during which there is no febrile phase or alterations in cerebrospinal fluid composition. The lesions of scrapie are limited to the central nervous system (CNS) and are concentrated in the cerebellum, where widespread neuronal degeneration and the prominent hypertrophy and proliferation of astrocytes are typical features (Adams, 1975).

Different theories have emerged during the 20th century regarding the nature of the etiological agent of scrapie, and a "slow-virus" hypothesis was predominant until the revolutionary "protein-only" proposal that suggested that scrapie could spread in the absence of DNA (Schneider et al., 2008;Prusiner, 1999;Griffith, 1967). Experiments in sheep demonstrating a lengthy incubation period enabled the proposal of the "slow-virus" hypothesis. The unknown agent presented some viral features, such as the ability to spread and cause disease in other sheep indefinitely. In addition, the infectious agent could be filtered and appeared to be self-replicating. Moreover, this agent had been detected in most tissues including brain, spinal cord, pituitary gland, adrenal gland, salivary glands, spleen, liver, and lymphatic glands (Schneider et al., 2008).

However, the initial experimental studies did not show evidence of the agent being present and active in tissue culture models or detectable via serology or electron microscopy (Adams, 1975). In these studies, the scrapie agent puzzled investigators with properties that challenged the current knowledge regarding viruses, such as its remarkable resistance to a number of physical and chemical treatments that destroy conventional viruses.

The possibility that the scrapie agent did not contain nucleic acids suggested that a hitherto unrecognized agent could be involved in this disease (Adams, 1975). In agreement with these findings, early evidence of an unconventional transmission of scrapie arose accidentally in 1930's in Scotland. In an attempt to vaccinate sheep against infectious encephalomyelitis caused by a virus (looping-ill virus), the animals received inoculums derived from the brain and spleen of affected animals that had been treated with formalin. The tissues used to produce the "inactivated virus" were, in fact, contaminated with scrapie, which caused the disease in a fraction of the animals that received the inoculum, suggesting that the agent involved in this disease was resistant to formalin treatment (Prusiner, 1999;Gordon, 1946).

Following the findings of experimental transmission of scrapie in sheep, little progress in the field was made until Carleton Gajdusek demonstrated that kuru, a human disease responsible for a high mortality in the Fore people from Papua, New Guinea, was a transmissible spongiform encephalopathy.

This story begins in 1955, after an invitation made by Vincent Zigas, a physician of the Fore region, to his colleague Carleton Gajdusek, who had a strong background in microbiology, to help understanding the increasing incidence of a strange disease the aborigines called kuru. At that time, approximately 10% of the Fore people were dying of kuru each year, and women and children were particularly affected (Zetterstrom, 2010) (Figure 1).

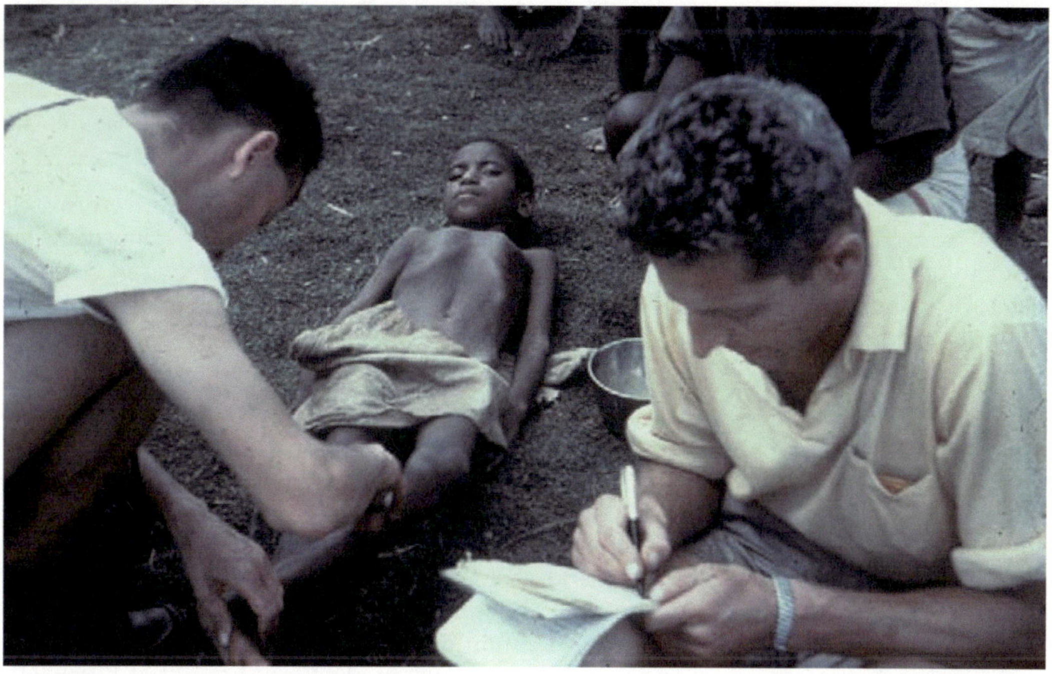

Fig. 1. Dr Carleton Gajdusek (left) and Dr Vincent Zigas study a child patient with kuru at Okapa in 1957. Reproduced with permission from Gajdusek in: Phil. Trans. R. Soc. B (2008) 363, 3636-3643 (Gajdusek, 2008).

Gajdusek and Zigas first described the clinical symptoms of kuru (the name means shivering or trembling in the Fore language) in 1957 (Zetterstrom, 2010). They described the disease as subacute and characterized by progressive cerebellar ataxia manifesting as athetoid movements that progresses to complete motor incapacity and, although cognition was generally unaffected, kuru was invariably fatal, patients typically died within 3-9 months after disease onset (Gajdusek and Zigas, 1957). However, the clinical and epidemiological profiles suggested that this was indeed a peculiar disease, as brains autopsies showed spongiform encephalopathy, suggesting that, like scrapie, kuru was an infectious disease (Gajdusek and Zigas, 1959; Zetterstrom, 2010; Harper, 1977).

A genetic explanation was initially proposed based in the apparent restriction of the disease to a particular tribal group and the remarkable familial clustering, with vertical transmission from generation to another (Harper, 1977). The elucidation of the causative factors of kuru came from the elegant experimental approaches and epidemiological studies carried out by Gajdusek and others (Harper, 1977;Zetterstrom, 2010). They demonstrated that ritual cannibalism of the brain and other parts of deceased relatives, practiced by the family, particularly by women and children, as an act of mourning and respect, provided the clue to the discovery that consumption of kuru-contaminated tissue was the means of transmitting the disease (Gajdusek, 1977). These findings led to the successful transmission of the disease to chimpanzees by the intracerebral inoculation of brain tissue from kuru patients (Harper, 1977;Gajdusek et al., 1966).

As in scrapie, the infectious agent of kuru accumulated in great quantities in the brain and did not have the features of a typical viral pathogen. These observations led Gajdusek to speculate that an unconventional type of virus might be the etiological agent of kuru, and this view was supported by the experimental transmission of kuru, scrapie and also Creutzfeldt-Jakob disease to chimpanzees during the 1960s and 1970s (Gajdusek et al., 1966).

These findings led to a new vision of the etiology of various neurodegenerative diseases, which garnered Gajdusek the Nobel Prize in 1976 (Zetterstrom, 2010). However, the "protein only" hypothesis came from the mind of J. S. Griffith, a mathematician (Griffith, 1967). He presented different models of transmission solely by protein particles with the ability to modify native proteins. The term "prion" was introduced in 1982 by Stanley Prusiner to describe an infectious proteinaceous particle (Prusiner, 1982).

The elucidation of the true chemical nature of prions occurred in the 1980s, following the isolation of infectious material from affected brains of Syrian hamsters (Bolton et al., 1982). This material was highly insoluble, with characteristics typical of amyloid aggregates (Prusiner et al., 1983), and was resistant to treatments that inactivate nucleic acid activity. Conversely, the infectious ability of prions was completely abrogated by moieties that modify protein activity and structure, such as proteases and detergents, strengthening the concept of the prion being an infectious "protein-only" agent. The isolation of prions permitted the characterization of a native protein synthesized by the host genome, termed the cellular prion protein (Oesch et al., 1985;Meyer et al., 1986). To characterize the infectious agent of transmissible spongiform encephalopathies, the prion protein gene was cloned from host cells by Dr. Prusiner, who went on to discover that changes in the three-dimensional structure of the native prion protein was the cause of these disorders. For this work, Dr. Prusiner was awarded the Nobel Prize in 1998 (Schneider et al., 2008).

The importance of these findings extended far beyond simply elucidating the means of transmission of a disease; they have broken a biology dogma that stated that information passing from one organism to another must be mediated by nucleic acids. From the discovery of prions, scientists knew that proteins were also able to transmit information from one organism to another.

2.2 The BSE epidemic and transmission to humans

Coincident with the period in which the elucidation prion biology was the focus of TSE studies came the "mad-cow disease." In the mid-1980s, an epidemic of bovine spongiform encephalopathy (BSE; commonly known as mad-cow disease) had a major impact on the human health policies as well as the economies of Europe, particularly the United Kingdom (UK), and Canada (Tyrrell and Taylor, 1996;Prusiner, 1999). In the UK, the incidence of BSE in cattle peaked at 370,000 cases in 1992, and has steadily diminished since (Zetterstrom, 2010). The incubation period of BSE varies from 2 to 8 years and thus affects adult cattle. Importantly, all breeds of cattle are equally susceptible to the infection (Chesebro, 2003).

Several pieces of evidence suggested that BSE was transmitted from sheep to cows via contaminated feed in the 1980's (Stack et al., 2006;Wells and Wilesmith, 1995). The epidemic began simultaneously at many geographic locations in England and was traced to the contamination of meat and bone meal derived from scrapie-infected sheep that was used in cattle feed. The spread of BSE was likely accelerated by the recycling of infected bovine tissues to manufacture feed, a practice halted following the recognition of BSE (Nathanson et al., 1997). The onset of the BSE epidemic was coincident with modifications in the process of extracting fat from meat and bone meal that unknowingly allowed prion particles to remain active (Wilesmith et al., 1991).

The BSE epidemic provoked much alarm in societies worldwide, as it had been associated with a new human disease, known as variant CJD (vCJD), that had been observed in individuals who had eaten infected cattle meat (Aguzzi, 2006;Aguzzi and Weissmann, 1996;Hill et al., 1997a). Despite concerns about a potential epidemic of vCJD, the total number of victims was relatively small (Valleron et al., 2001;Aguzzi, 2006). However, the risk of acquiring CJD is not limited to consumption of BSE-contaminated meat, as the transmission of prions has also been documented to occur during clinical procedures (iatrogenic transmission) (Aguzzi, 2006;Brown et al., 1992). Cases of CJD have been attributed to the transplantation of tissues or from pituitary hormone derived from deceased individuals that had unrecognized or asymptomatic TSE at the time of death. The contamination of medical instruments during neurosurgical interventions was also of concern, as patients with CJD were documented to have undergone invasive procedures, including brain biopsies (Will et al., 1999). Moreover, transmission of CJD was observed in patients submitted to depth electroencephalogram (EEG) recordings using electrodes that had previously been used in a CJD patient (Bernoulli et al., 1977). Evidence was also presented for prion transmission via human blood and derivatives; however, controversy still exists regarding the presence of CJD infectivity in human blood (Brown, 1995;Will et al., 1999).

3. Human forms of TSE

In humans, TSE has been classified into three subtypes: infectious (kuru, iatrogenic (i) CJD and variant (v) CJD), in which transmission has occurred because of human intervention, heritable familial (fCJD, GSS, and FFI) forms, and sporadic (sCJD) in which the disease cannot be linked to any of the previous forms of infection. In all three subgroups, the TSE can be transmitted to primates via ingestion or inoculation (Brown et al., 1994), thus fulfilling one of the main characteristics of TSE diseases, transmissibility.

Kuru was the first human neurodegenerative disease to be transmitted to laboratory primates (Gajdusek et al., 1966) and classified as a TSE. The most striking sign of the disease is a fine tremor of the head, trunk, and limbs that is associated with the insidious onset of ataxia. Both the ataxia and tremor become more pronounced as the disease progresses, and these signs are joined by other indicators of cerebellar pathology, as well as behavioral abnormalities (Gajdusek and Reid, 1961). Following the cessation of ritual cannibalism in the Fore people of Papua New Guinea, the incidence of kuru has steadily decreased to its current low levels (Collinge et al., 2006). The incubation period of this disease can be as long as 56 years, according to reports. Analysis of the PrP^C gene showed that most kuru patients were heterozygous for a polymorphism at codon 129 (presenting both a methionine and a valine at this position - M129V), a genotype associated with extended incubation periods and resistance to prion disease (Collinge et al., 2006).

Pathologically, kuru is characterized by a mild to moderate degree of neuronal vacuolation, an intense astrocytic gliosis, cerebellar degeneration, and the presence of numerous amyloid plaques that tend to be most common in the cerebellum, but can also be widely distributed in the brain.

CJD is the most common human TSE (the name Creutzfeldt-Jakob disease was coined by Spielmeyer in 1922), which has been shown to have familial (fCJD), infectious (iatrogenic/iCJD and variant/vCJD), and sporadic (sCJD) etiologies. Approximately 85% of all human prion diseases are sporadic forms of CJD, with incidences of 0.6-1.2 cases per million people per year distributed equally between men and women (Ladogana et al., 2005). The cause of sCJD is still unclear, although the spontaneous misfolding of PrP^{C} to PrP^{Sc} is a plausible hypothesis (Prusiner, 1989;Hsiao et al., 1991a). Alternate explanations include somatic mutations in the PrP^{C} gene that could lead to abnormal protein folding, even though no case of somatic mutations has been reported. However, the M129V polymorphism in the PrP^{C} gene appears to be associated with a lower risk (Palmer et al., 1991) and/or prolonged incubation time (Collinge et al., 2006). It remains possible that sCJD could be an acquired illness, as two case-control studies have reported prior surgery as a risk factor (Ward et al., 2002;Collins et al., 1999). However, evidence that these factors directly contribute to the etiology of sCJD is still lacking.

Unlike other diseases with dementia, such as Alzheimer's and Parkinson's diseases, in which incidence rises with age, the incidence of sCJD is primarily between 55 and 60 years of age, although patients as young as 14 (Murray et al., 2008) and as old as 86 (de et al., 1997) years of age have been reported. sCJD is a rapidly progressing dementia, and usually leads to death within a few weeks of the first symptoms. Initial symptoms include very rapid cognitive decline and dementia, sleep disturbances, and behavioral abnormalities consistent with proeminent cerebral atrophy (Figure 2). Cerebellar symptoms including ataxia and myoclonus are often present. Visual disturbances and ocular movement disorders, as well as extrapyramidal signs and hallucinations may also occur with sCJD. The final stages are characterized by an akinetic mute state (Murray, 2011). The rapidity of deterioration in sCJD usually allows the clinician to distinguish it from other dementias and neurodegenerative conditions. Pathological findings consist primarily of astrocytosis and spongiform changes associated with loss of neurons. The abnormal protease-resistant PrP^{Sc} can frequently be detected directly by immunohistochemistry in properly treated brain sections. Amyloid plaques containing PrP^{Sc} are also present in 5% of cases (Brown et al., 1994).

While variant CJD (vCJD) is associated with the consumption of BSE-infected meat, another CJD acquired by infection is iatrogenic CJD (iCJD), which is believed to result from the patient's exposure to prions by contact with contaminated human tissues. iCJD can be inadvertently transmitted during the course of medical or surgical procedures, either by the transplantation of tissues from patients with TSE or by neurosurgery using instruments incompletely sterilized following use on TSE patient (Aguzzi and Polymenidou, 2004). The first reported case of iCJD occurred in 1974 and was caused by the corneal transplantation of a graft derived from a patient suffering from sCJD (Duffy et al., 1974). Iatrogenic CJD is rare and is most often observed in individuals that have received cadaveric *dura mater* implants, human growth hormone, or were placed contaminated brain electrodes (Will, 2003).

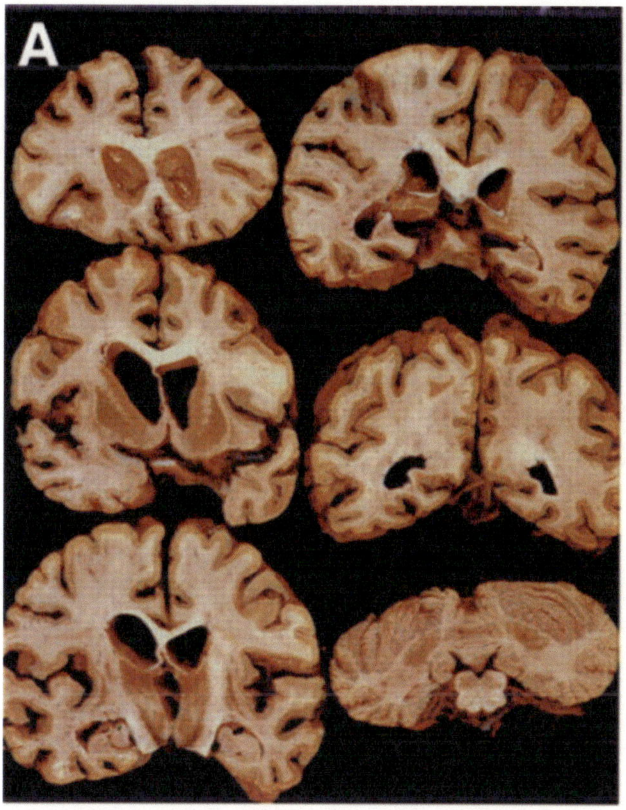

Fig. 2. Macroscopical aspect of a sporadic CJD brain with prominent cerebral, but not cerebellar, atrophy. Reproduced with permission from Budka, British Medical Bulletin 2003; 66: 121–130 (Budka, 2003).

The incubation period for iCJD is long, ranging from two to more than ten years. Additional evidence indicates that the route of prion exposure influences the clinical manifestation of CJD. For example, a predominantly ataxic phenotype is observed for *dura mater* or growth hormone-related cases, whereas cases in which prions were directly introduced into the CNS present with dementia as the initial symptom (Glatzel et al., 2005).

The newest version of human TSE, vCJD, was first reported in 1996 (Will et al., 1996) and was linked to the consumption of food contaminated with the BSE agent. In recent years, several studies regarding the biochemical, neuropathologic, and transmission characteristics of vCJD confirms that this disease represents the transmission of BSE prions to humans (Aguzzi, 1996;Aguzzi and Weissmann, 1996;Bruce et al., 1997;Hill et al., 1997a). In contrast to traditional forms of CJD, vCJD has affected younger patients (average age 19-39 years, as opposed to 65 years), has a relatively long duration of illness (median of 14 months as opposed to 4.5 months), and is strongly linked to exposure, probably through consumption, to cattle BSE (Will et al., 2000). The young age range of these patients and their distinctive pathology indicated that they represented a novel clinical TSE disease, combined with the initial occurrence of these patients in the UK, suggested an association with bovine BSE (Will et al., 1996). Subsequent laboratory experiments suggested that a strong similarity existed between BSE and vCJD on the basis of the lesion distribution in these disorders. Approximately 200 people have been diagnosed with vCJD world-wide, with most affected individuals being from the UK and France. Since 2001, the incidence vCJD in the UK appears to have stabilized (http://www.cjd.ed.ac.uk). The predominant clinical presentation for vCJD involves psychiatric symptoms, including behavioral changes, anxiety, and depression. These symptoms are followed, within weeks to months, by a cerebellar syndrome with ataxia and subsequent myoclonus. Later in the course of the disease, memory disturbances are evident, which progress to severe cognitive impairment and, finally, akinetic mutism. Neuropathological analyses have shown spongiform changes, neuronal loss, and astrogliosis, most prominently in the basal ganglia and thalamus. In addition, striking amyloid plaques containing PrP^{Sc} may be present throughout the cerebrum and cerebellum, and are often surrounded by vacuoles (Will et al., 1996).

The familial/inherited human prion diseases can be subdivided into three phenotypes, including fCJD, GSS, and FFI, according to the clinical symptoms presented. Familial prion diseases are far more rare than sCJD, and account for 10 to 20% of all TSE cases with an incidence of approximately 1 per 10 million. Familial TSEs are associated with an autosomal dominant alteration in the gene that encodes the PrP^{C} protein (Hsiao et al., 1989). To date, over 40 different mutations in this gene have been described to segregate with TSEs (Table 2).

Diseases	Mutations
GSS	P102L-129M
	P105L-129V
	A117V-129V
	G131V-129M
	Y145*-129M
	H187R-129V
	F189S-129V
	D202N-129V
	Q212P
	Q217R-129M
fCJD	D178N-129V
	V180I
	T188K
	T188R-129V
	E196K
	E200K
	V203I
	E208H
	V210I
	E211Q
	M232R
FFI	D178N-129M

Table 2. Summarizes known mutations that cause human TSEs. Point mutations found in patients with prion disease in the gene that codes for PrP^{C}. In some cases, the mutations are found in association with a polymorphism in codon 129, where methionine (M) or valine (V) are indicated. Amino acids are given in single-letter code. The asterisk indicates a stop codon; consequently, this mutation results in a truncated protein.

Several different mutations in the gene encoding PrP^C have been implicated in fCJD (Goldfarb et al., 1990;Hsiao et al., 1991b;Hsiao et al., 1991a;Bertoni et al., 1992). The clinicopathological phenotype of fCJD varies depending upon the mutation, as well as on the presence of a polymorphism at amino acid 129 (methionine (M) or valine(V)) (Kovacs et al., 2002). Highly variable symptoms may present even in affected members of the same family. The pattern of symptoms is sometimes similar to that observed for sCJD. Early symptoms may include depression, memory lapses, social withdrawal, and a lack of interest. However, the rapid progression to dementia and neurological symptoms are diagnostic. Within weeks, the patient may become unsteady on their feet, lack coordination, experience blurred vision or even blindness, rigidity in the limbs, and difficulty in speaking. In fCJD, the average age of onset symptoms is 52 years of age, compared to 65 years for sCJD.

A mutation in the gene encoding for PrP^C that results in an aspartate (D) to asparagine (N) substitution at amino acid 178 (D178N) can underlie either fCJD or FFI, depending on the polymorphism present at amino acid 129 (M or V). D178N coupled with V129 produces fCJD, in which patients present dementia and a widespread deposition of prion protein in the brain (Goldfarb et al., 1991a;Goldfarb et al., 1991b). When D178N is coupled with M129, the result is FFI.

The FFI diagnosis was first used in 1986 to describe an illness affecting five members of a large Italian family (Lugaresi et al., 1986). Over 20 kindred and seven nonfamilial (sporadic) cases of this unusual variety of prion disease have since been identified throughout the world. In the most characteristic presentation, the patient with FFI develops untreatable insomnia, sometimes for a prolonged period of weeks or months. Insomnia is followed by dysautonomia, ataxia, and variable pyramidal and extrapyramidal signs and symptoms, with a relative sparing of cognitive function until late in the disease course. The dysautonomias may include episodic alterations in blood pressure, heart rate, temperature, respiratory rate, and secretions. Electroencephalogram (EEG) recordings performed on these patients shows diffuse slowing, rather than periodic, discharges. Positron emission tomography (PET) reveals a reduction in metabolic activity in, or blood flow to, the thalamus relatively early in the disease (Padovani et al., 1998). The average age of onset for FFI is 50 years of age, with an average disease duration of 12 months.

The neuropathologic features of FFI include neuronal loss and astrogliosis within the thalamus and inferior olives and, to a lesser degree, the cerebellum. Vacuolation is minimal or absent in typical cases. Protease-resistant PrP^{Sc} is detectable in the brains of affected patients; however, it is usually present only in small amounts and is often restricted to specific regions such as the thalamus and temporal lobe (http://www.medscape.com/viewarticle/410863_4).

A specific mutation in the gene encoding PrP^C, which results in a proline (P) to leucine (L) substitution at amino acid 102 (P102L), was found to be present in patients with GSS. This was first detected in the original Austrian family described by Gerstmann, and was later observed in other cases (Hainfellner et al., 1996). This finding led to the unprecedented conclusion that prion diseases can have both genetic and infectious etiologies (Hsiao et al., 1989;Prusiner, 1989). This mutation has been found in unrelated families from several countries (Goldgaber et al., 1989;Kretzschmar et al., 1991) and other mutations causing GSS have also been identified. GSS is characterized by a slowly progressive cerebellar ataxia accompanied by cognitive decline (Ghetti et al., 1995). In contrast to other inherited human prion diseases, GSS has unique neuropathologic features that consist of widespread, multicentric PrP^{Sc} plaques in the cerebellar cortex. In families with GSS, symptoms usually begin in the fifth or sixth decade of life, but disease onset may occur as young as 25 years of age, with illness durations ranging from three months to 13 years (mean five to six years) (Chabry et al., 1999;Masters et al., 1981;Gajdusek, 1977;Hill et al., 1997a). Variation in the age of onset is associated with the presence of the P102L mutation (Deslys et al., 1996).

4. Transmission of prions

The most notorious means of prion transmission is via the ingestion of contaminated meat, although transmission by this route is actually highly inefficient. The concept of prion infectivity was presented to the general population during the rise of the mad-cow disease epidemic and the recognition of vCJD. vCJD was reported for the first time in 1996 as a disease having a clinical and pathological phenotype distinct from sCJD. Following many years of investigation, it became clear that vCJD is caused by consumption of BSE-contaminated meat products. Since 1996, 223 cases of vCJD have been reported, most occurring in the UK and France, although other countries have also reported cases (Table 3) (Ironside, 2010). The most likely period for transmission of BSE to humans was from 1984-89 and 1995-96 during the outbreak of BSE in cattle. Although a major portion of the UK population was likely exposed to BSE infectivity, a relatively small number of individuals have died from vCJD (Knight, 2010). Reasons for this low incidence may include a significant inter-species barrier, inefficiency of oral ingestion as a route of transmission, as well as difference in individual susceptibility.

Iatrogenic transmission of CJD is relatively rare. To date, iCJD has been reported in more than 400 patients who were exposed to prion transmission via contaminated neurosurgical instruments, intracerebral electroencephalographic electrodes, human pituitary hormone, corneal transplant, or *dura mater* graft. iCJD was first suggested in the case of a woman who died of CJD in 1974. She had received a corneal transplant 18 months before disease onset, derived from a patient who also died of CJD (Duffy et al., 1974). In 1997, a 45-year-old German woman developed CJD 30 years after corneal graft from a donor with confirmed CJD. Another eight cases of suspected contamination through corneal transplant have been reported, but the status of the donor in these cases has not been confirmed (Hamaguchi et al., 2009).

Country	**Number of cases (October 2011)**
United Kingdom	176
France	25
Spain	5
Ireland	4
Netherlands	3
United States of America	3
Portugal	2
Italy	2
Canada	1
Saudi Arabia	1
Japan	1

Table 3. Variant CJD cases worldwide.

The first case of *dura mater* graft-associated CJD (dCJD) was reported in the US in 1987(1987). Since then, 196 dCJD cases have been described, more than 50% of which occurred in Japan (Hamaguchi et al., 2009).

Another iatrogenic means of prion transmission resulted from the treatment of children with short stature with human growth hormone (hGH) that was derived from pituitary glands from the corpses of CJD-affected individuals. The process of purifying hGH did not eliminate prion infectivity causing this kind of contamination. To date, more than 190 patients worldwide have presented with iCJD following hGH treatment. More than 100 cases occurred in France (Hamaguchi et al., 2009), and others have been described in the UK, US, New Zealand, Brazil, and others (Brown et al., 2006). Although the use of recombinant GH began in 1985, cases of hGH-associated iCJD are still being observed due to the prolonged incubation period, up to 20 years, observed for these iCJD cases.

Thus, the length of the incubation period for the CJDs appears to be related to the means by which the prion particles were transmitted. Direct intracerebral exposure to prions via contaminated surgical material and the implantation of prion-contaminated *dura mater*, for example, have been associated with relatively short incubation periods (16-28 months). Peripheral exposure to prions, through the consumption of contaminated meat or exposure to contaminated hGH, results in longer incubation times that range from 5 to 30 years (Glatzel et al., 2005).

The occurrence of secondary transmission of CJD via blood transfusion has been reported. This route of human to human iCJD transmission has particularly important implications for public health, as relatively high infectivity has been observed in the lymphoid tissues of CJD patients. The existence of subclinical infected donors, combined with the high CJD infectivity of blood and the efficiency of blood as a route of transmissions, are key factors influencing the likelihood of acquiring iCJD via transfusion. To date, there are four confirmed cases of iCJD associated with the transfusion of non-leukoreduced red blood cells from an asymptomatic donor who subsequently died from vCJD (McCutcheon et al., 2011). The incubation time in the recipients was approximately 7 years after the contaminated transfusions (Ironside, 2010).

5. Diagnosis

Although a rapidly progressive dementia, myoclonus, and other neurological signs may lead the clinician to suspect a TSE, the definitive diagnostics in humans can only be confirmed by brain biopsy or necropsy followed by the histopathological and immunohistochemical examination of brain tissue. Cerebral biopsy in living patients is discouraged, unless its purpose is to achieve an alternative diagnosis of a treatable disorder.

The misfolded prion protein, PrP^{Sc}, is the single most significant marker for the TSE diseases, but its detection using standard serological methods is complicated by its antigenic similarity to the normal prion protein, PrP^{C}. Many research groups have tried to detect PrP^{Sc} outside of the brain in order to develop more accurate and less invasive diagnostic tools, but these attempts have so far been unsuccessful or are still in clinical trials. Electrophysiological examinations using EEG, or imaging exams using magnetic resonance imaging (MRI), combined with biochemical analysis, are among the methods currently used to probe for prion diseases, as discussed below (Venneti, 2010). In the following section we will present the main features of the diagnostic tools that have, to date, been in use.

5.1 Genetic investigations

DNA sequencing of the gene that encodes PrP^C can detect the inherited forms of prion diseases that are caused by point mutations. There have been 55 pathogenic mutations described in the gene that encodes PrP^C (Table 2) which include 24 missense point mutations, 27 insertion mutations, 2 deletions, and 2 nonsense mutation that result in the premature termination of the PrP^C protein. If DNA sequencing detects a mutation in a patient, the diagnosis of TSE can be confirmed (Figure 3). However, the absence of detectable mutations does not exclude the sporadic or iatrogenic forms of the disease (Gambetti et al., 1999).

Twelve polymorphisms that do not result in amino acid substitution have been described in the gene encoding for PrP^C (Gambetti et al., 1999). Four additional polymorphisms that do alter the amino acid sequence of PrP^C have also been reported. The polymorphism at amino acid 129 of PrP^C is of particular importance; compelling evidence from studies in genetically modified mice as well as from clinical studies indicate that homozygosity for the less common methionine at position 129 constitutes a risk factor for the development of prion disease. Notably, methionine homozygotes are overrepresented among patients with sCJD, and all individuals affected by vCJD are codon 129 methionine homozygotes. Besides constituting a risk factor for the development of prion diseases, this polymorphism has a considerable effect on the clinical, biochemical, and neuropathologic presentation of individuals with prion diseases (Glatzel et al., 2005). As described in previous sections, a mutation in PrP^C at amino acid 178, when combined with the presence of methionine at position 129, results in the development of CJD or FFI.

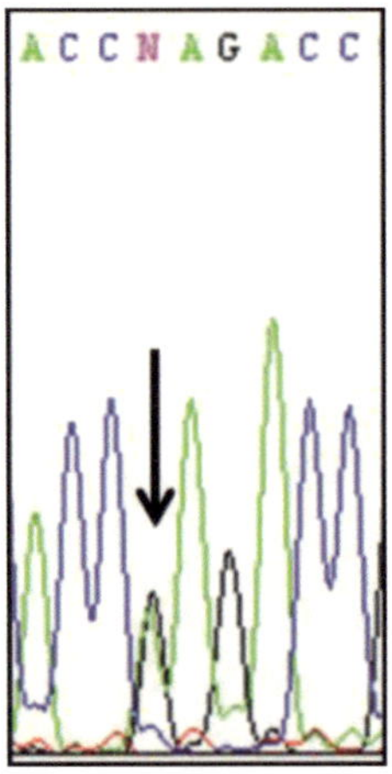

Fig. 3. Genomic sequencing of PrP^C encoding gene. This particular test shows a mutation (AAG to GAG) in heterozygosis that would code for amino acid 200, replacing a glutamate for a lysine (E200K).

5.2 EEG

EEG recording show periodic or pseudoperiodic paroxysms of triphasic or sharp waves of 0.5 to 2.0 Hz against a slow background in about two-thirds of sCJD patients. However, this EEG pattern is not specific to sCJD, and occurs in other conditions, such as metabolic diseases. In addition, at least 30% of cases may not demonstrate the typical features. There appears to be a temporal window of opportunity for the detection of abnormal EEG patterns in sCJD, as these patterns may not be evident either early or late in the disease course. Thus, a serial course of weekly or bi-weekly EEGs may be necessary to capture the characteristic periodic discharges (Will et al., 1999).

In iCJD, the EEG shows a slow wave pattern and, in FFI, the EEG displays diffuse slowing, rather than rather than the periodic triphasic discharges typical of sCJD (Will et al., 1999).

5.3 MRI

Although the use of MRI is not included in the exams recommended by the World Health Organization (WHO) (http://www.who.int/entity/zoonoses/diseases/Creutzfeldt.pdf), it can be useful for CJD diagnosis. In sCJD almost all cases present gray matter hyperintensities in the neocortical, limbic and subcortical areas. In 70% to 90% of patients, cortical ribboning is evident that may be accompanied by increased intensities in the putamen and caudate nuclei detectable with fluid-attenuated inversion-recovery sequences and diffusion-weighted imaging (DWI) MRI (Geschwind et al., 2008). In vCJD, a characteristic MRI pulvinar sign is evident as hyperintensity in the pulvinar - posterior thalamus relative to the anterior putamen in about 80% of patients(Glatzel et al., 2005). In prolonged courses of sCJD (more than one year), brain MRIs show significant atrophy with loss of DWI hyperintensity, particularly in areas that previously displayed restricted diffusion (Vitali et al., 2011).

In prion disorders associated with a high degree of amyloid deposition, such as GSS and other genetic variants, PET ligands that bind to prion-containing amyloid deposits, such as 2-(1-{6-[(2-[F-18]fluoroethyl) (methyl)amino]-2-naphthyl}ethylidene)malononitrile (FDDNP), may offer additional diagnostic opportunities (http://www.medscape.com/viewarticle/582032_7). As with EEG results, these signs can also be found in other diseases, complicating the definitive diagnosis of a prion disease.

5.4 14.3.3 detection

The 14.3.3 proteins are a group of cytosolic polypeptides whose abnormal presence in the cerebrospinal fluid (CSF) can be detected in many conditions including stroke, infection, inflammatory processes, epileptic seizures, and toxic metabolic conditions, and is a reliable marker of the rapid destruction of neurons characteristic of a number of progressive neurological disorders (Zanusso et al., 2011).

The use of 14.3.3 as a diagnosis for prion disease was suggested for the first time in 1996 (Hsich et al., 1996). Despite controversy regarding the specificity of this diagnostic tool, in 1999, 14.3.3 detection was included by the WHO in their guidelines for CJD diagnosis. The 14.3.3 protein can be detected in many clinical laboratories; however, this is considered to be an expensive and time-consuming test that generates often inconclusive data due to the difficulty with which the protein band patterns can be discerned (Satoh et al., 2010). In spite of these limitations, 14.3.3 tests are considered to be reliable diagnostic markers for CJD and present an approximately 90% specificity and sensitivity in the diagnosis of sCJD. In addition, the presence of 14.3.3 in the CSF occurs in around 90% of fCJD cases. However, the presence of 14.3.3 has not been reported in the CSF of patients suffering from FFI or GSS (Glatzel et al., 2005).

Other biochemical analyses of the CSF useful for CJD diagnosis are the presence of neuron-specific enolase (NSE) and S100 proteins, which have been shown to be increased in the CSF of patients with CJD. The presence of Tau proteins in the CSF has also been described to be diagnostic for CJD, but only in a small group of patients. Although the test for the presence of Tau is highly sensitive, it is not a differential diagnostic that can be used to distinguish CJD from other diseases (Otto et al., 2002).

5.5 Neuropathological analysis

The neuropathological hallmark of prion disease is the presence of the classical triad of spongiform changes, neuronal loss, and gliosis. As neuronal loss and gliosis are found in other neurodegenerative conditions, the spongiform changes in the brain are the most specific characteristic of prion disease. The spongiform changes may be mild, moderate, or severe, and are characterized by diffuse or clustered, small, round, or oval vacuoles in the neuropil (Budka, 2003) (Figure 4).

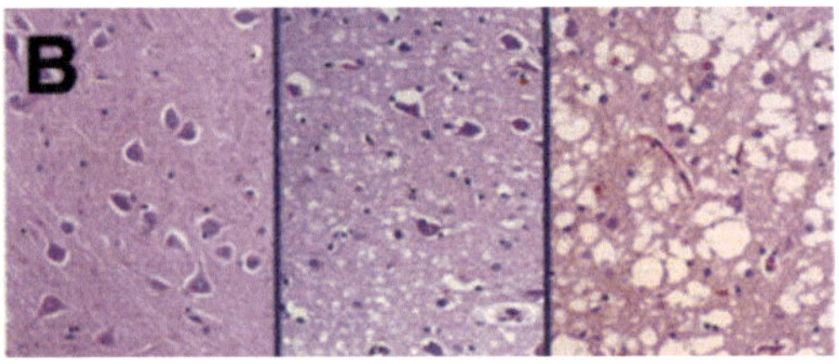

Fig. 4. Spongiform degeneration: In sporadic CJD, some brain areas may have no (hippocampal end plate, at left), mild (subiculum, at middle) or severe (temporal cortex, at right) spongiform change. Haematoxylin and eosin (H & E) stain. Reproduced with permission from Budka, British Medical Bulletin 2003; 66: 121–130 (Budka, 2003).

Other routine neuropathologic investigations include sampling from different regions of the CNS and the immunohistochemical detection of aggregated PrP^{Sc}. The type of PrP^{Sc} plaque deposition varies with the disease; synaptic-type deposits and unicentric PrP^{Sc} plaques occur in both CJD and GSS, while abundant multicentric plaques are peculiar to GSS. Plaque-like deposits are the only type of PrP^{Sc} deposits that extend to the subcortical white matter. Kuru plaques are present in a minority of sCJD cases and are most frequent in the cerebellar cortex (Budka, 2003) (Figure 5). GSS presents multicentric PrP^{Sc} plaques and thalamic degeneration, and also variable spongiform changes in cerebrum.

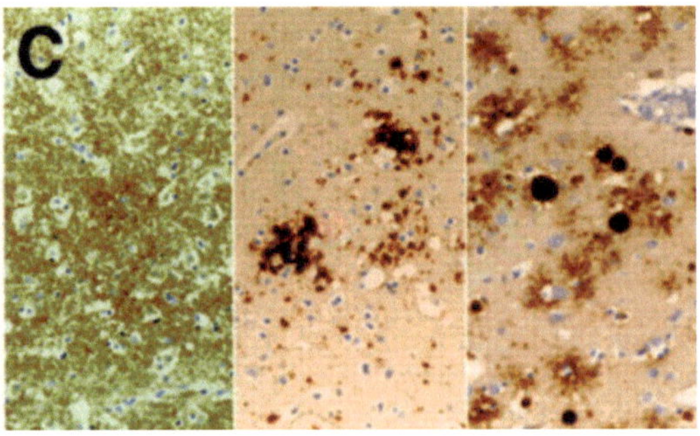

Fig. 5. Patterns of PrP^{Sc} deposition: Cortical sections immunostained for PrP^{Sc} in sporadic CJD: synaptic (at left), patchy/perivacuolar (at middle) or plaque type (at right) patterns of PrP^{Sc} deposition. Reproduced with permission from Budka, British Medical Bulletin 2003; 66: 121–130 (Budka, 2003).

In vCJD, a very particular pattern of PrP^{Sc} deposition is found. These depositions are composed of abundant multiple fibrillary PrP^{Sc} plaques surrounded by a halo of spongiform vacuoles called "florid" plaques or "daisy-like" plaques (Figure 6). Also present are amorphous pericellular and perivascular PrP^{Sc} deposits that are particularly prominent in the molecular layer of the cerebellum (Minor et al., 2004;Will et al., 1999;1997).

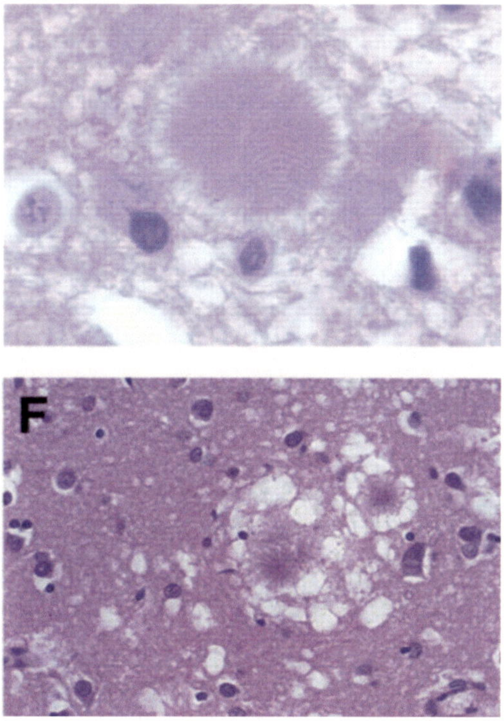

Fig. 6. Amyloid plaques in prion diseases. Upper panel - Large Kuru-type plaque, Hematoxylin and Eosin stain. Lower panel - Typical 'florid' plaques in vCJD, H & E stain. Reproduced with permission from Budka, British Medical Bulletin 2003; 66: 121–130 (Budka, 2003).

5.6 Tonsil biopsy

The presence of PrP^{Sc} in postmortem tonsillar tissue was first described in a 35 year old woman in 1997. The immunohistochemical and western blot findings in this suspected vCJD case showed an abnormal PrP^{Sc} immunoreactivity within tonsillar germinal centers that are not observed in sCJD, suggesting that tonsil biopsy may be applicable as a differential diagnostic tool (Hill et al., 1997b). The WHO does not recommend tonsil biopsy routinely in cases in which EEG findings are typical of sCJD, but the biopsy may be useful in cases where the clinical features are compatible with vCJD and the MRI does not show a high bilateral pulvinar signal.

5.7 Classification of sCJD and vCJD

According to all the above clinical signs and symptoms, and the use of the before mentioned diagnostic exams, the WHO classifies sCJD and vCJD according to the following criteria:

Possible sCJD

- Duration < two years
- Progressive dementia
- At least two of the following clinical features: myoclonus, visual or cerebellar disturbance, pyramidal, extrapyramidal dysfunction, akinetic mutism

Probable sCJD

- Duration < two years
- Progressive dementia
- At least two out of the following clinical features: myoclonus, visual or cerebellar disturbance, pyramidal, extrapyramidal dysfunction, akinetic mutism
- The presence of 14.3.3 immunoreactivity in the CSF, or typical EEG patterns of periodic triphasic sharp waves

Confirmed sCJD

- Spongiform changes in cerebral and/or cerebellar cortex and/or subcortical grey matter
- PrP^{Sc} immunoreactivity of the plaque and/or diffuse synaptic and/or patchy/ perivacuolar type

Although the clinical criteria for CJD are fairly comprehensive, neuropathological analysis is important in every suspected case. The above criteria do not cover all CJD cases, and approximately 17% of all confirmed CJD cases do not fulfill clinical criteria for probable or possible CJD (Hainfellner et al., 1996;Radbauer et al., 1998).

5.8 Variant CJD

vCJD cannot be diagnosed with certainty using clinical criteria alone; the diagnosis requires neuropathological confirmation. The following combinations of signs, symptoms, and clinical investigations serve to define possible, probable, and definite vCJD (Table 4):

(I)
Progressive psychiatric disorder
Clinical duration >6 months
Routine investigations do not suggest an alternative diagnosis
No history of potential iatrogenic exposure
No evidence of a familial form of TSE (transmissible spongiform encephalopathies).

(II)
Early psychiatric symptoms (depression, anxiety, apathy, withdrawal, delusions)
Persistent painful sensory symptoms (pain and/or dysaesthesia)
Ataxia
Chorea / dystonia or myoclonus
Dementia.

Possible vCJD

- A patient with the items in (I) and at least four items in (II)
- EEG is not typical of sCJD

Probable vCJD

- A patient with the items in (I) and at least four items in (II)
- High bilateral pulvinar signal on MRI brain scan
- EEG in not typical of sCJD, although generalized periodic complexes may occasionally be seen at the later stages of the disease.
- Or, a patient with the items in (I) and a positive tonsil biopsy.

Definite vCJD

- A patient with the items in (I)
- Neuropathological confirmation of vCJD

HUMAN PRION DISEASE	SPORADIC CJD	VARIANT CJD
Age at onset (range)	60-70y	26y (12-74)
Disease Duration (range)	6 mo (1-35)	14 mo (6-24)
Clinical Symptoms	Progressive dementia, myoclonus, cerebellar ataxia, visual problems, extrapyramidal symptoms	Early psychiatric symptoms, dysesthesia, later neurologic deficits and cognitive decline
CSF 14.3.3	Positive > 90%	Positive in 50%
EEG	PSWC 60-70%	Nonspecific alterations
MRI	Brain atrophy hyperintensities in basal ganglia and/or cortical in 67%	Hyperintensities in the posterior thalamus (pulvinar sign), 78%
Histopathologic Features	Spongiform changes, neuronal loss, astrogliosis, PrP deposition - various patterns	Spongiform changes, neuronal loss, astrogliosis, PrP deposition - florid plaques

Adapted from Glatzel et al, 2009.

Table 4. Clinical, Diagnostic and Neuropathologic Features in Sporadic CJD and Variant CJD.

Because of their potential infectious properties, the incidence of prion disease should be followed worldwide. The global surveillance of vCJD and other forms of CJD will lead to a better understanding of these diseases, including the potential causes of iCJD as well as the distribution of the various familial forms. Such epidemiology should also provide information useful for the protection of individuals against the risks of these diseases. The surveillance of CJD is recommended by the WHO and has been implemented in many countries including the UK, the US, Canada, Japan, Brazil, and many countries in Europe.

6. Therapies and perspectives

There are currently no effective means of curing or even ameliorating the symptoms of prion disease. There is currently a multitude of studies using different strategies aimed at finding effective treatments for these diseases (Rigter et al., 2010). The many attempts to achieve this goal are discussed in this section (Table 5).

Four types of studies have been conducted. These include the 1) *in vitro* observation of abnormal prions in a test tube, 2) the observation of cultured cells infected with prions, 3) studies involving prion-infected animals or 4) actual patients affected by the disease. No drug has shown efficacy in the treatment of animal models after the onset of symptoms, although several compounds have been shown to delay the onset of disease if given before symptoms are evident.

The physiological functions of PrP^{C}, as well as the exact molecular processes underlying its conversion into PrP^{Sc}, are not completely understood. Nevertheless, a number of compounds and techniques have been investigated for their therapeutic potential against prion disease. Current therapeutic strategies are focused upon preventing the accumulation of PrP^{Sc} in the nervous system. This can be accomplished by lowering PrP^{C} availability, thus preventing PrP^{Sc} spread in the CNS, or by increasing PrP^{Sc} clearance. Additional non-specific therapeutic strategies, such as stem cell therapy or the use of neurotrophic factors to prevent neuronal death, which have been tried in other protein conformational diseases such as AD, are emerging amongst prion researchers.

The most direct strategy of inhibiting PrP^{Sc} conversion is to render PrP^{C} unavailable. This may be accomplished by lowering the cellular amounts of PrP^{C}. In mice, genetic deletion of PrP^{C} confers resistance to prion diseases (Bueler et al., 1993). In humans, the ablation of PrP^{C} may be possible via the recently-developed technology of interference RNA (RNAi). The transcription of DNA constructs that contain an antisense sequence to PrP^{C} would produce an RNA molecule complementary to PrP^{C} mRNA. This results in the annealing of both strands and the formation of a double-stranded RNA molecule, which activates a cellular mechanism of RNA degradation, thus preventing the translation and expression of PrP^{C}. In cells, this technique was successful in inhibiting normal amounts of PrP^{C} and its conversion to PrP^{Sc} (Daude et al., 2003). In mice inoculated with prions and allowed to incubate the disease until early neuropathology was established, a single injection of viral particles containing RNAi to PrP^{C} prevented the onset of early behavioral and cognitive deficits, reduced PrP^{Sc} deposition and spongiosis, and resulted in the significantly increased survival of the animals (White and Mallucci, 2009).

A potential drawback to the use of therapeutic RNAi in neurodegenerative diseases is the need to overcome the blood-brain-barrier (BBB); this would require either the transient disruption of the BBB's impermeability or direct injection into the brain. However, in animal studies the efficacy of the viral delivery was restricted to the sites of injection. Therefore, protection against the formation of PrP^{Sc} in multiple areas of the brain would depend on several brain injections (White et al., 2008). Another caveat to the use of RNAi *in vivo* is the need to avoid silencing of unintended genes, cytotoxicity, activation of interferon responses, and interference with the processing of endogenous micro RNAs due to an over-loading of the RNAi pathway.

In the treatment of prion disease, even a partial reduction of PrP^{C} expression would likely be beneficial; thus low doses of RNAi should be sufficient, minimizing the potential for unintended side effects. An additional caveat of this strategy is that, since PrP^{C} has many described functions, there may be undesirable side effects from its ablation. However, if a reversible process for gene silencing is developed, the physiological functions of PrP^{C} could be restored following treatment.

Therapeutic Strategy	*In vitro*	*In vivo*	Human trials
PrPc depletion by interference RNA	Yes	Yes	n.d.
Heterologous PrP	Yes	Yes	n.d
Amiloydogenic motif peptide	Yes	n.d.	n.d.
Dendritic Follicular Cell inhibition of differentiation	Yes	Yes	n.d.
Branched Polyamines	Yes	Yes	n.d.
β-breaker peptides	Yes	Yes	n.d.
Quinacrine	Yes	Limited efficacy	Underway
Active immunization	n.d.	Yes	n.d.
Passive immunization	n.d.	Yes	n.d.
Dextran Sulfate	n.d.	Yes	n.d.
Pentosan Polysulfate	Yes	Yes	Not conclusive
Heparin mimetic	Yes	Not conclusive	n.d
Congo red analogues	Yes	Yes	n.d.
Suramin analogues	Yes	Yes	n.d.
Poryphyrines/phtalocyanines	Yes	Yes	n.d.
Quinine/biquinoline	Yes	Some	n.d.
Tetracycline	Yes	Yes	Underway

n.d. - not determined. Adapted from: Vaccine 28 (2010) 7810–7823.

Table 5. Overview of therapeutic strategies designed so far.

A different strategy for reduction of PrP^{Sc} conversion is based upon the need for compatibility between the host PrP^{C} and infectious PrP^{Sc} proteins for efficient conversion. Incompatibilities in PrP^{C} between species, or from amino acid substitutions, may even block the conversion of compatible PrP^{C} (Horiuchi et al., 2000). For example, treatment of prion-infected mice with viral particles expressing PrP^{C} containing specific mutations increased survival time, even when treatment was started at a late stage of infection (Toupet et al., 2008). In this manner, the expression of incompatible PrP^{C} may be a viable therapeutic strategy in prion disease, without the drawback of impairing normal PrP^{C} functions. This approach has been applied to sheep in the Netherlands, where the preferential breeding of resistant phenotypes has been widely and effectively implemented. The difficulties of this treatment rely on the need of a continuous means of delivery for the resistant PrP^{C} forms that would also efficiently spread this molecule throughout the brain.

In addition to conversion-resistant PrP^{C} proteins, the introduction of peptides from a conserved region of PrP^{C} are also able to block conversion (Chabry et al., 1999). Even though peptides are easily synthesized, they have the disadvantage of being sensitive to proteolytic degradation and, like the PrP^{C} protein, the difficulties in crossing the BBB requires intracranial injections.

Alternatively, the prevention of PrP^{Sc} migration to the CNS can block the progression of the disease without the need of bypassing the BBB. In cases where infection is acquired, PrP^{Sc} must spread to the nervous system. Studies suggest that PrP^{Sc} first accumulates on follicular dendritic cells, from where neuronal invasion occurs. The experimental impairment of dendritic cell maturation was shown to inhibit prion neuroinvasion. However, this approach was most successful when treatment was administered prior to scrapie inoculation (Mabbott et al., 2003;Montrasio et al., 2000), and would not be effective against the familial prion diseases.

The study of the mechanisms by which PrP^{Sc} induces neurodegeneration also promises new therapeutic strategies. For example, the calcium-dependent phosphatase calcineurin (CaN) was shown to be hyperactivated as a result of PrP^{Sc} formation. Prion-infected mice treated with the CaN inhibitor FK506 at the clinical phase of the disease exhibited reduced severity of the clinical abnormalities and increased survival times. These animals also displayed a reduced degree of neurodegeneration that was independent of the amount of PrP^{Sc}, suggesting that inhibition of PrP^{Sc} formation may not be necessary for therapeutic effects with FK506 (Mukherjee et al., 2010).

At the current time, no protein conformational disorder has a highly effective therapy. Many studies using AD animal models have shown that immunotherapeutic approaches can reduce both amyloid and tau-related pathology, leading to cognitive rescue. Partly because of success observed in AD models, similar experiments with anti-PrP antibodies were initiated. In tissue culture studies, anti-PrP antibodies and antigen-binding fragments directed against PrP have been shown to inhibit prion replication. Administering specific anti-PrP monoclonal antibodies directly following the inoculation of mice with prions, resulted in prolonged survival in treated animals (Sigurdsson et al., 2003) and continuous treatment with antibodies delayed the incubation period (White et al., 2003). Passive immunization of extra-cerebrally infected mice with an anti-PrP antibody resulted in the effective suppression of PrP^{Sc} replication in the linforeticular system, effectively preventing prion invasion into the CNS (Sadowski et al., 2009). In a different approach, the artificial expression of the anti-PrP antibody 6H4 protected mice from prion disease following prion inoculation (Heppner et al., 2001).

Potential complications of this immunotherapy approach can arise from the fact that *in vivo* cross-linking with PrP^{C}-specific antibodies has been shown to trigger rapid and extensive apoptosis in neurons (Solforosi et al., 2004). Additionally, passive immunization has not been found to be effective when administered close to the clinically symptomatic stages of prion infection. Additionally, this approach would be too costly for the treatment of prion diseases in animals.

Active immunization (vaccination) was also shown to prolong the survival of infected mice, especially when vaccination occurred prior to prion exposure (Sigurdsson et al., 2002; Schwarz et al., 2003). Full-length PrP^{C}, or a peptide sequence of PrP^{C}, were expressed in mice using viral particles resulting in the production of high-affinity antibodies able to inhibit PrP^{Sc} formation in prion-infected cells (Nikles et al., 2005;Handisurya et al., 2007). Trials using this methodology to prevent Chronic Wasting Disease in mule deer are ongoing.

A drawback of active immunization is that endogenous PrP^{C} functionality would be indefinitely impaired in the treated animal. Additionally, immunomodulation to target prions must overcome the body's natural tolerance to endogenous PrP^{C} at the same time that humoral or cellular autoimmune cytotoxic effects should be avoided or minimized (Wisniewski and Goni, 2010).

Preventing the accumulation of PrP^{Sc} is also a viable therapeutic strategy, and a number of compounds have been examine for this purpose. Branched polyamines were shown to disaggregate prion aggregates, rendering PrP^{Sc} susceptible to proteolysis. Although the mechanisms are not clear, these compounds appear to interact with PrP^{Sc}, resulting in the blockade of de novo PrP^{Sc} formation and increased PrP^{Sc} clearance. However, the *in vitro* susceptibility of PrP^{Sc} to polyamine treatment was strain-dependent, limiting its application (Supattapone et al., 2001;Solassol et al., 2004). Peptides that disrupt protein β-sheets also can increase the susceptibility of PrP^{Sc} to protease degradation. A peptide capable of disrupting β-sheet structure was shown to reverse the inherent protease resistance of PrP^{Sc}, preventing prion formation in infected cultured cells and increasing the survival of mice inoculated with PrP^{Sc} (Soto et al., 2000). In this case, the same drawbacks described for other peptide treatments, namely BBB penetrability and protease susceptibility, still apply.

A number of other classes of compounds have also been tested for the ability to inhibit PrP^{Sc} accumulation. Polyanionic glycans, such as sulphated glycans, are known to non-specifically and indirectly inhibit the entry of viruses in cells and were first tested when prions were thought to be an unconventional virus. Pentosan polysulfate (PPS) showed promise as a therapeutic when administered directly into the cerebral ventricular system of a vCJD patient (Todd et al., 2005); however, these results were not replicated in other patients (Whittle et al., 2006). A recent monitoring study of seven British patients treated with PPS showed that, in spite of complications related to the administration itself, some of the patients treated with PPS appear to have survived for long periods (Bone et al., 2008) (http://www.prion.ucl.ac.uk/clinic-services/research/drug-treatments). It cannot be concluded, however, that the PPS treatment itself had a beneficial effect, as it was impossible to make direct comparisons with similar, but untreated, patients. It is also very difficult to determine exactly the time of disease onset, and this obviously affects the estimation of survival time. An drawback of polyanions is that their penetration of the BBB is minimal, again requiring direct brain administration.

Heparan mimetics (Congo Red, porphyrins and phtalocyanins) are among the first compounds identified as capable of binding to PrP^{C} and preventing PrP^{Sc} production (Caughey and Race, 1992). Congo Red displayed an ability to inhibit PrP^{Sc}, but is also limited in its ability to pass the BBB. Additionally, Congo Red can be cleaved in the mammalian gut and intestines to release highly carcinogenic benzidine. Curcumin shares many properties of Congo Red without its toxicity, and was demonstrated to share its properties as an effective inhibitor of PrP^{Sc} formation (Caughey et al., 2003). Curcumin treatment in mice was shown to result in a significantly prolonged survival time (Riemer et al., 2008).

Porphyrins and phtalocyanines are classes of compounds that were shown to prophylactically inhibit PrP^{Sc} formation and prolong survival in hamsters. Nevertheless, treatment at the onset of clinical symptoms did not result in significantly prolonged survival rates (Priola et al., 2000). Recently, poly-L-lysine polymers were also shown to strongly inhibit PrP^{Sc} propagation *in vitro*, in cell culture, and in mouse models of prion disease (Ryou et al., 2011).

Acridine and phenothiazine derivatives, which include the antimalarial and antipsychotic drug quinacrine, can pass the BBB and are effective inhibitors of PrP^{Sc} formation both *in vitro* and in cultured cells (Barret et al., 2003;Doh-ura et al., 2004). Even though quinacrine did not show anti-prion effects in infected rodents, this drug has been used extensively as an experimental treatment in CJD patients (Nakajima et al., 2004;Martinez-Lage et al., 2005). Although treatment sometimes resulted in slight improvement in patients' condition, this improvement was temporary and quinacrine treatment did not significantly delay disease progression. Following reports of improvement after quinacrine administration, two clinical trials were initiated. PRION-1 was led by Drs. Collinge and Darbyshire at the National Prion Clinic in the UK (http://www.prion.ucl.ac.uk/clinic-services/research/drug-treatments). The headline-making results of PRION-1 were published in 2009 and unfortunately showed no survival benefit of quinacrine (Collinge et al., 2009). A separate trial based in San Francisco, US, is currently active, led by Dr. Michael Geshwind (http://clinicaltrials.gov/ct2/show/NCT00183092?term=prion&rank=2). In addition, newer compounds with structures similar to quinacrine, trimipramine, and fluphenazine, have been shown to prolong the asymptomatic incubation period of prion infection, as well as to significantly reduce the degree of spongiosis, astrocytosis, and PrP^{Sc} levels in the brains of treated mice (Chung et al., 2011).

Tetracyclines also have been tested in prion therapy. Tetracycline efficiently crosses the BBB and can interact with amyloid fibrils that mimic the central features of the proteinase-resistant core of PrP^{Sc}. Incubation of tetracycline with purified PrP^{Sc} results in diminished proteinase resistance. Doxycycline administration leads to prolonged survival when administered 30 days after prion inoculation in mice. Preliminary data from observational studies in humans, in which doxycycline is administered for compassionate reasons, show to significantly prolong the survival of CJD patients, confirming the anti-prion activity of tetracyclines in humans. A drug vs. placebo clinical study is currently underway (Rigter et al., 2010) (http://www.prion.ucl.ac.uk/clinic-services/research/drug-treatments).

Interestingly, compounds that block amyloid aggregation may reach the clinic for the treatment of systemic amyloidoses long before amyloid-targeted drugs for neurodegenerative disorders, as these systemic disorders do not require compounds that cross the BBB. For example, transthyretin amyloidosis (ATTR) is caused by the deposition of transthyretin (TTR) amyloid fibrils in various tissues. The hereditary form of ATTR is caused by amyloidogenic mutations leading to abnormally folded monomers that self-assemble to amyloid fibrils. These TTR amyloid fibrils are then deposited extracellularly in various tissues. Two such compounds for the treatment of ATTR amyloidosis (Tafamidis from Pfizer and Scyllo-inositol from Elan) are currently in Phase III clinical trials (Aguzzi and O'Connor, 2010).

Alternative to the strategies aimed at reducing PrP^{Sc} accumulation, temptative therapies involving regeneration of the damaged tissues are also in progress. Cell therapy, which has been in trials for other neurodegenerative disorders, such as AD, is beginning to emerge as a viable option for prion diseases. In prion disease, intracerebral transplantation of fetal neural stem cells significantly extended both the incubation and survival time in mice, suggesting that stem cell therapy may be an effective possibility for human prion diseases (Relano-Gines et al., 2011).

The above mentioned therapeutic strategies all focus on impairing neurodegeneration engendered by these conditions. Nonetheless, for some neurodegenerative diseases, it has been proposed that compromised synaptic function is one of the earliest symptoms. Synaptic connectivity between neurons is critical for their survival and thus loss of synapses, spines, and dendrites precedes the loss of neuronal cell bodies. On the other hand, while synapses have an intrinsic plasticity and can be potentially replaced, neuronal loss is thus far irreversible. This knowledge means that the early stages of disease represent a highly attractive target for treatment. In prion diseases, it was recently demonstrated that mice experimentally infected with prions show changes in motivational behaviors long before the emergence of motor signs, and that these behavioral changes correlate with synaptic loss. Further, preventing neuronal death, but not synaptic dysfunction, does not halt the development of clinical disease in mice (Moreno et al., 2003; White and Mallucci, 2009; Verity and Mallucci, 2011). Many of the proposed therapies, therefore, may prove effective if administered at the time of synapse loss, rather than at the later stage of neuronal death. Thus, the identification of early dysfunction would help to direct therapies towards the earlier stages of disease, when rescue may still be possible. This may reflect a critical window for neuronal rescue that depends upon the kinetics of prion spread. The pre-clinical diagnosis of TSE is therefore of importance in the improvement and development of new therapies.

Ideally, a successful prion disease therapy should be able to cross the BBB or be delivered to the CNS, be non-toxic and effective at physiological concentrations, be efficient even after PrP^{Sc} accumulation, and would either not compromise PrP^{C} functionality or would allow for its restoration. Unfortunately, current therapeutic strategies are either only useful as a prophylactic or their applicability *in vivo* remains to be determined.

There are currently only a small number of clinical trials for treatment of CJD patients. Most reports include a single patient, and very few studies have been conducted under strict conditions. Due to the rarity of these diseases, studies usually contain a mixture of patients with different prion diseases with the assumption than the treatment may be effective for all of them. This is not necessarily true, as different prion strains may exhibit different sensitivities to drug treatments.

In the future, a combination of therapies aimed lowering the amount of PrP^{C} available for conversion with other strategies may prove the most effective. For example, the combination of RNAi against the PrP^{C} mRNA with a drug to increase endogenous clearance of PrP^{Sc} may be likely to delay disease progression. Hence, potential therapies need not aim for the total ablation of aberrant protein expression, but instead could have the lowering levels of expression below the cellular threshold for clearance as their goal. Of course, from a public health perspective, the elimination of neurotoxicity without abolishing prion replication maintains infectivity, leaving open the possibility of prion transmission.

While the ablation of PrP^{C} expression in adult mice is well tolerated, the consequences of reducing PrP^{C} in humans remain unknown. It may be that the risk-benefit ratio of the possible adverse effects of PrP^{C} loss against the potential for improved survival and protection against neuronal loss will determine future therapies for prion and other neurodegenerative disorders.

7. Concluding remarks

Prion diseases have represented a challenge to researchers and clinicians since the discovery of scrapie and kuru. The determination that scrapie, kuru, and CJD are related diseases and that they are both hereditary and transmissible, was a task that took many decades to resolve.

The discovery of the nature of the etiological agent responsible for these diseases also represented a breakthrough in the traditional concepts of molecular biology, and modified the paradigm that stated that flow of genetic information was mediated only by nucleic acids. A small number of proteins, particularly in yeast, are now known to have prion properties and are able to transmit information to their offspring (Uptain and Lindquist, 2002). Even more impressive, other neurodegenerative diseases, such as taupathies, have recently been demonstrated to be transmissible in transgenic mouse models (Clavaguera et al., 2009).

Although much progress has been made in the understanding of prion disease, many unanswered questions remain. For example, the exact molecular mechanism by which the PrP^{C} alteration leads to neurodegeneration is unknown. As a consequence, no effective therapy against these diseases has been developed. Also lacking is a precise, low-cost, high-throughput diagnostic tool, and an advance in this aspect could contribute to the chances of a successful therapy, due to the possibility of detecting the illness before the onset of clinical symptoms.

The realization that diseases characterized by protein conformational disorders have many aspects in common is also a recent development. The presence of soluble oligomeric forms of the proteins responsible for these different diseases is currently recognized as the most likely entities to induce neuronal damage, and plaques and proteinaceous aggregates are now though to play potentially protective roles in sequestering toxic oligomeric proteins. Thus, successful diagnostic or therapeutic strategies directed at one of these diseases will likely open new fields for all the others.

8. References

(1987) Rapidly progressive dementia in a patient who received a cadaveric dura mater graft. MMWR Morb Mortal Wkly Rep 36:49-50, 55.

(1997) Medicinal and other products and human and animal transmissible spongiform encephalopathies: memorandum from a WHO meeting. Bull World Health Organ 75:505-513.

Adams JM (1975) Persistent or slow viral infections and related diseases. West J Med 122:380-393.

Aguzzi A (1996) Pathogenesis of spongiform encephalopathies: an update. Int Arch Allergy Immunol 110:99-106.

Aguzzi A (2006) Prion diseases of humans and farm animals: epidemiology, genetics, and pathogenesis. J Neurochem 97:1726-1739.

Aguzzi A, Montrasio F, Kaeser PS (2001) Prions: health scare and biological challenge. Nat Rev Mol Cell Biol 2:118-126.

Aguzzi A, O'Connor T (2010) Protein aggregation diseases: pathogenicity and therapeutic perspectives. Nat Rev Drug Discov 9:237-248.

Aguzzi A, Polymenidou M (2004) Mammalian prion biology: one century of evolving concepts. Cell 116:313-327.

Aguzzi A, Weissmann C (1996) Spongiform encephalopathies: a suspicious signature. Nature 383:666-667.

Barret A, Tagliavini F, Forloni G, Bate C, Salmona M, Colombo L, De LA, Limido L, Suardi S, Rossi G, Auvre F, Adjou KT, Sales N, Williams A, Lasmezas C, Deslys JP (2003) Evaluation of quinacrine treatment for prion diseases. J Virol 77:8462-8469.

Bernoulli C, Siegfried J, Baumgartner G, Regli F, Rabinowicz T, Gajdusek DC, Gibbs CJ, Jr. (1977) Danger of accidental person-to-person transmission of Creutzfeldt-Jakob disease by surgery. Lancet 1:478-479.

Bertoni JM, Brown P, Goldfarb LG, Rubenstein R, Gajdusek DC (1992) Familial Creutzfeldt-Jakob disease (codon 200 mutation) with supranuclear palsy. JAMA 268:2413-2415.

Bolton DC, McKinley MP, Prusiner SB (1982) Identification of a protein that purifies with the scrapie prion. Science 218:1309-1311.

Bone I, Belton L, Walker AS, Darbyshire J (2008) Intraventricular pentosan polysulphate in human prion diseases: an observational study in the UK. Eur J Neurol 15:458-464.

Brown P (1995) Can Creutzfeldt-Jakob disease be transmitted by transfusion? Curr Opin Hematol 2:472-477.

Brown P, Brandel JP, Preece M, Sato T (2006) Iatrogenic Creutzfeldt-Jakob disease: the waning of an era. Neurology 67:389-393.

Brown P, Gibbs CJ, Jr., Rodgers-Johnson P, Asher DM, Sulima MP, Bacote A, Goldfarb LG, Gajdusek DC (1994) Human spongiform encephalopathy: the National Institutes of Health series of 300 cases of experimentally transmitted disease. Ann Neurol 35:513-529.

Brown P, Preece MA, Will RG (1992) "Friendly fire" in medicine: hormones, homografts, and Creutzfeldt-Jakob disease. Lancet 340:24-27.

Bruce ME, Will RG, Ironside JW, McConnell I, Drummond D, Suttie A, McCardle L, Chree A, Hope J, Birkett C, Cousens S, Fraser H, Bostock CJ (1997) Transmissions to mice indicate that 'new variant' CJD is caused by the BSE agent. Nature 389:498-501.

Budka H (2003) Neuropathology of prion diseases. Br Med Bull 66:121-130.

Bueler H, Aguzzi A, Sailer A, Greiner RA, Autenried P, Aguet M, Weissmann C (1993) Mice devoid of PrP are resistant to scrapie. Cell 73:1339-1347.

Caughey B, Race RE (1992) Potent inhibition of scrapie-associated PrP accumulation by congo red. J Neurochem 59:768-771.

Caughey B, Raymond LD, Raymond GJ, Maxson L, Silveira J, Baron GS (2003) Inhibition of protease-resistant prion protein accumulation in vitro by curcumin. J Virol 77:5499-5502.

Chabry J, Priola SA, Wehrly K, Nishio J, Hope J, Chesebro B (1999) Species-independent inhibition of abnormal prion protein (PrP) formation by a peptide containing a conserved PrP sequence. J Virol 73:6245-6250.

Chesebro B (2003) Introduction to the transmissible spongiform encephalopathies or prion diseases. Br Med Bull 66:1-20.

Chung E, Prelli F, Dealler S, Lee WS, Chang YT, Wisniewski T (2011) Styryl-based and tricyclic compounds as potential anti-prion agents. PLoS One 6:e24844.

Clavaguera F, Bolmont T, Crowther RA, Abramowski D, Frank S, Probst A, Fraser G, Stalder AK, Beibel M, Staufenbiel M, Jucker M, Goedert M, Tolnay M (2009) Transmission and spreading of tauopathy in transgenic mouse brain. Nat Cell Biol 11:909-913.

Collinge J, Gorham M, Hudson F, Kennedy A, Keogh G, Pal S, Rossor M, Rudge P, Siddique D, Spyer M, Thomas D, Walker S, Webb T, Wroe S, Darbyshire J (2009) Safety and efficacy of quinacrine in human prion disease (PRION-1 study): a patient-preference trial. Lancet Neurol 8:334-344.

Collinge J, Whitfield J, McKintosh E, Beck J, Mead S, Thomas DJ, Alpers MP (2006) Kuru in the 21st century--an acquired human prion disease with very long incubation periods. Lancet 367:2068-2074.

Collins S, Law MG, Fletcher A, Boyd A, Kaldor J, Masters CL (1999) Surgical treatment and risk of sporadic Creutzfeldt-Jakob disease: a case-control study. Lancet 353:693-697.

Collins SJ, Lawson VA, Masters CL (2004) Transmissible spongiform encephalopathies. Lancet 363:51-61.

Daude N, Marella M, Chabry J (2003) Specific inhibition of pathological prion protein accumulation by small interfering RNAs. J Cell Sci 116:2775-2779.

de SR, Findlay C, Awad I, Harries-Jones R, Knight R, Will R (1997) Creutzfeldt-Jakob disease in the elderly. Postgrad Med J 73:557-559.

Deslys JP, Lasmezas CI, Billette d, V, Jaegly A, Dormont D (1996) Creutzfeldt-Jakob disease. Lancet 347:1332.

Doh-ura K, Ishikawa K, Murakami-Kubo I, Sasaki K, Mohri S, Race R, Iwaki T (2004) Treatment of transmissible spongiform encephalopathy by intraventricular drug infusion in animal models. J Virol 78:4999-5006.

Duffy P, Wolf J, Collins G, DeVoe AG, Streeten B, Cowen D (1974) Letter: Possible person-to-person transmission of Creutzfeldt-Jakob disease. N Engl J Med 290:692-693.

Gajdusek DC (1977) Unconventional viruses and the origin and disappearance of kuru. Science 197:943-960.

Gajdusek DC (2008) Early images of kuru and the people of Okapa. Philos Trans R Soc Lond B Biol Sci 363:3636-3643.

Gajdusek DC, Gibbs CJ, Alpers M (1966) Experimental transmission of a Kuru-like syndrome to chimpanzees. Nature 209:794-796.

Gajdusek DC, REID LH (1961) Studies on kuru. IV. The kuru pattern in Moke, a representative Fore village. Am J Trop Med Hyg 10:628-638.

Gajdusek DC, ZIGAS V (1957) Degenerative disease of the central nervous system in New Guinea; the endemic occurrence of kuru in the native population. N Engl J Med 257:974-978.

Gajdusek DC, ZIGAS V (1959) Kuru; clinical, pathological and epidemiological study of an acute progressive degenerative disease of the central nervous system among natives of the Eastern Highlands of New Guinea. Am J Med 26:442-469.

Gambetti P, Petersen RB, Parchi P, Chen SG, Capellari S, Goldfarb L, Gabizon R, Montagna P, Lugaresi E, Piccardo P, Ghetti B (1999) Inherited Prion Diseases. In: Prion Biology and Diseases (Prusiner S, ed), pp 509-583. Cold Spring Harbor Laboratory Press.

Geschwind MD, Shu H, Haman A, Sejvar JJ, Miller BL (2008) Rapidly progressive dementia. Ann Neurol 64:97-108.

Ghetti B, Dlouhy SR, Giaccone G, Bugiani O, Frangione B, Farlow MR, Tagliavini F (1995) Gerstmann-Straussler-Scheinker disease and the Indiana kindred. Brain Pathol 5:61-75.

Gibbs CJ, Jr., Gajdusek DC, Asher DM, Alpers MP, Beck E, Daniel PM, Matthews WB (1968) Creutzfeldt-Jakob disease (spongiform encephalopathy): transmission to the chimpanzee. Science 161:388-389.

Glatzel M, Stoeck K, Seeger H, Luhrs T, Aguzzi A (2005) Human prion diseases: molecular and clinical aspects. Arch Neurol 62:545-552.

Goldfarb LG, Brown P, McCombie WR, Goldgaber D, Swergold GD, Wills PR, Cervenakova L, Baron H, Gibbs CJ, Jr., Gajdusek DC (1991a) Transmissible familial Creutzfeldt-Jakob disease associated with five, seven, and eight extra octapeptide coding repeats in the PRNP gene. Proc Natl Acad Sci U S A 88:10926-10930.

Goldfarb LG, Brown P, Mitrova E, Cervenakova L, Goldin L, Korczyn AD, Chapman J, Galvez S, Cartier L, Rubenstein R, . (1991b) Creutzfeldt-Jacob disease associated with the PRNP codon 200Lys mutation: an analysis of 45 families. Eur J Epidemiol 7:477-486.

Goldfarb LG, Mitrova E, Brown P, Toh BK, Gajdusek DC (1990) Mutation in codon 200 of scrapie amyloid protein gene in two clusters of Creutzfeldt-Jakob disease in Slovakia. Lancet 336:514-515.

Goldgaber D, Goldfarb LG, Brown P, Asher DM, Brown WT, Lin S, Teener JW, Feinstone SM, Rubenstein R, Kascsak RJ, . (1989) Mutations in familial Creutzfeldt-Jakob disease and Gerstmann-Straussler-Scheinker's syndrome. Exp Neurol 106:204-206.

Gordon WS (1946) Advances in veterinary research. Vet Rec 58:516-525.

Griffith JS (1967) Self-replication and scrapie. Nature 215:1043-1044.

Hainfellner JA, Jellinger K, Diringer H, Guentchev M, Kleinert R, Pilz P, Maier H, Budka H (1996) Creutzfeldt-Jakob disease in Austria. J Neurol Neurosurg Psychiatry 61:139-142.

Hamaguchi T, Noguchi-Shinohara M, Nozaki I, Nakamura Y, Sato T, Kitamoto T, Mizusawa H, Yamada M (2009) The risk of iatrogenic Creutzfeldt-Jakob disease through medical and surgical procedures. Neuropathology 29:625-631.

Handisurya A, Gilch S, Winter D, Shafti-Keramat S, Maurer D, Schatzl HM, Kirnbauer R (2007) Vaccination with prion peptide-displaying papillomavirus-like particles induces autoantibodies to normal prion protein that interfere with pathologic prion protein production in infected cells. FEBS J 274:1747-1758.

Harper PS (1977) Mendelian inheritance or transmissible agent? The lesson Kuru and the Australia antigen. J Med Genet 14:389-398.

Heppner FL, Musahl C, Arrighi I, Klein MA, Rulicke T, Oesch B, Zinkernagel RM, Kalinke U, Aguzzi A (2001) Prevention of scrapie pathogenesis by transgenic expression of anti-prion protein antibodies. Science 294:178-182.

Hill AF, Desbruslais M, Joiner S, Sidle KC, Gowland I, Collinge J, Doey LJ, Lantos P (1997a) The same prion strain causes vCJD and BSE. Nature 389:448-50, 526.

Hill AF, Zeidler M, Ironside J, Collinge J (1997b) Diagnosis of new variant Creutzfeldt-Jakob disease by tonsil biopsy. Lancet 349:99-100.

Horiuchi M, Priola SA, Chabry J, Caughey B (2000) Interactions between heterologous forms of prion protein: binding, inhibition of conversion, and species barriers. Proc Natl Acad Sci U S A 97:5836-5841.

Hsiao K, Baker HF, Crow TJ, Poulter M, Owen F, Terwilliger JD, Westaway D, Ott J, Prusiner SB (1989) Linkage of a prion protein missense variant to Gerstmann-Straussler syndrome. Nature 338:342-345.

Hsiao K, Meiner Z, Kahana E, Cass C, Kahana I, Avrahami D, Scarlato G, Abramsky O, Prusiner SB, Gabizon R (1991a) Mutation of the prion protein in Libyan Jews with Creutzfeldt-Jakob disease. N Engl J Med 324:1091-1097.

Hsiao KK, Cass C, Schellenberg GD, Bird T, Devine-Gage E, Wisniewski H, Prusiner SB (1991b) A prion protein variant in a family with the telencephalic form of Gerstmann-Straussler-Scheinker syndrome. Neurology 41:681-684.

Hsich G, Kenney K, Gibbs CJ, Lee KH, Harrington MG (1996) The 14-3-3 brain protein in cerebrospinal fluid as a marker for transmissible spongiform encephalopathies. N Engl J Med 335:924-930.

Ironside JW (2010) Variant Creutzfeldt-Jakob disease. Haemophilia 16 Suppl 5:175-180.

Knight R (2010) The risk of transmitting prion disease by blood or plasma products. Transfus Apher Sci 43:387-391.

Kovacs GG, Zerbi P, Voigtlander T, Strohschneider M, Trabattoni G, Hainfellner JA, Budka H (2002) The prion protein in human neurodegenerative disorders. Neurosci Lett 329:269-272.

Kretzschmar HA, Honold G, Seitelberger F, Feucht M, Wessely P, Mehraein P, Budka H (1991) Prion protein mutation in family first reported by Gerstmann, Straussler, and Scheinker. Lancet 337:1160.

Ladogana A, Puopolo M, Poleggi A, Almonti S, Mellina V, Equestre M, Pocchiari M (2005) High incidence of genetic human transmissible spongiform encephalopathies in Italy. Neurology 64:1592-1597.

Llewelyn CA, Hewitt PE, Knight RS, Amar K, Cousens S, Mackenzie J, Will RG (2004) Possible transmission of variant Creutzfeldt-Jakob disease by blood transfusion. Lancet 363:417-421.

Lugaresi E, Medori R, Montagna P, Baruzzi A, Cortelli P, Lugaresi A, Tinuper P, Zucconi M, Gambetti P (1986) Fatal familial insomnia and dysautonomia with selective degeneration of thalamic nuclei. N Engl J Med 315:997-1003.

Mabbott NA, Young J, McConnell I, Bruce ME (2003) Follicular dendritic cell dedifferentiation by treatment with an inhibitor of the lymphotoxin pathway dramatically reduces scrapie susceptibility. J Virol 77:6845-6854.

Martinez-Lage JF, Rabano A, Bermejo J, Martinez PM, Guerrero MC, Contreras MA, Lunar A (2005) Creutzfeldt-Jakob disease acquired via a dural graft: failure of therapy with quinacrine and chlorpromazine. Surg Neurol 64:542-5, discussion.

Masters CL, Gajdusek DC, Gibbs CJ, Jr. (1981) Creutzfeldt-Jakob disease virus isolations from the Gerstmann-Straussler syndrome with an analysis of the various forms of amyloid plaque deposition in the virus-induced spongiform encephalopathies. Brain 104:559-588.

McCutcheon S, Alejo Blanco AR, Houston EF, de WC, Tan BC, Smith A, Groschup MH, Hunter N, Hornsey VS, MacGregor IR, Prowse CV, Turner M, Manson JC (2011) All clinically-relevant blood components transmit prion disease following a single blood transfusion: a sheep model of vCJD. PLoS One 6:e23169.

Medori R, Montagna P, Tritschler HJ, LeBlanc A, Cortelli P, Tinuper P, Lugaresi E, Gambetti P (1992a) Fatal familial insomnia: a second kindred with mutation of prion protein gene at codon 178. Neurology 42:669-670.

Medori R, Tritschler HJ, LeBlanc A, Villare F, Manetto V, Chen HY, Xue R, Leal S, Montagna P, Cortelli P, . (1992b) Fatal familial insomnia, a prion disease with a mutation at codon 178 of the prion protein gene. N Engl J Med 326:444-449.

Meyer RK, McKinley MP, Bowman KA, Braunfeld MB, Barry RA, Prusiner SB (1986) Separation and properties of cellular and scrapie prion proteins. Proc Natl Acad Sci U S A 83:2310-2314.

Minor P, Newham J, Jones N, Bergeron C, Gregori L, Asher D, van EF, Stroebel T, Vey M, Barnard G, Head M (2004) Standards for the assay of Creutzfeldt-Jakob disease specimens. J Gen Virol 85:1777-1784.

Montrasio F, Frigg R, Glatzel M, Klein MA, Mackay F, Aguzzi A, Weissmann C (2000) Impaired prion replication in spleens of mice lacking functional follicular dendritic cells. Science 288:1257-1259.

Moreno CR, Lantier F, Lantier I, Sarradin P, Elsen JM (2003) Detection of new quantitative trait Loci for susceptibility to transmissible spongiform encephalopathies in mice. Genetics 165:2085-2091.

Mukherjee A, Morales-Scheihing D, Gonzalez-Romero D, Green K, Taglialatela G, Soto C (2010) Calcineurin inhibition at the clinical phase of prion disease reduces neurodegeneration, improves behavioral alterations and increases animal survival. PLoS Pathog 6:e1001138.

Murray K (2011) Creutzfeldt-Jacob disease mimics, or how to sort out the subacute encephalopathy patient. Pract Neurol 11:19-28.

Murray K, Ritchie DL, Bruce M, Young CA, Doran M, Ironside JW, Will RG (2008) Sporadic Creutzfeldt-Jakob disease in two adolescents. J Neurol Neurosurg Psychiatry 79:14-18.

Nakajima M, Yamada T, Kusuhara T, Furukawa H, Takahashi M, Yamauchi A, Kataoka Y (2004) Results of quinacrine administration to patients with Creutzfeldt-Jakob disease. Dement Geriatr Cogn Disord 17:158-163.

Nathanson N, Wilesmith J, Griot C (1997) Bovine spongiform encephalopathy (BSE): causes and consequences of a common source epidemic. Am J Epidemiol 145:959-969.

Nikles D, Bach P, Boller K, Merten CA, Montrasio F, Heppner FL, Aguzzi A, Cichutek K, Kalinke U, Buchholz CJ (2005) Circumventing tolerance to the prion protein (PrP): vaccination with PrP-displaying retrovirus particles induces humoral immune responses against the native form of cellular PrP. J Virol 79:4033-4042.

Oesch B, Westaway D, Walchli M, McKinley MP, Kent SB, Aebersold R, Barry RA, Tempst P, Teplow DB, Hood LE, . (1985) A cellular gene encodes scrapie PrP 27-30 protein. Cell 40:735-746.

Otto M, Wiltfang J, Cepek L, Neumann M, Mollenhauer B, Steinacker P, Ciesielczyk B, Schulz-Schaeffer W, Kretzschmar HA, Poser S (2002) Tau protein and 14-3-3 protein in the differential diagnosis of Creutzfeldt-Jakob disease. Neurology 58:192-197.

Padovani A, D'Alessandro M, Parchi P, Cortelli P, Anzola GP, Montagna P, Vignolo LA, Petraroli R, Pocchiari M, Lugaresi E, Gambetti P (1998) Fatal familial insomnia in a new Italian kindred. Neurology 51:1491-1494.

Palmer MS, Dryden AJ, Hughes JT, Collinge J (1991) Homozygous prion protein genotype predisposes to sporadic Creutzfeldt-Jakob disease. Nature 352:340-342.

Priola SA, Raines A, Caughey WS (2000) Porphyrin and phthalocyanine antiscrapie compounds. Science 287:1503-1506.

Prusiner S (1999) An Introduction to Prion Biology and Diseases. In: Prion Biology and Disease (Prusiner S, ed), pp 1-66. Cold Spring Harbor Laboratory Press.

Prusiner SB (1982) Novel proteinaceous infectious particles cause scrapie. Science 216:136-144.

Prusiner SB (1989) Creutzfeldt-Jakob disease and scrapie prions. Alzheimer Dis Assoc Disord 3:52-78.

Prusiner SB, McKinley MP, Bowman KA, Bolton DC, Bendheim PE, Groth DF, Glenner GG (1983) Scrapie prions aggregate to form amyloid-like birefringent rods. Cell 35:349-358.

Radbauer C, Hainfellner JA, Jellinger K, Pilz P, Maier H, Kleinert R, Budka H (1998) [Epidemiology of transmissible spongiform encephalopathies (prion diseases) in Austria]. Wien Med Wochenschr 148:101-106.

Relano-Gines A, Lehmann S, Bencsik A, Herva ME, Torres JM, Crozet CA (2011) Stem cell therapy extends incubation and survival time in prion-infected mice in a time window-dependant manner. J Infect Dis 204:1038-1045.

Riemer C, Burwinkel M, Schwarz A, Gultner S, Mok SW, Heise I, Holtkamp N, Baier M (2008) Evaluation of drugs for treatment of prion infections of the central nervous system. J Gen Virol 89:594-597.

Rigter A, Langeveld JP, van Zijderveld FG, Bossers A (2010) Prion protein self-interactions: a gateway to novel therapeutic strategies? Vaccine 28:7810-7823.

Ryou C, Titlow WB, Mays CE, Bae Y, Kim S (2011) The suppression of prion propagation using poly-L-lysine by targeting plasminogen that stimulates prion protein conversion. Biomaterials 32:3141-3149.

Sadowski MJ, Pankiewicz J, Prelli F, Scholtzova H, Spinner DS, Kascsak RB, Kascsak RJ, Wisniewski T (2009) Anti-PrP Mab 6D11 suppresses PrP(Sc) replication in prion infected myeloid precursor line FDC-P1/22L and in the lymphoreticular system in vivo. Neurobiol Dis 34:267-278.

Satoh K, Tobiume M, Matsui Y, Mutsukura K, Nishida N, Shiga Y, Eguhchi K, Shirabe S, Sata T (2010) Establishment of a standard 14-3-3 protein assay of cerebrospinal fluid as a diagnostic tool for Creutzfeldt-Jakob disease. Lab Invest 90:1637-1644.

Schneider K, Fangerau H, Michaelsen B, Raab WH (2008) The early history of the transmissible spongiform encephalopathies exemplified by scrapie. Brain Res Bull 77:343-355.

Schwarz A, Kratke O, Burwinkel M, Riemer C, Schultz J, Henklein P, Bamme T, Baier M (2003) Immunisation with a synthetic prion protein-derived peptide prolongs survival times of mice orally exposed to the scrapie agent. Neurosci Lett 350:187-189.

Shastry BS (2003) Neurodegenerative disorders of protein aggregation. Neurochem Int 43:1-7.

Sigurdsson EM, Brown DR, Daniels M, Kascsak RJ, Kascsak R, Carp R, Meeker HC, Frangione B, Wisniewski T (2002) Immunization delays the onset of prion disease in mice. Am J Pathol 161:13-17.

Sigurdsson EM, Sy MS, Li R, Scholtzova H, Kascsak RJ, Kascsak R, Carp R, Meeker HC, Frangione B, Wisniewski T (2003) Anti-prion antibodies for prophylaxis following prion exposure in mice. Neurosci Lett 336:185-187.

Solassol J, Crozet C, Perrier V, Leclaire J, Beranger F, Caminade AM, Meunier B, Dormont D, Majoral JP, Lehmann S (2004) Cationic phosphorus-containing dendrimers reduce prion replication both in cell culture and in mice infected with scrapie. J Gen Virol 85:1791-1799.

Solforosi L, Criado JR, McGavern DB, Wirz S, Sanchez-Alavez M, Sugama S, DeGiorgio LA, Volpe BT, Wiseman E, Abalos G, Masliah E, Gilden D, Oldstone MB, Conti B, Williamson RA (2004) Cross-linking cellular prion protein triggers neuronal apoptosis in vivo. Science 303:1514-1516.

Soto C (2003) Unfolding the role of protein misfolding in neurodegenerative diseases. Nat Rev Neurosci 4:49-60.

Soto C, Kascsak RJ, Saborio GP, Aucouturier P, Wisniewski T, Prelli F, Kascsak R, Mendez E, Harris DA, Ironside J, Tagliavini F, Carp RI, Frangione B (2000) Reversion of prion protein conformational changes by synthetic beta-sheet breaker peptides. Lancet 355:192-197.

Stack M, Jeffrey M, Gubbins S, Grimmer S, Gonzalez L, Martin S, Chaplin M, Webb P, Simmons M, Spencer Y, Bellerby P, Hope J, Wilesmith J, Matthews D (2006) Monitoring for bovine spongiform encephalopathy in sheep in Great Britain, 1998-2004. J Gen Virol 87:2099-2107.

Supattapone S, Wille H, Uyechi L, Safar J, Tremblay P, Szoka FC, Cohen FE, Prusiner SB, Scott MR (2001) Branched polyamines cure prion-infected neuroblastoma cells. J Virol 75:3453-3461.

Todd NV, Morrow J, Doh-ura K, Dealler S, O'Hare S, Farling P, Duddy M, Rainov NG (2005) Cerebroventricular infusion of pentosan polysulphate in human variant Creutzfeldt-Jakob disease. J Infect 50:394-396.

Toupet K, Compan V, Crozet C, Mourton-Gilles C, Mestre-Frances N, Ibos F, Corbeau P, Verdier JM, Perrier V (2008) Effective gene therapy in a mouse model of prion diseases. PLoS One 3:e2773.

Tyrrell DAJ, Taylor K (1996) Handling the BSE Epidemic in Great Britain. In: Prion Diseases (Baker HF, Ridley RM, eds), pp 175-198. Humana Press.

Uptain SM, Lindquist S (2002) Prions as protein-based genetic elements. Annu Rev Microbiol 56:703-741.

Valleron AJ, Boelle PY, Will R, Cesbron JY (2001) Estimation of epidemic size and incubation time based on age characteristics of vCJD in the United Kingdom. Science 294:1726-1728.

Venneti S (2010) Prion diseases. Clin Lab Med 30:293-309.

Verity NC, Mallucci GR (2011) Rescuing neurons in prion disease. Biochem J 433:19-29.

Vitali P, Maccagnano E, Caverzasi E, Henry RG, Haman A, Torres-Chae C, Johnson DY, Miller BL, Geschwind MD (2011) Diffusion-weighted MRI hyperintensity patterns differentiate CJD from other rapid dementias. Neurology 76:1711-1719.

Ward HJ, Everington D, Croes EA, Alperovitch A, Delasnerie-Laupretre N, Zerr I, Poser S, van Duijn CM (2002) Sporadic Creutzfeldt-Jakob disease and surgery: a case-control study using community controls. Neurology 59:543-548.

Wells GA, Wilesmith JW (1995) The neuropathology and epidemiology of bovine spongiform encephalopathy. Brain Pathol 5:91-103.

White AR, Enever P, Tayebi M, Mushens R, Linehan J, Brandner S, Anstee D, Collinge J, Hawke S (2003) Monoclonal antibodies inhibit prion replication and delay the development of prion disease. Nature 422:80-83.

White MD, Farmer M, Mirabile I, Brandner S, Collinge J, Mallucci GR (2008) Single treatment with RNAi against prion protein rescues early neuronal dysfunction and prolongs survival in mice with prion disease. Proc Natl Acad Sci U S A 105:10238-10243.

White MD, Mallucci GR (2009) RNAi for the treatment of prion disease: a window for intervention in neurodegeneration? CNS Neurol Disord Drug Targets 8:342-352.

Whittle IR, Knight RS, Will RG (2006) Unsuccessful intraventricular pentosan polysulphate treatment of variant Creutzfeldt-Jakob disease. Acta Neurochir (Wien) 148:677-679.

Wilesmith JW, Ryan JB, Atkinson MJ (1991) Bovine spongiform encephalopathy: epidemiological studies on the origin. Vet Rec 128:199-203.

Will RG (2003) Acquired prion disease: iatrogenic CJD, variant CJD, kuru. Br Med Bull 66:255-265.

Will RG, Alpers MP, Dormont D, Schonberger LB, Tateishi J (1999) Infectious and Sporadic Prion Diseases. In: Prion Biology and Diseases (Prusiner S, ed), pp 465-507. Cold Spring Harbor Laboratory Press.

Will RG, Ironside JW, Zeidler M, Cousens SN, Estibeiro K, Alperovitch A, Poser S, Pocchiari M, Hofman A, Smith PG (1996) A new variant of Creutzfeldt-Jakob disease in the UK. Lancet 347:921-925.

Will RG, Zeidler M, Stewart GE, Macleod MA, Ironside JW, Cousens SN, Mackenzie J, Estibeiro K, Green AJ, Knight RS (2000) Diagnosis of new variant Creutzfeldt-Jakob disease. Ann Neurol 47:575-582.

Wisniewski T, Goni F (2010) Immunomodulation for prion and prion-related diseases. Expert Rev Vaccines 9:1441-1452.

Zanusso G, Fiorini M, Ferrari S, Gajofatto A, Cagnin A, Galassi A, Richelli S, Monaco S (2011) Cerebrospinal fluid markers in sporadic creutzfeldt-jakob disease. Int J Mol Sci 12:6281-6292.

Zetterstrom R (2010) The discovery of misfolded prions as an infectious agent. Acta Paediatr 99:1910-1913.

9

Cognitive Impairments in Drug Addicts

Fred Nyberg
Department of Pharmaceutical Biosciences, Uppsala University
Sweden

1. Introduction

Recent work exploring the effects of abusing alcohol, central stimulants, and opiates on the central nervous system (CNS) have demonstrated a variety of adverse effects related to mental health. In several laboratories and clinics substantial damages of brain function are seen to result from these drugs. Among the harmful effects of the abusing drugs on brain are those contributing to accelerated obsolescence. These putative aging effects including inhibition of neurogenesis and enhanced apoptosis underline the dark side of drug addiction and will doubtlessy be a challenge for future research (Carvalho, 2009). An observation that has received special attention during recent years is that chronic drug users display pronounced impairment in brain areas associated with executive and memory function (Ersche et al., 2006).

Addiction to drugs is characterized as a compulsive behavior, including drug seeking, drug use, and drug cravings but it is also considered as a disorder of altered cognition (Gould, 2010). Indeed, brain areas and processes involved in drug addiction substantially overlap with those known to be of relevance for cognitive functions. Studies have indicated that abusing drugs may alter the normal structure in these regions and influence functions that induce cognitive shifts and promote continued drug use. Processes during early stages of drug abuse is suggested to promote strong maladaptive connections between use of drugs and environmental input underlying future cravings and drug-seeking behaviors. Continued drug use causes cognitive deficits that aggravate the difficulty of establishing sustained abstinence (Gould, 2010). In fact, drug addiction has been characterized as a disease of "pathological learning" by several investigators (Hyman, 2005; Gould, 2010).

In earlier days abusing drugs were considered only to induce non-specific effects on the brain. Today, it is widely believed that they may produce selective adaptations in very specific brain regions. These neuroadaptations have been extensively examined in order to clarify mechanisms underlying the development and maintenance of addiction to find strategies for relevant treatment. The hippocampus is an area included in the limbic structures that is of particular interest, as it is found to be essential for several aspects related to the addictive process. A remarked neuroadaptation caused by addictive drugs, such as alcohol, central stimulants and opiates involves diminished neurogenesis in the subgranular zone (SGZ) of the hippocampus. Indeed, it has been proposed that decreased adult neurogenesis in the SGZ could modify the hippocampal function in such a way that it contributes to relapse and a maintained addictive behavior (Arguello et al., 2008). It also raises the possibility that decreased neurogenesis may contribute to cognitive deficits elicited by these abusing drugs.

In addition to hippocampal structures the prefrontal cortex and its different subregions have also been hypothesized to represent this cognitive control system (George et al., 2010; Ridderinkhof et al., 2004). Neurons in the dorsolateral prefrontal cortex are suggested to be involved in activity that in delayed matching to sample tasks persists throughout the delay period (Weiss and Disterhoft, 2011). Moreover, age-related changes in the prefrontal cortex microcolumnar organization are shown to correlate with age-related declines in cognition. Activity that persists beyond the induction of a specific stimulus is believed to mediate working memory processes, and disruption of those processes is related to memory deficits that often accompany the aging process. The prefrontal cortex is known as an area with enhanced vulnerability to alcohol-induced damage. It is suggested that inhibition of adult neurogenesis may be a factor that underlie alcohol-mediated cognitive dysfunction, which in turn may be a cause to decreased behavioral control over consumption (Nixon and McClain, 2010). Also, an influence of opioids and stimulant drugs on hippocampal neurogenesis in adults has been confirmed (Eisch et al., 2000). Exposure to psychotropic drugs is suggested to regulate the rate of neurogenesis in the adult brain, suggesting a possible role for neurogenesis in the drug-induced impairments seen in cognitive functions (Duman et al., 2001).

This article is aimed to provide a comprehensive collocation of the impact of abusing drugs on cognitive functions. It describes adverse effects on learning and memory of selected drugs and how these compounds interact with neuronal circuits involved in these behaviors. Possible approaches to deal with these drug-induced damages from the pharmacological point of view will also be discussed.

2. Memory and learning

Memory is described as a multi-system phenomenon in the brain. Each system has been associated with a separate memory function targeting different neurological substrates. For example, declarative memory is attributed to a function of retaining conscious memories of facts and sights. The establishment of new declarative memories is related to structures in the diencephalon and the medial temporal lobe, and it has been proposed that these memory imprints are generated in specific areas of the cerebral cortex. For example, brain areas implicated in deficits in declarative memory include the prefrontal cortex and the hippocampus. The frontal cortex is recognized as an important substrate for features related to reasoning and memory content of the declarative memory (Samuelson, 2011; Weiss and Disterhoft, 2011). Classical conditioning, skill learning and repetition learning, i.e. nondeclarative forms of memory, are documented through changes in the way they are carried out and are not considered to involve conscious recollection. The functional anatomy of these nondeclarative forms of memory are believed to comprise the basal ganglia, cerebellum and cerebral cortex.

A concept of synaptic plasticity essential for the storage of long-term memory (LTM) at the cellular level is the long-term potentiation (LTP). LTP is shown to enhance the signal transmission between neighboring neurons over a long period of time and it can be induced by high-frequency stimulation of the synapse, and at this level it represents an important target for studies of memory enhancement. LTP is an attractive candidate for explanation of cellular mechanisms underlying learning and memory as it shares many features with LTM. Both LTP and LTM are triggered rapidly, and each of them seems to be dependent on the biosynthetic process for protein formation and the proteins, which are formed, are belived to have a role in associative memory and have been suggested to last over a long period of time. Furthermore, LTP is found to be linked to a number of different types of learning, and these are shown to include the simple classical conditioning observed in experimental animals as well as the more complex, higher-level cognition that is experienced by humans (Cooke and Bliss, 2006).

Although LTP is not demonstrated in all brain regions it has been clearly seen in many areas, including amygdala, hippocampus, nucleus accumbens and prefrontal cortex, i.e. regions involved in drug reward but also in memory and learning (Kenney and Gould, 2008). For instance, enhanced activity in amygdala and enhanced amygdala-hippocampus connectivity leading to long-lasting, non-temporary memory alterations has been described (Edelson et al., 2011). It was further indicated that the hippocampus is essential for the transfer of short-term memories to LTMs (Santini et al., 2001; Glannon, 2006). In addition, clinical investigations including neuropsychological patients as well as studies using experimental animals have suggested that, in addition to its critical role in the LTM formation, the hippocampal structure is essential for the integrating and processing of spatial and coherent information (Kim and Lee, 2011).

The molecular mechanism underlying memory potentiation is suggested to involve the excitatory amino acid glutamate (Abel and Lattal, 2001). Glutamate binding activates both the N-methyl-D-aspartyl (NMDA) and the α-amino-3-hydroxy-5-methyl-4-isoxazole propionic acid (AMPA) receptors located on the cell membrane of the nerve cells. These events lead to the opening of calcium and sodium channels into the nerve cells. The calcium influx activates the enzyme adenylate cyclase, which in turn converts ATP to cAMP. Subsequent to this event the cAMP actuates a sequential activation of protein kinase A, mitogen-activated protein kinase/extracellular signal-regulated protein kinase, as well as the cAMP response element-binding factor (CREB). The activated CREB attaches to DNA and induces transcription and subsequently an increased production of proteins essential for the construction of new synapses (Abel and Lattal, 2001).

Regarding the NMDA receptor it has been shown in experimental animal models that the organization of the receptor subunits NR1, NR2A, NR2B and NR2D is essential for the memory promoting effect of glutamate. For instance, transgenic mice overexpressing the NR2B subunit exhibit improved performance in memory tests (Tang et al., 1999). Also the ratio of the NR2B to NR2A ratio has been shown as a relevant marker on cognitive functioning in the rat. Increased ratio of NR2B/NR2A has been seen to increase LTP (Le Grevès et al., 2002; Le Grevés et al., 2006; Zhao et al., 2005).

A considerable amount of evidence supports an important role for glutamate and its ligand-gated ionotropic receptors (i.e. NMDA, AMPA, and kainic acid (KA) subtypes) in mediating addictive behaviors have been collected over the years (Wolf, 1998; Tzschentke and Schmidt, 2003; Kalivas, 2004; Gass and Olive, 2009). However, the role of metabotropic glutamate (mGlu) receptors in the neural mechanisms underlying drug addiction has become apparent only within the latest decades (Olive, 2010). Evidence for a role of Group I ($mGlu_1$ and

$mGlu_5$) receptors in regulating drug intake, reward, reinforcement, and reinstatement of drug-seeking behavior have emerged from recent pharmacological and genetic studies (Olive, 2009) . However, these kind of mGlu receptors is also suggested to mediate cognitive processes including learning and memory, behavioral flexibility, and extinction (Moghaddam, 2004; Simonyi et al., 2005; Gravius et al., 2006; Gass and Olive, 2009) and deficits in these expressions of cognition are frequently observed in drug addicts.

3. Drug effects on cognitive function

As mentioned above drug addiction is seen as a chronic relapsing disorder with persistent brain alterations associated with cognitive, motivational and emotional alterations and studies have indicated the presence of extensive cognitive alterations in many individuals diagnosed with substance use disorders (Goldstein and Volkow, 2002; Fernández-Serrano et al., 2010). Thus, over the past decades the influence of abusing drugs on cognitive capabilities in addicts has been the subject for many studies in various clinical and basic science laboratories. Although it has been known for long that alcoholism is connected with deficient memory and learning and seems to accelerate aging processes, negative effects of chronic use of narcotics on cognitive functions have become evident during more recent times. This section focuses on adverse effects induced by some frequently used drugs, including alcohol, central stimulants, and opioids. All these substances have been reported to affect many aspects of memory and learning.

3.1 Alcohol-induced effects on memory and cognition

Emerging data from past and current research provide evidence for cognitive impairments of alcohol-dependent patients, particularly regarding their ability to perform tasks sensitive to frontal lobe function. This fact has brought up the importance of a significant abstinence allowing individuals with these impairments to recover (Glass et al., 2009; Loeber et al., 2009).

The adverse effect of alcohol on cognitive function is typified by the well-known Wernicke-Korsakoff syndrome (WKS). This disorder is a neurological disturbance and it is caused by the lack of thiamine (vitamin B_1) in the brain. Its onset is linked to mal nutrition or to alcoholism. In Western countries WKS is perhaps the most common alcohol-induced memory disturbance. It is characterized by neuropathological changes in the diencephalon, including the anterior part of the thalamus, and the mammillary body caused by thiamine deficiency (Kopelman et al., 2009). The most characteristic neuropsychological feature of WKS is a marked decline in memory capabilities, whereas other intellectual abilities are relatively preserved. Alcohol-related dementia is generally defined as alcohol-induced dementia in the Diagnostic and Statistical Manual of Mental Disorders IV- Text Revision (DSM-IV- TR). It has been described as an organic brain syndrome induced by over-consumption of alcohol, which causes severe cognitive impairment, including executive dysfunction, lack of emotional control and disturbances in memory function (Asada et al., 2010).

Evidence that emerges from experimental studies has shown that early exposure to alcohol sensitizes the neurocircuitry of addiction and affects chromatin remodeling. These events could give rise to altered plasticity in reward-related cognitive processes that contribute to vulnerability to drug addiction in adolescents (Guerri and Pascual, 2010). There are potential mechanisms by which alcohol affects brain development and causes brain impairments including cognitive and behavioral dysfunctions but also neurochemical processes underlying the adolescent-specific vulnerability to drug addiction (Guerri and Pascual, 2010).

Moreover, in heavy episodic drinkers reduced psychomotor speed and a decline in accuracy when performing tasks of attention, working memory, implicit memory as well as associate learning and memory have been reported (Cairney et al., 2007). For instance, among the population of Aboriginal Australians, who were heavy episodic alcoholic users, specific cognitive abnormalities that suggest frontostriatal abnormalities have been observed in association with chronic alcoholism (Cairney et al., 2007).

In the brains of alcoholics the frontal lobes, with significant neuronal losses in the superior frontal cortex, are shown to be the most insulted areas (Kubota et al., 2001; Sullivan and Pfefferbaum, 2005). These lobes are known to regulate complex cognitive skills including working memory, attention, temporal ordering, mood, motivation, risk taking and wanting as well as discrimination and reversal learning that underlie judgment. Studies have revealed that a complicated mechanism may underlie alcohol-induced damage to the brain. Also, the mechanism underlying the abstinence-induced regeneration seems to be complex. The magnitude of neurodegeneration and the potential for recovery and regeneration vary between different regions of the brain and seem to be dependent on several factors, such as pattern of intake, age and genetics (Crews and Nixon, 2009). Moreover, binge ethanol exposure of rats is seen to reduce hippocampal neurogenesis (Nixon and Crews, 2002) and brain degeneration in the binge ethanol treatment model is generally widely circulated and diffused, in similarity to what is observed in human alcoholics.

A recent study performed in order to investigate the harmful effects of binge alcohol on the hippocampal neurogenesis in adolescent non-human primates suggested that the liquid drug may interfere with the migration and distribution of hippocampal preneuronal progenitors (Taffe et al., 2010). Furthermore, the decreased neurogenesis induced by alcohol in the hippocampus was seen to be paralleled by an increase in neural degeneration thought to be mediated by non-apoptotic pathways. This effect remained for quite a long time following alcohol discontinuation and it was suggested to cause the deterioration in hippocampus-associated cognitive tasks that are frequently seen in alcoholics (Taffe et al., 2010).

Regarding the mechanism underlying alcohol-induced neurodegeneration and cognitive impairment the involvement of glutamatergic neurotransmission seems well documented, however, many details of the underlying mechanism remains unknown. Studies have been focused both on the NMDA receptor system and the group II metabotropic glutamate receptor. A recent study examined the effect of the agonist LY379268 on its ability to prevent neuronal death and learning deficits in a rat model of binge-like exposure to alcohol (Cippitelli et al., 2010). It was found that neurodegeneration was most extensive in the ventral hippocampus and the entorhinal cortex (EC) and the glutamate receptor agonist was potently neuroprotective in the EC but not in the dentate gyrus of the hippocampus. In additional experiments, binge alcohol exposure suppressed the expression of transforming growth factor beta (TGF-beta) expression in both the EC and dentate gyrus, while the glutamate agonist increased TGF-beta in the EC only. It was further reported that the neuroprotective effects of the glutamate agonist were paralleled with prevention of deficits in spatial reversal learning. These data was considered to give support for a protective role of TGF-beta and group II metabotropic glutamate receptor agonists in alcohol-induced neurodegeneration (Cippitelli et al., 2010).

However, studies have confirmed that alcohol may damage specific regions both in the adult and the adolescent brain (Alfonso-Loeches and Guerri, 2011). The mechanisms behind this damage is suggested to involve excitotoxicity, free radical formation and neuroinflammatory destructions caused by activation of the immune system and mediated through Toll-like receptor 4 (TLR4 receptor). Alcohol is also shown to act on specific cell surface receptors, e.g. the NMDA, GABA-A receptors and on certain ion channels, like L-type Ca^{2+} channels and GIRKs but the drug is also found to interact with various signaling pathways, e.g. PKA and PKC signaling. All these multi-targets are belived to underlie the wide variety of behavioral effects seen to result from chronic intake of ethanol (Alfonso-Loeches and Guerri, 2011).

Several effects of alcohol seems to involve the endogenous opioid systems (EOS). Opioid peptides, including beta-endorphin, have a role in mediating the reward effect of the drug. However, also some adverse effects are mediated through the EOS. A recent study on human alcohol-dependent subjects investigated whether the EOS is altered in brain areas involved in cognitive control of addiction. Human post-mortem brain specimens, including the dorsolateral prefrontal cortex (dl-PFC), orbitofrontal cortex (OFC) and hippocampus, from alcoholic and control subjects were examined. The expression of the prodynorphin gene transcript and dynorphin peptides in dl-PFC, the κ-opioid peptide (KOP) receptor message in OFC and dynorphins in hippocampus were all up-regulated in alcoholics. No significant changes in expression of other EOS gene transcripts were reported. Activation of the KOP receptor by the up-regulated dynorphin peptides in alcoholic brains was suggested to at least partly underlie neurocognitive dysfunctions relevant for addiction and disrupted inhibitory control (Bazov et al., 2011). In a subsequent study focused on genetic, epigenetic and environmental factors and their influence on the risk for alcoholism the result was indicative of a causal link between alcoholism-associated prodynorphin 3'-UTR CpG-SNP methylation, activation of prodynorphin transcription and vulnerability of individuals with the C, non-risk allele(s) to develop alcohol dependence (Taqi et al., 2011).

A study highlighting the specific attentional processes impaired in alcoholics concluded that a representative sample of alcoholics show specific deficits of attention as opposed to a general decline of attention at treatment intake. It was thus reported that sober alcoholics appear to be as efficient as controls at selecting on the basis of location, however, when they are required to select on the basis of semantic information or required to respond to two independent sources of information they are at a deficit (Tedstone and Coyle, 2004).

Taking together it appears that chronic alcohol intake under a variety of condiditions impairs cognitive factors including various aspects of memory and learning, attention, risk taking, motivation, mood and wanting. Specific brain areas targeted by the drug in this context includes hippocampus and frontal cortex. The mechanisms underlying the effects of ethanol involve inhibition of neurogenesis and interaction with a number of signal pathways, including glutamate, monoamines and endogenous opioids.

3.2 Effects of central stimulants on cognition

Epidemiological studies have confirmed a high prevalence of stimulant drugs and that these drugs are being used increasingly over the past decades (Gonzales et al., 2010; Ciccarone, 2011; Vardakou et al., 2011). They have been taken in order to enhance social or cognitive performance but also to induce euphoria and wellbeing. However, chronic use of these drugs has been associated with substantial deficits in learning and verbal memory. Thus the harmful consequences of long-term stimulant abuse also seem to include neurodegenerative effects leading to cognitive disabilities (Ciccarone, 2011; McKetin and Mattik, 1997; Krasnova et al., 2005).

3.2.1 Amphetamine

The psychostimulant amphetamine is shown to improve cognition in healthy subjects but also in attention-deficit hyperactivity disorder as well as in other neuropsychiatric disorders. However, at higher doses the stimulant may induce impaired cognitive function (Reske et al., 2010), particularly those mediated by the prefrontal cortex (Xu et al., 2010). Also, chronic use of amphetamine induces significantly impaired performance in cognitive tests (Ornstein et al., 2000). Data has indicated that amphetamine as well as other psychostimulants affects the capacity of the brain to stimulate neurogenesis, and that their effects also include disruption of the blood-brain barrier (BBB) (Silva et al., 2010). Thus, in chronic use the psychostimulatory effect of amphetamine is not only connected with reward and euphoria but also with impairments in attention and memory. These cognitive deficits have been suggested to be related to neurotoxic effects of the drug (Krasnova et al., 2005). Amphetamine injection is shown to affect dopaminergic terminals in striatal cells and to increase levels of cleaved caspase-3, a marker of apoptosis. Furthermore, the stimunlant is also demonstrated to increase the expression of p53 and Bax at both transcriptional and protein levels, whereas it decreased the levels of the Bcl-2 protein, all these events in agreement with increased apopotosis (Krasonova et al., 2005). Amphetamine is also shown to affect dopamine circuits in the prefrontal cortex (Dunn and Killcross, 2007; Fletcher et al., 2007) and thereby inducing impaired cognitive function.

3.2.2 Cocaine

Long-lasting memory deficits have been seen in individuals chronically abused to cocaine (Beatty et al., 1995; Bolla et al., 1999), although some ambiguities in respect to the specificity of this impairment remain to be fully clarified. Also, in studies using preclinical models of addiction it was demonstrated that stress and mechanisms related to the HPA-axis may contribute to impaired learning (Ehninger and Kempermann, 2006). In a more recent study it was shown that the deficiences in learning and memory seen in individuals addicted to cocaine are associated with increased levels of cortisol but also with the outcomes of cocaine use after inpatient treatment (Fox et al., 2009). Learning-related deficits was found to include poor immediate and retardent verbal recall and recognition as well as a selective reduction in working memory. These findings were seen to be in congruence with studies implicating that neuroadaptations in cocaine addicts affects learning and memory function, which in turn, appeared to affect the outcomes of drug use (Fox et al., 2009).

Sudai and collaborators investigated the effects of cocaine on cell proliferation and neurogenesis in the hippocampal dentate gyrus of adult rats (Sudai et al., 2011). The influence of the stimulant drug on working memory during abstinence was examined using the water T-maze test. Results suggested that cocaine, in addition to its effects on the reward system, also may inhibit the generation and development of new cells in the hippocampus, and thereby reduce the capacity of the working memory (Sudai et al., 2011).

In studies on mechanisms underlying the effects of cocaine on memory function several laboratories have focused on brain circuits and transmitter substances known to be involved in stress and memory formation. Muriach and collaborators described a study on nuclear factor kappa B (NFKappaB). NFKappaB is known as a sensor of oxidative stress and it is demonstrated to have a role in memory formation that could be involved in addiction mechanisms. They reported a mechanistic role of NFKappaB in alterations induced by cocaine and observed memory disabilities that was impaired and correlated negatively with the NFkappaB activity in the frontal cortex (Muriach et al., 2010). Cocaine has also been shown to induce neuroadaptive effects in hippocampal regions by enhancing LTP through interaction with the dopamine transporter and a subsequent enhancement of dopamine (Thomson et al., 2005). Subsequent studies have confirmed that endogenous dopamine in the presence of cocaine facilitates the elevation of basal hippopcampal LTP (Stramiello and Wagner, 2010). Cocaine may also induce impairments in working memory by action on dopaminergic circuits in the prefrontal cortex (George et al., 2008).

3.2.3 Methamphetamine, ecstasy and mephedrone

In addition to amphetamine, during the past years chronic use of several stimulant drugs with similar structure have been shown to impair cognitive functions. Among these compounds are methamphetamine, ecstasy and perhaps also cathinones (Gouzoulis-Mayfrank and Daumann, 2009; Rogers et al., 2009; Hoffman and Al'Absi, 2010). All these substances are not in clinical use and are classified as illegal drugs. They are easily accessible at internet and are misused in many countries. Regarding their mechanism of action ecstasy was shown to cause selective and persistent damages on central serotonergic nerve terminals, while methamphetamine produces lesions in both the serotonergic and dopaminergic systems. Also mephedrone seems to affect both transmitter systems (Kehr et al., 2011).

Chronic methamphetamine is shown to cause persisting cognitive deficits in human addicts as well as in animals exposed to this central stimulant (Reichel et al., 2011). Recent findings suggest that methamphetamine may induce a hypofunction in cortical areas that are important for executive function that in turn underlies the cognitive control deficits seen in individuals dependent on this drug (Nestor et al., 2011).

Methamphetamine-induced changes in the serotonin transporter SERT function in areas associated with cognition may underlie memory deficits independently of overt neurotoxic effects (Reichel et al., 2011). Moreover, data has indicated that also the σ receptors may be implicated in various acute and subchronic effects of methamphetamine. These include locomotor stimulation, development of sensitization and neurotoxicity, effects that may be attenuated by σ receptor antagonists. The σ receptors are also suggested to be involved in methamphetamine-induced deficits in cognitive and motor function (Kaushal and Masumoto, 2011).

Abuse of methamphetamine has also been seen to result in impaired adult hippocampal neurogenesis, and effects of this stimulant drug on neural progenitor cells is suggested to be mediated by protein nitration (Venkatesan et al., 2011). This observation was considered to open for new strategies regarding design and development of therapeutic approaches for methamphetamine-abusing individuals with neurologic dysfunction or even for other disorders with impaired hippocampal neurogenesis.

Use of ecstasy is shown to reduce cognitive functioning by reducing levels of dopamine and serotonin in CNS areas of importance for memory and learning (Gouzoulis-Mayfrank and Daumann, 2009; Chummun et al., 2011). Ecstasy is an abusing drug related to amphetamine and can act as a stimulant producing euphoria by enhancing dopamine levels in the nucleus accumbens in conformity to but to a lesser extent than amphetamine and cocaine. However, ecstasy may also interact with serotonergic payhways and long term exposure to this drug results in decreased activity in both serotonin and dopamine neurons (Kehr et al., 2011). The reduction in these transmitter systems is seen as dose-related impairments in cognitive function, in particular regarding complex cognitive skills. The decreased serotonergic and dopaminergic activity is also believed to cause changes in mood, hallucinations, altered perception and memory loss. Previous and current research demonstrate that abusing ecstasy is strongly associated with deteriorated working memory, and that this worsening correlates to the total lifetime of ecstasy consumption. These findings stresses the long-term, cumulative behavioral manifestations linked to ecstasy use in humans (Nulsen et al., 2010). Ecstasy users often show decreased levels of serotonin, its metabolite 5-HIAA, tryptophan hydroxylase and SERT density during abstinence. They also display functional impairments in learning and memory but also in higher cognitive processing, as well as sleep disturbance and deficits related appetite and reduced psychiatric wellbeing (Canales, 2010). These psychobiological impairments appeared most pronounced in heavy ecstasy users and may reflect losses in serotonergic axones in certain brain regions, in particular the frontal lobes, temporal lobes and hippocampus. These complications seem to last long after cessation of ecstasy use, suggesting that these drug-induced neurological impairments may be permament. It is believed that at least some of the harmful effects on memory of ecstasy abuse could result from its neurotoxic actions on adult hippocampal neurogenesis. Evidence suggests that stimulant abuse negatively affects cognitive functions that are regulated and influenced by adult hippocampal neurogenesis, including contextual memory, spatial memory, working memory and cognitive flexibility (Canales, 2010).

4-methylmethcathinone (mephedrone) represents a designer stimulant that is among the most popular of the naturally occurring psychostimulant cathinone derivatives. A web-based survey has shown that mephedrone users consider the effects of this drug to compare best with those of ecstasy (Carhart-Harris et al., 2011), which agrees with research studies comparing the effects of mephedrone and ecstasy on brain 5HT and dopamine (Kehr et al., 2011). This cathinone has been readily available for purchase both online and in the streets and has been promoted by aggressive web-based marketing. Its abuse in many western countries has been described as a serious public health concern (Hadlock et al., 2011). In conformity with ecstasy, metamphetamine and methcathinone, repeated mephedrone injections causes a rapid decrease in the striatal dopamine and in the hippocampal 5HT transporter function. Mephedrone is also shown to inhibit both synaptosomal dopamine and 5HT reuptake. Similar to ecstasy but unlike methamphetamine or methcathinone, repeated mephedrone also causes persistent serotonergic, but not dopaminergic, deficits (Hadlock et al., 2011, Kehr et al., 2011). No studies on learning and memory impairments in mephedrone abusers has yet been published, however, due to similarieties with ecstasy and methamphetamine research investigating the actual domains of cognition in chronic and abstinent mephedrone users seems to be warranted in the future.

4. Opioid-induced adverse effects on cognitive functions

A variety of neuropathologic adaptations have been detected in the brains of heroin addicts. These include pathology caused by bacterial infections, viral infections, such as HIV-1 infection, but also complications such as hypoxic–ischemic *encephalopathy* with cerebral edema, ischemic neuronal damage and neuronal loss (Büttner et al., 2000). However, chronic exposure to opiates, such as heroin, morphine and to some extent also methadone are shown to impair cognitive function (Mintzer and Stiltzer, 2002; Gruber et al., 2007; Soyka et al., 2011). Heroin is characterized as one of the most frequently abused illegal drugs, and addiction to this drug is linked to significant attention deficits and inadequate performance on memory tasks (Guerra et al., 1987). Furthermore, chronic exposure to morphine is also shown to cause vigilance and attention impairments in chronic pain patients (Mao et al., 2002) and impairs acquisition of reference memory in rats (Spain and Newsom, 1991; Lu et al., 2010). Also addicts in methadone maintenance programs or chronic pain patients treated with methadone are shown to display cognitive impairmats (Mitzler and Stitzer, 2002; Soyka et al., 2010). These findings suggest an effect of chronic opiates on brain regions related to learning and memory, such as the frontal cortex (Ornstein et al., 2000; Yang et al., 2009) and the hippocampus (Lu et al., 2010)

Regarding the mechanisms by which opioids induce cognitive impairments through action on hippocampal and prefrontal cortex structures it is shown that these drugs may enhance apoptosis and inhibted neurogenesis. An opioid-induced attenuation of neurogenesis in hippocampus was earlier seen in male rats exposed to morphine (Eisch et al., 2000). Thus, opiates, such as morphine, is seen to reduce neurogenesis in the adult hippocampal subgranular zone (SGZ), suggesting that a waning neurogenesis contributes to opioid-induced deficits in cognitive function (Arguello et al., 2008). Enhanced apoptosis following exposure to opioids was reported to involve an upregulation of the proapoptotic caspase-3 and Bax proteins following NMDA receptor activation (Mao et al., 2002). Also, chronic methadone have been shown to up-regulate several pro-apoptotic proteins in the cortex and hippocampus, indicating activation of both the NMDA-receptor and mitochondrial apoptotic pathways (Tramullas et al., 2007). In addition, morphine-induced expression of the Toll-like receptor 9 (TLR9) and microglia apoptosis was suggested to involve the μ-opioid peptide receptor, MOP (He et al., 2011). It was further suggested that inhibition of the TLR9 and/or blockage of the MOP receptor may be a possible route for preventing opioid-induced brain damage.

The opiate elicited apoptosis in human fetal microglia and neurons (Hu et al., 2002), was also associated with morphine tolerance (Mao et al., 2002). The apoptotic effect of morphine is blocked by the opioid receptor antagonist naloxone (Hu et al., 2002), indicating an opioid receptor mechanism involved in this effect. The effect of morphine is known to be mediated mainly through the MOP receptor although, at high concentrations, this opiate is known also to interact with both the delta-opioid peptide (DOP) and the KOP receptors. Furthermore, it appears that the opioid receptor subtypes (MOP, DOP, and KOP) may regulate different aspects of neuronal development (Hauser et al., 2000). Evidence suggesting that the MOP receptor could play an important role in regulating progenitor cell survival has recently been described (Harburg et al., 2007). In addition, morphine was earlier shown to promote anomal programmed cell death by increasing the expression of the proapoptotic Fas receptor protein and decreasing the expression of the antiapoptotic Bcl-2 oncoprotein by maintaining the activation of opioid receptors (Boronat et al., 2001). Studies also indicated that opiate-induced alteration of hippocampal function most likely results from inhibited neurogenesis (Eisch and Harburg, 2006).

5. Reversal of drug-induced impairments of abusing drugs

It is obvious from the above that chronic use of many addictive drugs may elicit pronounced effects on brain structures associated with cognitive functions leading to impaired learning and memory capabilities. It is not yet clarified whether the effects are reversible or persist over the life time. However, it seems that for many individual addicts these drug-induced damages may contribute to accelerated senescence. Many attempts to develop therapeutic strategies to deal with this complication have been reported. Indeed, attempts to design molecules that may counteract these deficits and enhance cognitive capabilities have been reported over the past decade. Several approaches to reverse cognitive impairmnts induced by central stimulanta have been reported. In the following this article will describe attempts to reverse morphine-induced damage in the hippocampus with the far aim to reconstitute cognitive abilities in experimental animals exposed to opioids.

5.1 Attempts to reverse of opioid-induced impairments on cognition

In a previous study we demonstrated that a single dose of morphine may affect the expression of the growth hormone (GH) receptor as well as the GH binding protein (GHBP) in the rat hippocampus. The gene transcripts were significantly attenuated 4 h following drug injection but was restored after 24 h (Thörnwall-LeGreves et al., 2001). In rats chronically treated with morphine, a decrease in GH binding was observed during the acute phase but this alteration was restored when animals were tolerant to the drug (Zhai et al., 1995).

As mentioned above, chronic morphine may reduce neurogenesis in the granule cell layer of hippocampus in the adult rat and a similar effect was seen in male rats after chronic self-administration of heroin (Eisch et al., 2000). Furthermore, studies have shown that opioid effects on nerve cell regeneration is not mediated through interactions with the HPA-axis, as similar effects were found also in rats subjected to adrenalectomy and subsequent corticosterone replacement. These observations suggest that the opioid regulation of neurogenesis in the adult rat hippocampus may be mediated by direct effects of the opioid drugs on the hippocampal function. The recent study by Arguello and co-workers, as mentioned above, demonstrated that chronic morphine attenuates neurogenesis in the SGZ by impeding cell-dividing, primarily in the S-phase, and inhibiting progenitor cell progression to a more mature stage (Arguello et al., 2008). In order to find strategies to reverse the opioid-induced damage to the hippocampal function it is essential to look for agents that may stimulate hippocampal progenitors and thereby increase neurogenesis and regeneration of nerve cells. The above mentioned opioid effects on GH and its receptor suggest that the somatotrophic axis may be of importance in this regard. Indeed, both GH and its mediator insulin-like growth factor-I (IGF-I) have been reported to induce neuroprotective effects and also stimulate neurogenesis (Isgaard et al., 2007; Nyberg, 2009).

5.1.1 The impact of the somatotrophic axis on neuroprotection

Data indicating a substantial impact of the somatotrophic axis on nerve cell regeneration has been reported (Isgaard et al., 2007). IGF-I treatment was found to promote cell genesis in the brains of adult GH- and IGF-1-deficient rodents (Anderson et al., 2002; Aberg et al, 2009). In the hippocampus, treatment with bovine GH (bGH) induced an increase in the number of BrdU/NeuN-positive cells proportionally to the recorded increase in the number of BrdU-positive cells. In vitro incorporation of ^{3}[H]-labeled thymidine demonstrated that short-time exposure to bGH enhanced the cell proliferation in adult hippocampal progenitor cells. This observation demonstrated that peripherally administrated GH may increase the number of new cells in the brain of adult rats and that the hormone may exert a direct proliferative effect on neuronal progenitor cells (Aberg et al., 2006; Aberg et al., 2009).

Positive effects of GH on neurogenesis have been observed in several laboratories. A study by Harvey and co-workers showed that the hormone is produced in the retinal ganglion cells of embryonic chicks, in which GH stimulates cell survival during neurogenesis. The mechanism underlying this action was investigated in neural retina explants collected from 6-8 days-old embryos. These explants were allowed to incubate with GH for some days and the hormone was seen to reduce the number of spontaneous apoptotic cells. This anti-apoptotic action of the hormone was accompanied by a reduction in the expression of the apoptotic marker caspase-3 but also by a reduced expression of the caspase independent apoptosis inducing factor-1. These actions were considered specific, since other constituents known to be involved in apoptotic signaling, such as bcl-2, bcl-x and bid, remained unaffected. The result from this study was suggested to indicate that GH-induced retinal cell survival involved pathways dependent and independent on caspase activity (Harvey et al., 2006).

Studies over the past decades have clearly demonstrated that GH targets many areas of the CNS (for reviews, see Nyberg, 2000; 2007), and that GH deficits has been associated with cognitive impairments, memory loss, as well as diminished well being (Bengtsson et al., 1993: Burman and Deijen, 1998). GH replacement therapy in GH-deficient patients was demonstrated to ameliorate several adverse symptoms seen in these patients (Bengtsson et al., 1993: Burman and Deijen, 1998; McMillan et al., 2003). The hormone was also found to prevent neuronal loss in the aged rat hippocampus, confirming a neuroprotective effect of GH in old animals (Azcoitia et al, 2005). Decreased levels of circulating GH with age (van Dam et al., 2002) declining density of GH-binding sites with aging was found in several areas of the human brain, including the hippocampus (Lai et al., 1993). GH was also seen to enhance the expression of the rat hippocampal gene transcript of the NMDA receptor subunit NR2B (Le Greves et al., 2002). This receptor subunit is known to enhance memory and cognitive capabilities in an age-dependent manner while overexpressed (Tang et al., 1999). In addition, studies showed that GH replacement in hypophysectomized male rats may improve spatial performance and increase the hippocampal gene transcript levels of some of the NMDA receptor subunits as well as the postsynaptic density protein 95 (Le Greves et al., 2006; 2011). All together, these observations were considered to indicate a link between decreased GH levels in elderly and deterioration of cognitive functions, with a clear indication that the hormone may improve memory and cognitive capabilities and this may be compatible with increased neurogenesis as a result of GH administration.

The mechanism by which GH induces its beneficial effects on memory and cognition is still not clarified in all its details. However, GH is shown to promote nerve cell regeneration as well as gliogenesis during the development of the fetal rat brain (Ajo et al., 2003), presumably through local production of IGF-1. Peripheral administrated GH reaching the CNS may induce a release of IGF-1 in the brain and this factor may in turn account for the mediation of brain effects of GH. However, local production of both GH and IGF-1 in certain areas of the brain has been suggested, as mice with decreased levels of circulating GH and IGF-1 exhibit normal levels of the corresponding gene transcripts in the hippocampus (Sun et al., 2005). Also, GH is shown to be produced in the hippocampal formation, where it is suggested to be involved in functions associated with his region, such as learning and response to stress (Donahue et al., 2006). Effects on these behaviors may be caused by the action of GH-induced release of IGF-1 as this mediator is also shown to affect hippocampal related behaviors. In fact, intracerebroventricular administration of IGF-1 was found to attenuate the age-related decline in hippocampal neurogenesis in rats (Lichtenwalner et al., 2001). Moreover, peripheral infusions of IGF-1 were seen to induce neurogenesis in the hippocampus of the adult rat (Aberg et al., 2000) and overexpression of IGF-1 promotes neurogenesis during the postnatal development (O'Kusky et al., 2000).

5.1.2 Reversal of opioid-induced impairments by growth hormone

In addition, a recent study showed that chronic morphine significantly and dose-dependently attenuates neuronal cell density in cultured hippocampal cells from murine fetus (Svensson et al., 2008). The ability of morphine as well as other opioids to inhibit cell growth and induce apoptosis is already known from previous work as described earlier in this section (see section 4). Therefore, the decline observed in neurite outgrowth in the mouse hippocampal primary cell cultures (Nyberg, 2009; Svensson et al., 2008) was expected, and a consequence of this decline should be that markers of apoptosis, such as lactate dehydrogenase (LDH) and caspase 3, will be affected. In fact, the activity and level of these enzymes were found to be significantly enhanced (Svensson et al., 2008). The enhanced activity of LDH in morphine-treated hippocampal cells strongly indicates that morphine may induce apoptosis in cells of this brain area. LDH, a mitochondrial dehydrogenase, is known to represent a critical component of the astrocyte–neuron lactate shuttle. It regulates the formation of lactate and influences its turnover within the cells. Caspase-3 is another enzyme that serves as a marker of apoptosis and cleaved caspase-3 represents an activated form of this enzyme that acts as a lethal protease at the most distal stage of the apoptotic pathway (Kuribayashi et al., 2006). This enzyme was also investigated in order to clarify whether the reduction seen in the hippocampal cell density involves elements related to apoptosis. It was noted that the level of cleaved caspase-3, measured by Western blot analysis, was significantly enhanced by chronic morphine (Svensson et al., 2008).

As noted above, the hippocampus represents a brain area localized within the limbic system and is well known as an important brain substrate required for the acquisition of declarative or explicit memory (Benfenati, 2007). From the literature cited above, it is evident that chronic administration of opiates may counteract cell growth and stimulate apoptosis, but it is also demonstrated that opiate-induced toxicity may include impaired neurogensis (Hauser et al., 2000; He et al., 2002; Mao et al., 2002; Eisch and Harburg, 2006). An impact of adult-generated neurons on learning and memory was earlier suggested as training on associative learning tasks was found to double these neurons in the rat brain dentate gyrus (Kenney and Gould, 2008; Gould, 2010). Consequently, memory dysfunctions induced by chronic exposure to opiates could result from decreased adult neurogenesis as these drugs may inhibit neurogenesis in the adult hippocampus (Eisch and Harburg, 2006; Eisch et al., 2000). This inhibition might well reflect a decreased number of neural precursors caused by increased apoptosis of the newborn neurons. However, in recent years, several factors that may promote and enhance neurogenesis from preexisting neuronal precursors have been reported. Among them are GH and its mediator IGF-1 in addition to several other growth factors. IGF-1 is shown to be essential for hippocampal neurogenesis (Aberg et al., 2000, 2006). As mentioned above, this factor is regulated through the somatotrophic axis, where GH has an important role as an activator and releaser of IGF-1 as well as its binding proteins.

In order to investigate whether GH may reverse opiate-induced apoptosis or inhibition of neurogenesis, we examined the effect of human GH on murine primary hippocampal neuronal cell cultures exposed to morphine (Svensson et al., 2008). We observed that GH could significantly reverse the morphine-induced inhibition of neurite outgrowth and that cell density was restored after treatment with the hormone. The effect of GH was evident both when the hormone was added with morphine and when it was added after the opiate had induced its damaging effect. We also noted that GH reversed the morphine-induced effects on the apoptopic markers LDH and caspase-3 activity (Svensson et al., 2008). Thus, combining these observations with the effects of GH seen on memory and spatial performance in rats (Le Greves et al., 2006,; 2011) it appears that the hormone may be useful for the reversal of the adverse effects of morphine or other opiates on brain cells.

These data opens for future attemps also to use IGF-1 in order to reverse opioid-induced damage on the brain to improve cognitive capabilities. It also opens for the possibility to stimulate the somatotrophic axis to reverse cognitive impairments induced by other drugs of abuse. Actually, as can be seen below, growth factors have been used in attempt to counteract brain damages induced by alcohol.

5.2 Attempts to reverse alcohol-induced impairments in cognition

Studies on the reversal of the adverse effects induced by various drugs have shown that certain growth factors may be useful in attempts to counteract drug-induced cell damage and apoptosis. For instance, it was demonstrated (Gibson et al. 2002) that stimulation of human embryonic kidney cells HEK 293 and the breast cancer cell line MDA MB 231 with epidermal growth factor (EGF) effectively and dose-dependently protected these cells from tumor necrosis factor-related apoptosis-inducing ligand (TRAIL)-induced apoptosis. This stimulatory effect was shown to reduce apoptosis by blocking both TRAIL-mediated mitochondrial release of cytochrome c and activation of caspase-3. It was further shown that the survival response of EGF involved the activation of the protein kinase Akt. Activation of Akt was found to be sufficient for inibition of the TRAIL-induced apoptosis, and the expression of kinase-inactive Akt abolished the protective effect of EGF. In contrast, inhibition of the stimulatory effect of EGF on the extracellular-regulated kinase (ERK) activity did not affect EGF protection. From these findings it was concluded that activation of the EGF receptor generates a survival response against TRAIL-induced apoptosis by blocking the release of cytochrome c from the mitochondria, which, in turn, is mediated by the activation of Akt in epithelial-derived cells.

The effects of estrogens and certain growth factors subsequent to ethanol treatment were recently examined in order to assess the potential of these hormones to reverse the effects of ethanol-induced damage (Barclay et al., 2005). The result of these studies indicated that both IGF-I and bovine basic fibroblast growth factor (bFGF) reduced toxic effect of the drug on neuronal survival, whereas estrogen, bFGF, and nerve growth factor (NGF) seemed to increase the total neurite length after ethanol treatment (Barclay et al., 2005). In addition, heparin-binding epidermal growth factor (HB-EGF), also a member of the EGF family of growth factors, has been reported to prevent apoptosis and differentiation and, in a very recent study, it was shown that stimulation with HB-EGF could reverse alcohol-induced apoptosis in human embryonic stem cells (Nash et al., 2009). Another possibility for reversing alcohol-induced cell damage involves brain-derived neurotrophic factor (BDNF). BDNF signaling plays an important role in neural survival and differentiation and studies have shown that alcohol significantly reduces BDNF signaling in neuronal cells (Climent et al., 2002). Also, the antiproliferative action of ethanol can be modulated by changing the sensitivity of the autophosphorylation of the IGF-1 receptor to ethanol (Seiler et al., 2000). This raised the question of whether IGF-1 could counteract the antiproliferative effects induced by alcohol. In fact, studies have shown that alcohol inhibits differentiation of the neural stem and that this effect is reduced by both IGF-1 and BDNF (Tateno et al., 2004). These results suggest the possibility that stimulation of neurotrophic factor signaling can reverse apoptosis induced by alcohol exposure.

6. Conclusions

It is evident from studies reviewed in this article that most drugs of abuse may induce adverse effects on brain structures associated with cognitive functions. In most cases these effects seem to impact brain circuits linked to important aspects of cognition, such as memory and learning, attention, risk taking, motivation, mood and wanting. The deficits induced on these behaviors by alcohol and opioids are well documented, whereas those of central stimulants and other abusing drugs are less well characterized. As mentioned in this article an important issue is the approach to find strategies to reverse the drug-induced deficits and in the case of damages induced by alcohol and opioid abuse it seems that certain growth factors may be useful and open for new methods for successful therapy.

7. Acknowledgment

This work was supported by the Swedish Medical Research Council (Grant 9459) and by the Swedish Council for Working Life and Social Research.

8. References

Abel T, Lattal KM (2001). Molecular mechanisms of memory acquisition, consolidation and retrieval. Curr Opin Neurobiol. 11:180-187. Review.

Aberg MA, Aberg ND, Hedbäcker H, Oscarsson J, Eriksson PS (2000). Peripheral infusion of IGF-I selectively induces neurogenesis in the adult rat hippocampus. J Neurosci. 20:2896-2903.

Aberg ND, Brywe KG, Isgaard J (2006). Aspects of growth hormone and insulin-like growth factor-I related to neuroprotection, regeneration, and functional plasticity in the adult brain. ScientificWorld Journal. 6:53-80.

Aberg ND, Johansson I, Aberg MA, Lind J, Johansson UE, Cooper-Kuhn CM, Kuhn HG, Isgaard J (2009). Peripheral administration of GH induces cell proliferation in the brain of adult hypophysectomized rats. J Endocrinol. 201:141-150.

Ajo R, Cacicedo L, Navarro C, Sanchez-Franco F (2003). Growth hormone action on proliferation and differentiation of cerebral cortical cells from fetal rat. Endocrinology. 144:1086-1097.

Alfonso-Loeches S, Guerri C (2011). Molecular and behavioral aspects of the actions of alcohol on the adult and developing brain. Crit Rev Clin Lab Sci. 48:19-47.

Anderson MF, Aberg MA, Nilsson M, Eriksson PS (2002). Insulin-like growth factor-I and neurogenesis in the adult mammalian brain. Brain Res Dev Brain Res. 134:115- 122.

Arguello AA, Harburg GC, Schonborn JR, Mandyam CD, Yamaguchi M, Eisch AJ (2008). Time course of morphine's effects on adult hippocampal subgranular zone reveals preferential inhibition of cells in S phase of the cell cycle and a subpopulation of immature neurons. Neuroscience. 157:70-79.

Asada T, Takaya S, Takayama Y, Yamauchi H, Hashikawa K, Fukuyama H (2010). Reversible alcohol-related dementia: a five-year follow-up study using FDG-PET and neuropsychological tests. Intern Med. 49:283-287.

Azcoitia I, Perez-Martin M, Salazar V, Castillo C, Ariznavarreta C, Garcia-Segura LM, Tresguerres JA (2005). Growth hormone prevents neuronal loss in the aged rat hippocampus. Neurobiol Aging. 26:697-703.

Barclay DC, Hallbergson AF, Montague JR, Mudd LM (2005). Reversal of ethanol toxicity in embryonic neurons with growth factors and estrogen. Brain Res Bull. 67:459- 465.

Bazov I, Kononenko O, Watanabe H, Kuntić V, Sarkisyan D, Taqi MM, Hussain MZ, Nyberg F, Yakovleva T, Bakalkin G (2011). The endogenous opioid system in human alcoholics: molecular adaptations in brain areas involved in cognitive control of addiction. Addict Biol. 2011 Sep 28. doi: 10.1111/j.

Beatty WW, Katzung VM, Moreland VJ, Nixon SJ (1995). Neuropsychological performance of recently abstinent alcoholics and cocaine abusers. Drug Alcohol Depend. 37:247-253.

Benfenati F (2007). Synaptic plasticity and the neurobiology of learning and memory. Acta Biomed. 78 Suppl 1:58-66.

Bengtsson BA, Edén S, Lönn L, Kvist H, Stokland A, Lindstedt G, Bosaeus I, Tölli J, Sjöström L, Isaksson OG (1993). Treatment of adults with growth hormone (GH) deficiency with recombinant human GH. J Clin Endocrinol Metab. 76:309-317.

Blagrove M, Seddon J, George S, Parrott AC, Stickgold R, Walker MP, Jones KA, Morgan MJ (2011). Procedural and declarative memory task performance, and the memory consolidation function of sleep, in recent and abstinent ecstasy/MDMA users. J Psychopharmacol. 25:465-477

Bolla KI, Rothman R, Cadet JL (1999). Dose-related neurobehavioral effects of chronic cocaine use. J Neuropsychiatry Clin Neurosci. 11:361–369.

Boronat MA, García-Fuster MJ, García-Sevilla JA (2001). Chronic morphine induces up-regulation up-regulation of the pro-apoptotic Fas receptor and down-regulation of the anti-apoptotic Bcl-2 oncoprotein in rat brain. Br J Pharmacol. 134:1263-1270.

Burman P, Deijen JB (1998). Quality of life and cognitive function in patients with pituitary insufficiency. Psychother Psychosom. 67:154-167.

Büttner A, Mall G, Penning R, Weis S (2000). The neuropathology of heroin abuse. Forensic Sci Int. 2000 Sep 11;113(1-3):435-42.

Cairney S, Clough A, Jaragba M, Maruff P (2007). Cognitive impairment in Aboriginal people with heavy episodic patterns of alcohol use. Addiction.102:909-915.

Canales JJ (2010). Comparative neuroscience of stimulant-induced memory dysfunction: role for neurogenesis in the adult hippocampus. Behav Pharmacol. 21:379-393.

Carhart-Harris RL, King LA, Nutt DJ (2011). A web-based survey on mephedrone. Drug Alcohol Depend. 118:19-22.

Carvalho F (2009). How bad is accelerated senescence in consumers of drugs of abuse? Adicciones. 21:99-104. English, Spanish.

Chummun H, Tilley V, Ibe J (2010). 3,4-methylenedioxyamfetamine (ecstasy) use reduces cognition. Br J Nurs. 19:94-100.

Ciccarone D (2011). Stimulant abuse: pharmacology, cocaine, methamphetamine, treatment, attempts at pharmacotherapy. Prim Care. 38:41-58.

Cippitelli A, Damadzic R, Frankola K, Goldstein A, Thorsell A, Singley E, Eskay RL, Heilig M (2010). Alcohol-induced neurodegeneration, suppression of transforming growth factor-beta, and cognitive impairment in rats: prevention by group II metabotropic glutamate receptor activation. Biol Psychiatry. 67:823-830.

Climent E, Pascual M, Renau-Piqueras J, Guerri C (2002). Ethanol exposure enhances cell death in the developing cerebral cortex: role of brain-derived neurotrophic factor and its signaling pathways. J Neurosci Res. 68:213-225.

Cooke SF, Bliss TV (2005). Long-term potentiation and cognitive drug discovery. Curr Opin Investig Drugs. 6:25-34.

Crews FT, Nixon K (2009). Mechanisms of neurodegeneration and regeneration in alcoholism. Alcohol Alcohol. 44(2):115-127.

Donahue CP, Kosik KS, Shors TJ (2006). Growth hormone is produced within the hippocampus where it responds to age, sex, and stress. Proc Natl Acad Sci U S A. 103:6031-6036.

Duman RS, Malberg J, Nakagawa S (2001). Regulation of adult neurogenesis by psychotropic drugs and stress. J Pharmacol Exp Ther. 299:401-407.

Dunn MJ, Killcross S (2007). Medial prefrontal cortex infusion of alpha-flupenthixol attenuates systemic d-amphetamine-induced disruption of conditional discrimination performance in rats.Psychopharmacology (Berl).192:347-355.

Edelson M, Sharot T, Dolan RJ, Dudai Y (2011). Following the crowd: brain substrates of long-term memory conformity. Science. 333:108-11.

Ehninger D, Kempermann G (2008). Neurogenesis in the adult hippocampus. Cell Tissue Res. 331:243-250.

Eisch AJ, Harburg GC (2006). Opiates, psychostimulants, and adult hippocampal neurogenesis: Insights for addiction and stem cell biology. Hippocampus. 16:271-286.

Eisch AJ, Barrot M, Schad CA, Self DW, Nestler EJ (2000). Opiates inhibit neurogenesis in the adult rat hippocampus. Proc Natl Acad Sci U S A. 97:7579-7584.

Ersche KD, Clark L, London M, Robbins TW, Sahakian BJ (2006). Profile of executive and memory function associated with amphetamine and opiate dependence. Neuropsychopharmacology. 31:1036-1047.

Fernández-Serrano MJ, Lozano O, Pérez-García M, Verdejo-García A (2010). Impact of severity of drug use on discrete emotions recognition in polysubstance abusers. Drug Alcohol Depend. 109:57-64.

Fletcher PJ, Tenn CC, Sinyard J, Rizos Z, Kapur S (2007). A sensitizing regimen of amphetamine impairs visual attention in the 5-choice serial reaction time test: reversal by a D1 receptor agonist injected into the medial prefrontal cortex. Neuropsychopharmacology. 32:1122-1132.

Fox HC, Jackson ED, Sinha R (2009). Elevated cortisol and learning and memory deficits in cocaine dependent individuals: relationship to relapse outcomes. Psychoneuroendocrinology. 34:1198-1207.

Gass JT, Olive MF (2009). Positive allosteric modulation of mGluR5 receptors facilitates extinction of a cocaine contextual memory. Biol Psychiatry. 65:717-720.

George O, Mandyam CD, Wee S, Koob GF (2008). Extended access to cocaine self-administration produces long-lasting prefrontal cortex-dependent working memory impairments. Neuropsychopharmacology. 33:2474-2482.

Gibson EM, Henson ES, Haney N, Villanueva J, Gibson SB (2002). Epidermal growth factor protects epithelial-derived cells from tumor necrosis factor-related apoptosis-inducing ligand-induced apoptosis by inhibiting cytochrome c release. Cancer Res. 62:488-496.

Glannon W (2006). Psychopharmacology and memory. J Med Ethics. 32:74-78. Review.

Glass JM, Buu A, Adams KM, Nigg JT, Puttler LI, Jester JM, Zucker RA (2009). Effects of alcoholism severity and smoking on executive neurocognitive function. Addiction. 104:38-48.

Goldstein, R.Z., Volkow, N.D. (2002). Drug addiction and its underlying neurobiologi- cal basis: neuroimaging evidence for the involvement of the frontal cortex. Am J Psychiatry. 159:1642-1652.

Gould TJ (2010). Addiction and cognition. Addict Sci Clin Pract. 5:4-14.

Gouzoulis-Mayfrank E, Daumann J (2009). Neurotoxicity of drugs of abuse--the case of methylenedioxyamphetamines (MDMA, ecstasy), and amphetamines. Dialogues Clin Neurosci.11:305-317.

Gonzales R, Mooney L, Rawson RA (2010). The methamphetamine problem in the United States. Annu Rev Public Health. 31:385-398.

Gravius A, Pietraszek M, Schmidt WJ, Danysz W (2006). Functional interaction of NMDA and group I metabotropic glutamate receptors in negatively reinforced learning in rats. Psychopharmacology (Berl). 185:58-65.

Gruber SA, Silveri MM, Yurgelun-Todd DA (2007). Neuropsychological consequences of opiate use. Neuropsychol Rev. 17:299-315.

Guerra D, Solé A, Camí J, Tobeña A (1987). Neuropsychological performance in opiate addicts after rapid detoxification. Drug Alcohol Depend. 20:261-270.

Guerri C, Pascual M (2010). Mechanisms involved in the neurotoxic, cognitive, and neurobehavioral effects of alcohol consumption during adolescence. Alcohol. 44:15-26.

Hadlock GC, Webb KM, McFadden LM, Chu PW, Ellis JD, Allen SC, Andrenyak DM, Vieira-Brock PL, German CL, Conrad KM, Hoonakker AJ, Gibb JW, Wilkins DG, Hanson GR, Fleckenstein AE (2011). 4-Methylmethcathinone (mephedrone): neuropharmacological effects of a designer stimulant of abuse. J Pharmacol Exp Ther. 339:530-536.

Harburg GC, Hall FS, Harrist AV, Sora I, Uhl GR, Eisch AJ (2007). Knockout of the mu opioid receptor enhances the survival of adult-generated hippocampal granule cell neurons. Neuroscience. 144:77-87

Harvey S, Baudet ML, Sanders EJ (2006). Growth hormone and cell survival in the neural retina: caspase dependence and independence. Neuroreport. 17:1715-1718.

Hauser KF, Houdi AA, Turbek CS, Elde RP, Maxson W 3rd (2000). Opioids intrinsically inhibit the genesis of mouse cerebellar granule neuron precursors in vitro: differential impact of mu and delta receptor activation on proliferation and neurite elongation. Eur J Neurosci. 12:1281-1293.

He L, Li H, Chen L, Miao J, Jiang Y, Zhang Y, Xiao Z, Hanley G, Li Y, Zhang X, LeSage G, Peng Y, Yin D (2011). Toll-like receptor 9 is required for opioid-induced microglia apoptosis. PLoS One. 2011 Apr 29;6(4):e18190.

Hoffman R, Al'Absi M (2010). Khat use and neurobehavioral functions: suggestions for future studies. J Ethnopharmacol. 132:554-563

Hu S, Sheng WS, Lokensgard JR, Peterson PK (2002). Morphine induces apoptosis of human microglia and neurons. Neuropharmacology. 42:829-836.

Hyman SE (2005). Addiction: a disease of learning and memory. Am J Psychiatry. 162:1414-1422.

Isgaard J, Aberg D, Nilsson M (2007). Protective and regenerative effects of the GH/IGF-I axis on the brain. Minerva Endocrinol. 32:103-113.

Kaushal N, Matsumoto RR (2011). Role of sigma receptors in methamphetamine-induced neurotoxicity. Curr Neuropharmacol. 9:54-57.

Kalivas PW (2004). Glutamate systems in cocaine addiction. Curr Opin Pharmacol. 4:23- 29. Review.

Kehr J, Ichinose F, Yoshitake S, Goiny M, Sievertsson T, Nyberg F, Yoshitake T (2011). Mephedrone, compared with MDMA (ecstasy) and amphetamine, rapidly increases both dopamine and 5-HT levels in nucleus accumbens of awake rats. Br J Pharmacol. 164:1949-1958.

Kenney JW, Gould TJ (2008). Modulation of hippocampus-dependent learning and synaptic plasticity by nicotine. Mol Neurobiol. 38:101-121

Kim J, Lee I (2011). Hippocampus is necessary for spatial discrimination using distal cue-configuration. Hippocampus. 21:609-621.

Kopelman MD, Thomson AD, Guerrini I, Marshall EJ (2009). The Korsakoff syndrome: clinical aspects, psychology and treatment. Alcohol Alcohol. 44:148-154

Krasnova IN, Ladenheim B, Cadet JL (2005). Amphetamine induces apoptosis of medium spiny striatal projection neurons via the mitochondria-dependent pathway. FASEB J. 19:851-853 Psychiatry 159, 1642–1652.

Kubota M, Nakazaki S, Hirai S, Saeki N, Yamaura A, Kusaka T (2001). Alcohol consumption and frontal lobe shrinkage: study of 1432 non-alcoholic subjects. J Neurol Neurosurg Psychiatry. 71:104-106.

Kuribayashi K, Mayes PA, El-Deiry WS (2006). What are caspases 3 and 7 doing upstream of the mitochondria? Cancer Biol Ther. 5:763-765.

Lai Z, Roos P, Zhai O, Olsson Y, Fholenhag K, Larsson C, Nyberg F (1993). Age-related reduction of human growth hormone-binding sites in the human brain. Brain Res. 621:260-266.

Le Greves M, Steensland P, Le Greves P, Nyberg F (2002). Growth hormone induces age-dependent alteration in the expression of hippocampal growth hormone receptor and N-methyl-D-aspartate receptor subunits gene transcripts in male rats. Proc Natl Acad Sci U S A. 99:7119-7123.

Le Greves M, Zhou Q, Berg M, Le Greves P, Fholenhag K, Meyerson B, Nyberg F (2006). Growth hormone replacement in hypophysectomized rats affects spatial performance and hippocampal levels of NMDA receptor subunit and PSD-95 gene transcript levels. Exp Brain Res. 173:267-273.

Le Grevès M, Enhamre E, Zhou Q, Fhölenhag K, Berg M, Meyerson B, Nyberg F (2011). Growth Hormone Enhances Cognitive Functions in Hypophys-Ectomized Male Rats Am. J. Neuroprotec. Neuroregen. 3:53-58.

Lichtenwalner RJ, Forbes ME, Bennett SA, Lynch CD, Sonntag WE, Riddle DR (2001). Intracerebroventricular infusion of insulin-like growth factor-I ameliorates the age-related decline in hippocampal neurogenesis. Neuroscience. 107:603-613

Loeber S, Duka T, Welzel H, Nakovics H, Heinz A, Flor H, Mann K (2009). Impairment of cognitive abilities and decision making after chronic use of alcohol: the impact of multiple detoxifications. Alcohol Alcohol. 44:372-381.

Lu G, Zhou QX, Kang S, Li QL, Zhao LC, Chen JD, Sun JF, Cao J, Wang YJ, Chen J, Chen XY, Zhong DF, Chi ZQ, Xu L, Liu JG (2010). Chronic morphine treatment impaired hippocampal long-term potentiation and spatial memory via accumulation of extracellular adenosine acting on adenosine A1 receptors. J Neurosci. 30:5058- 5070.

Mao J, Sung B, Ji RR, Lim G (2002). Neuronal apoptosis associated with morphine tolerance: Evidence for an opioid-induced neurotoxic mechanism. J Neurosci. 22:7650–7661.

McKetin, R., and Mattick, R. P. (1997) Attention and memory in illicit amphetamine users. Drug Alcohol Depend. 48:235–242.

McMillan CV, Bradley C, Gibney J, Healy ML, Russell-Jones DL, Sönksen PH (2003). Psychological effects of withdrawal of growth hormone therapy from adults with growth hormone deficiency. Clin Endocrinol (Oxf). 59:467-475.

Mintzer MZ, Stitzer ML (2002). Cognitive impairment in methadone maintenance patients. Drug Alcohol Depend. 67:41-51.

Muriach M, López-Pedrajas R, Barcia JM, Sanchez-Villarejo MV, Almansa I, Romero FJ (2010). Cocaine causes memory and learning impairments in rats: involvement of nuclear factor kappa B and oxidative stress, and prevention by topiramate. J Neurochem. 114:675-684.

Moghaddam B (2004). Targeting metabotropic glutamate receptors for treatment of the cognitive symptoms of schizophrenia. Psychopharmacology (Berl). 174:39-44.

Nash RJ, Heimburg-Molinaro J, Nash RJ (2009). Heparin binding epidermal growth factor-like growth factor reduces ethanol-induced apoptosis and differentiation in human embryonic stem cells. Growth Factors. 27:362-369.

Nestor LJ, Ghahremani DG, Monterosso J, London ED (2011). Prefrontal hypoactivation during cognitive control in early abstinent methamphetamine-dependent subjects. Psychiatry Res. 194(:287-295

Nixon K, Crews FT (2002). Binge ethanol exposure decreases neurogenesis in adult rat hippocampus. J Neurochem. 83:1087-1093.

Nixon K, McClain JA (2010). Adolescence as a critical window for developing an alcohol use disorder: current findings in neuroscience. Curr Opin Psychiatry. 23:227-232.

Nulsen CE, Fox AM, Hammond GR (2010). Differential effects of ecstasy on short-term and working memory: a meta-analysis. Neuropsychol Rev. 20:21-32.

Nyberg F (2000). Growth hormone in the brain: characteristics of specific brain targets for the hormone and their functional significance. Front Neuroendocrinol. 21:330-348.

Nyberg F (2007). Growth hormone and brain function. In Ranke MB, Price DA, Reiter EO (eds.) Growth Hormone Therapy in Pediatrics. 20 years of KIGS. Karger, Basel, pp 450-460.

Nyberg F (2009). The role of the somatotrophic axis in neuroprotection and neuroregeneration of the addictive brain. Int Rev Neurobiol. 88:399-427.

O'Kusky JR, Ye P, D'Ercole AJ (2000). Insulin-like growth factor-I promotes neurogenesis and synaptogenesis in the hippocampal dentate gyrus during postnatal development. J Neurosci. 20:8435-8442.

Olive MF (2009). Metabotropic glutamate receptor ligands as potential therapeutics for addiction. Curr Drug Abuse Rev. 2:83-98.

Olive MF (2010). Cognitive effects of Group I metabotropic glutamate receptor ligands in the context of drug addiction. Eur J Pharmacol. 639:47-58.

Ornstein TJ, Iddon JL, Baldacchino AM, Sahakian BJ, London M, Everitt BJ, Robbins TW (2000). Profiles of cognitive dysfunction in chronic amphetamine and heroin abusers. Neuropsychopharmacology. 23:113-126

Parrott AC, Lasky J (1998). Ecstasy (MDMA) effects upon mood and cognition: before, during and after a Saturday night dance. Psychopharmacology (Berl). 139:261-268.

Reichel CM, Ramsey LA, Schwendt M, McGinty JF, See RE (2011). Methamphetamine-induced changes in the object recognition memory circuit. Neuropharmacology. 2011 Nov 18. [Epub ahead of print].

Reske M, Eidt CA, Delis DC, Paulus MP (2010). Nondependent stimulant users of cocaine and prescription amphetamines show verbal learning and memory deficits. Biol Psychiatry. 68:762-769.

Ridderinkhof KR, van den Wildenberg WP, Segalowitz SJ, Carter CS (2004). Neurocognitive mechanisms of cognitive control: the role of prefrontal cortex in action selection, response inhibition, performance monitoring, and reward-based learning. Brain Cogn. 56:129-140.

Rogers G, Elston J, Garside R, et al. (2009) The harmful health effects of recreational ecstasy: A systematic review of observational evidence. Health Technol Assess 13: 1–315.

Samuelson KW (2011). Post-traumatic stress disorder and declarative memory functioning: a review. Dialogues Clin Neurosci. 13:346-351.

Santini E, Muller RU, Quirk GJ (2001). Consolidation of extinction learning involves transfer from NMDA-independent to NMDA-dependent memory. J Neurosci. 21:9009-9017.

Seiler AE, Ross BN, Green JS, Rubin R (2000). Differential effects of ethanol on insulin- like growth factor-I receptor signaling. Alcohol Clin Exp Res. 24:140-148.

Silva AP, Martins T, Baptista S, Gonçalves J, Agasse F, Malva JO (2010). Brain injury associated with widely abused amphetamines: neuroinflammation, neurogenesis and blood-brain barrier. Curr Drug Abuse Rev. 3:239-254

Simonyi A, Schachtman TR, Christoffersen GR (2005).The role of metabotropic glutamate receptor 5 in learning and memory processes. Drug News Perspect. 18:353-361.

Soyka M, Limmer C, Lehnert R, Koller G, Martin G, Küfner H, Kagerer S, Haberthür A (2011). A comparison of cognitive function in patients under maintenance treatment with heroin, methadone, or buprenorphine and healthy controls: an open pilot study. Am J Drug Alcohol Abuse. 37:497-508.

Spain JW, Newsom GC (1991). Chronic opioids impair acquisition of both radial maze and Y-maze choice escape. Psychopharmacology (Berl). 105:101-106

Stramiello M, Wagner JJ (2010). Cocaine enhancement of long-term potentiation in the CA1 region of rat hippocampus: lamina-specific mechanisms of action. Synapse. 64:644-648.

Sudai E, Croitoru O, Shaldubina A, Abraham L, Gispan I, Flaumenhaft Y, Roth-Deri I, Kinor N, Aharoni S, Ben-Tzion M, Yadid G (2011). High cocaine dosage decreases neurogenesis in the hippocampus and impairs working memory. Addict Biol. 16:251-260.

Sullivan EV, Pfefferbaum A (2005). Neurocircuitry in alcoholism: a substrate of disruption and repair. Psychopharmacology (Berl). 180:583-594.

Sun LY, Al-Regaiey K, Masternak MM, Wang J, Bartke A (2005). Local expression of GH and IGF-1 in the hippocampus of GH-deficient long-lived mice. Neurobiol Aging. 26:929-937.

Svensson AL, Bucht N, Hallberg M, Nyberg F (2008). Reversal of opiate-induced apoptosis by human recombinant growth hormone in murine foetus primary hippocampal neuronal cell cultures. Proc Natl Acad Sci U S A. 105:7304-7308.

Taffe MA, Kotzebue RW, Crean RD, Crawford EF, Edwards S, Mandyam CD (2010). Long-lasting reduction in hippocampal neurogenesis by alcohol consumption in adolescent nonhuman primates. Proc Natl Acad Sci U S A.107:11104-11109.

Tang YP, Shimizu E, Dube GR, Rampon C, Kerchner GA, Zhuo M, Liu G, Tsien JZ (1999). Genetic enhancement of learning and memory in mice. Nature. 401:63-69.

Taqi MM, Bazov I, Watanabe H, Sheedy D, Harper C, Alkass K, Druid H, Wentzel P, Nyberg F, Yakovleva T, Bakalkin G (2011). Prodynorphin CpG-SNPs associated with alcohol dependence: elevated methylation in the brain of human alcoholics. Addict Biol. 16:499-509.

Tateno M, Ukai W, Ozawa H, Yamamoto M, Toki S, Ikeda H, Saito T (2004). Ethanol inhibition of neural stem cell differentiation is reduced by neurotrophic factors. Alcohol Clin Exp Res. 2004 Aug;28(8 Suppl Proceedings):134S-138S.

Tedstone D, Coyle K (2004). Cognitive impairments in sober alcoholics: performance on selective and divided attention tasks. Drug Alcohol Depend. 75:277-286.

Thompson AM, Swant J, Wagner JJ (2005). Cocaine-induced modulation of long-term potentiation in the CA1 region of rat hippocampus. Neuropharmacology. 49:185–194.

Thornwall-Le Greves M, Zhou Q, Lagerholm S, Huang W, Le Greves P, Nyberg F (2001). Morphine decreases the levels of the gene transcripts of growth hormone receptor and growth hormone binding protein in the male rat hippocampus and spinal cord. Neurosci Lett. 304:69-72

Tramullas M, Martínez-Cué C, Hurlé MA (2007). Chronic methadone treatment and repeated withdrawal impair cognition and increase the expression of apoptosis-related proteins in mouse brain. Psychopharmacology (Berl). 193:107-120.

Tzschentke TM, Schmidt WJ (2003). Glutamatergic mechanisms in addiction. Mol Psychiatry. 8:373-382.

van Dam PS, Aleman A, de Vries WR, Deijen JB, van der Veen EA, de Haan EH, Koppeschaar HP (2000). Growth hormone, insulin-like growth factor I and cognitive function in adults. Growth Horm IGF Res. 10 Suppl B:S69-73.

Vardakou I, Pistos C, Spiliopoulou Ch (2011). Drugs for youth via Internet and the example of mephedrone. Toxicol Lett. 201:191-195.

Venkatesan A, Uzasci L, Chen Z, Rajbhandari L, Anderson C, Lee MH, Bianchet MA, Cotter R, Song H, Nath A (2011). Impairment of adult hippocampal neural progenitor proliferation by methamphetamine: role for nitrotyrosination. Mol Brain. 2011 Jun 27;4:28.

Weiss C, Disterhoft JF (2011). Exploring prefrontal cortical memory mechanisms with eyeblink conditioning. Behav Neurosci. 125:318-326.

Wolf ME (1998). The role of excitatory amino acids in behavioral sensitization to psychomotor stimulants. Prog Neurobiol. 54:679-720. Review

Xu TX, Ma Q, Spealman RD, Yao WD (2010). Amphetamine modulation of long-term potentiation in the prefrontal cortex: dose dependency, monoaminergic contributions, and paradoxical rescue in hyperdopaminergic mutant. J Neurochem. 115:1643-1654.

Yang Z, Xie J, Shao YC, Xie CM, Fu LP, Li DJ, Fan M, Ma L, Li SJ (2009). Dynamic neural responses to cue-reactivity paradigms in heroin-dependent users: an fMRI study. Hum Brain Mapp. 30:766-775.

Zhai QZ, Lai Z, Yukhananov R, Roos P, Nyberg F (1995). Decreased binding of growth hormone in the rat hypothalamus and choroid plexus following morphine treatment. Neurosci Lett. 23;184:82-85

Zhao MG, Toyoda H, Lee YS, Wu LJ, Ko SW, Zhang XH, Jia Y, Shum F, Xu H, Li BM, Kaang BK, Zhuo M. Roles of NMDA NR2B subtype receptor in prefrontal long- term potentiation and contextual fear memory. Neuron. 2005; 47:859-872.

10

Brain Restoration: A Function of Sleep

Eva Acosta-Peña, Juan Carlos Rodríguez-Alba and Fabio García-García
Departamento de Biomedicina, Instituto de Ciencias de la Salud, Universidad Veracruzana
México

1. Introduction

Several hypotheses have been suggested in order to answer the question about the biological function of sleep, and although this question is still in discussion, all theories share the proposal that sleep plays a transcendental role for both physical and brain development.

It is well known that sleep deprivation impairs cognitive processes (Drummond & Brown, 2001; Nilsson et al., 2005; Smith et al., 2002), total time of rapid eye movements sleep (REM sleep) is increased after stress condition (Rampin et al., 1991), a brief nap during the day improves mood, memory consolidation and alertness during wakefulness (Backhaus & Junghanns, 2006; Hayashi et al., 1999), and also sleep promotes motor recovery following cerebral stroke (Gómez Beldarrain et al., 2008; Siengsukon & Boyd, 2008, 2009a, 2009b). For these reasons, it has been suggested that sleep preserves the brain in optimal conditions to support the damage occurred in different situations throughout the day. Although the exact way by which this occurs in the brain remains unknown, it is possible that sleep could do it by improving the functioning of antioxidant systems, the maintenance of cellular integrity through the synthesis of molecules involved in cellular structure or regulation of cell cycle, as well as improving synaptic efficiency. The purpose of this chapter is to summarize the main studies that demonstrate the role of sleep in brain restoration and, as a result, in body functioning.

2. Biology of sleep-wake cycle

Sleep is a biological phenomenon of reversible nature, which is generated and regulated by several complex systems of neuronal networks and neurotransmitters (García-García & Corona-Morales, 2008; Markov & Goldman, 2006; Stenberg, 2007). Behaviorally, sleep is described as a state of rest characterized by a reduction in mobility and low response to sensory stimuli (Stenberg, 2007). However, the detailed study of sleep involves recording of electrographic parameters, such as: electroencephalogram (EEG), electrooculogram (EOG) and electromyogram (EMG).

During the wakefulness period reactivity to sensorial stimuli is high, beta waves (frequency > 13 Hz) are present during all EEG recording (figure 1). Nevertheless, when a subject begins to fall asleep, the brain electrical activity is reduced and alpha waves (8-13 Hz) appear (figure 1) (Dobato-Ayuso et al., 2002). At this point the transition from wakefulness to sleep begins. According to behavioral and polysomnographic parameters, sleep is divided in two main stages: slow wave sleep (SWS) (sometimes denominated non-REM sleep) and REM sleep.

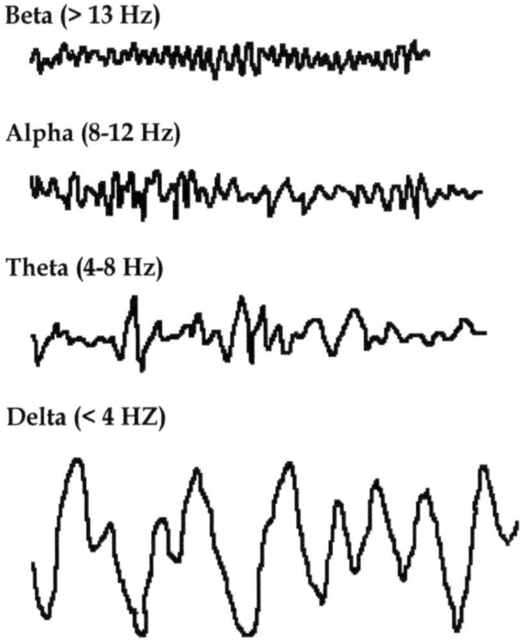

Fig. 1. Schematic representation of main different cerebral waves observed in EEG. Four wave types are organized according to brain activity, from fast to slow. Frequency (Hz) is directly related to brain activation whereas wave amplitude is opposite to this. During wakefulness beta waves prevail in EEG recordings. Alpha and delta waves are present in slow wave sleep (N1-N3 stages) and theta activity is characteristic of REM sleep.

2.1 Slow Wave Sleep

During this period, brain waves recorded in the EEG are synchronous due to reduction of frequency and increase in amplitude, until become very slow waves (figure 1) (Dobato-Ayuso et al., 2002). During this sleep stage vital functions (including respiratory and heart rates) are at the minimum and muscle tone in the EMG is very relaxed (Carskadon & Dement, 2005). At the beginning of this stage only a few slow ocular movements can be observed in the EOG, once that sleep depth is increased these movements disappear (Carskadon & Dement, 2005). In humans SWS is usually subdivided in three phases (NI-N3), in which the depth of the slow waves is gradually increased (Silber et al., 2007).

Cerebral activity recorded during SWS is the result of a decrease in firing frequency of cortical neurons, which were active during wakefulness, by action of GABA-ergic neurons in preoptical ventrolateral area (Steriade, 2001). Therefore; slow waves registered during SWS are result of the prolonged hyperpolarization of cortical neurons (Steriade, 2001).

2.2 REM sleep

During REM sleep brain activity is characterized by waves of low amplitude and high frequency (figure 1). Markedly rhythmical theta waves and series of beta waves less than 10 s of duration appear in the EEG recording (Carskadon & Dement, 2005; Dobato-Ayuso et al., 2002; Fuller et al., 2006). The muscle tone is at the minimum or absent (except in eyes and respiratory muscles) (Chase & Morales, 1990). Fast ocular movements in both horizontal and vertical direction are recorded by the EOG (Aserinsky & Kleitman, 2003); the presence of these ocular movements gives the name to this sleep stage.

Neuronal groups mainly in the peduncle pontine (PPT) and laterodorsal tegmental (LDT) nucleus increase their firing frequency producing cortical desincronization. Particularly, these neurons fire exclusively during REM sleep period and are therefore called REM-on cells. In addition, these neurons are also responsible for the loss of muscle tone characteristic of this sleep stage, due to the inhibition of motoneurons in the spinal cord (Aloe et al., 2005; Sakai et al., 2001; Sakai & Koyama, 1996). An additional component of REM sleep is the occurrence of ponto-geniculate-occipital waves (PGO); which are transitory waves that have their origin in the pons and they later propagate towards the lateral geniculate nucleus into the thalamus and towards the occipital cortex (Datta & Siwek, 2002).

During the course of one night, all different stages of sleep and wakefulness alternate between them generating the called sleep-wake cycle, with a frequency of 4 to 6 cycles per night (≈90-120 minutes each) (figure 2) (Carskadon & Dement, 2005). The sleep pattern every night can also be changed by experiences that occur during the previous day (Drucker-Colín, 1995; García-García et al., 1998).

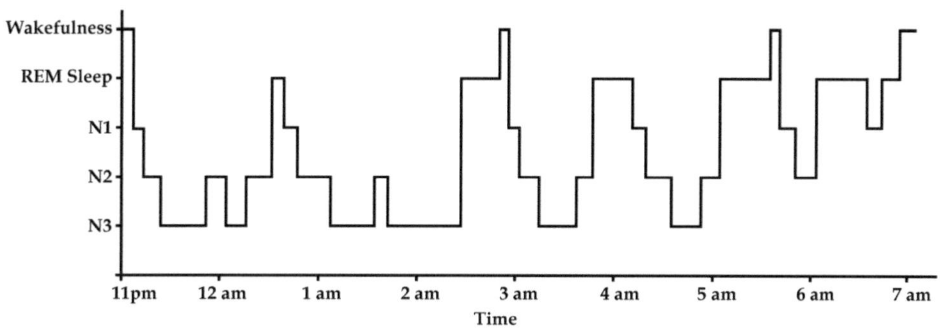

Fig. 2. Hypnogram of normal sleep-wake cycle of a human adult during a sleep night. First sleep cycle generally starts in wakefulness, followed by slow wave sleep (N1-N3) and REM sleep; in subsequent cycles, sleep stages could be randomly distributed. Overnight, 4-6 sleep cycles from 90-120 minutes of duration each can be recorded. There is a N2 and N3 predominance on the first part of night whereas N1 and REM sleep appear most frequently towards dawn. Commonly, some brief wakefulness periods may appear throughout night; however, they do not affect the sleep quality.

3. Biological function of sleep

In physiology, to know and study the function of some particular organ, this one is removed from the organism (generally in animal models) and changes produced due to its absence are observed. Sleep is not the exception since most methods used for the study of its function consists in suppressing it, manipulation known as sleep deprivation (SD).

Total sleep deprivation (TSD) in rats, by a period of three weeks, produces a significant physical deterioration: ulcerations in skin, tail and legs as well as an increase in food intake accompanied by excessive loss of weight that finally causes the death of the animal (Everson et al., 1989). In addition to physical deterioration, cognitive processes are severely affected by sleep deprivation; TSD or prolonged sleep fragmentation produces a decrease in cellular proliferation (Guzmán-Marín et al., 2003) and neurogenesis (García-García et al., 2011; Guzmán-Marín et al., 2007; Guzmán-Marín et al., 2005) in the hippocampus of adult rats. Furthermore, differentiation and survival of new cells in this region are affected by SD (García-García et al., 2011; Roman et al., 2005). In humans, insomnia or chronic loss of sleep is associated with excessive diurnal sleepiness and a decrease in psychomotor performance; being also affected the mood and functions of immune system (Malik & Kaplan, 2005). In this same way, in both animals and humans, it has been demonstrated that sleep, subsequent to a training period, improves execution of test (Stickgold et al., 2000) as well as memory consolidation (Fischer et al., 2002; Rauchs et al., 2004) whereas TSD or selective REM sleep deprivation (REMSD) impairs it considerably (Drummond & Brown, 2001; Nilsson et al., 2005; Smith et al., 2002). Although the exact way by which loss of sleep produces these negative cerebral effects is still unknown; it has been suggested that neuronal activity generated during prolonged periods of wakefulness can damage nervous cells and even induce cellular death (Inoué et al., 1995; Mamelak, 1997; Reimund, 1994).

4. Brain restoration as a sleep function

During high neuronal activity periods, glucose oxidation and oxygen requirements are increased due to high cost involved in the maintenance of bipotentials (Attwell & Laughlin, 2001), consequently, there is an increase in the intracellular production of reactive oxygen species (ROS), such as superoxide anions, hydroxyl radicals and hydrogen peroxide (Finkel & Holbrook, 2000). Usually, ROS levels in nervous system are regulated by several antioxidant mechanisms among which are glutathione, glutathione peroxidase and superoxide dismutase (SOD) (Attwell & Laughlin, 2001; Young & Woodside, 2001). Nevertheless, when intracellular amount of ROS is increased to the level that antioxidant systems are unable to maintain the cellular homeostasis, occurs a phenomenon known as oxidative stress (Finkel & Holbrook, 2000). It has been demonstrated that oxidative stress can damage cellular structure inducing destruction of different cellular components, including lipids, proteins and nucleic acids (Kannan & Jain, 2000).

One of the suggested functions of sleep is the role that it has on regulation of oxidative stress into the brain (Reimund, 1994). For example, it has been demonstrated that the induction of brain oxidation (through the injection of an organic hydroperoxide that promotes ROS production without cause cellular damage) during wakefulness promotes sleep (Ikeda et al., 2005). In addition, TSD or REMSD induces oxidative stress in different cerebral regions, mainly in the thalamus, hypothalamus and hippocampus, by increasing the concentration of oxidized glutathione forms (Komoda et al., 1990), reducing levels of reduced glutathione (D'Almeida et al., 1998; Singh et al., 2008), increasing lipid peroxidation (Komoda et al., 1990) as well as the decline of SOD activity (Ikeda et al., 2005; Ramanathan et al., 2002) (figure 3). However, some studies have reported that both TSD (8 hours or 14 days) and 96 hours of REMSD do not induced significant changes in the morphology and number of neurons in the brain of adult rats (Cirelli et al., 1999; Hipolide et al., 2002). In contrast, TSD > 45 hours reduces the cellular membrane integrity in neurons on supraoptic nucleus (Eiland et al., 2002). Furthermore, 6 days of REMSD affect both size and shape of neurons present in locus ceruleus (LC) and PPT/LDT nucleus, regions involved in REM sleep regulation (Majumdar & Mallick, 2005), there is also an increase in neuronal expression of pro-apoptotic genes (i.e. Bax) and a decrease in actin and tubulin levels (Biswas et al., 2006).

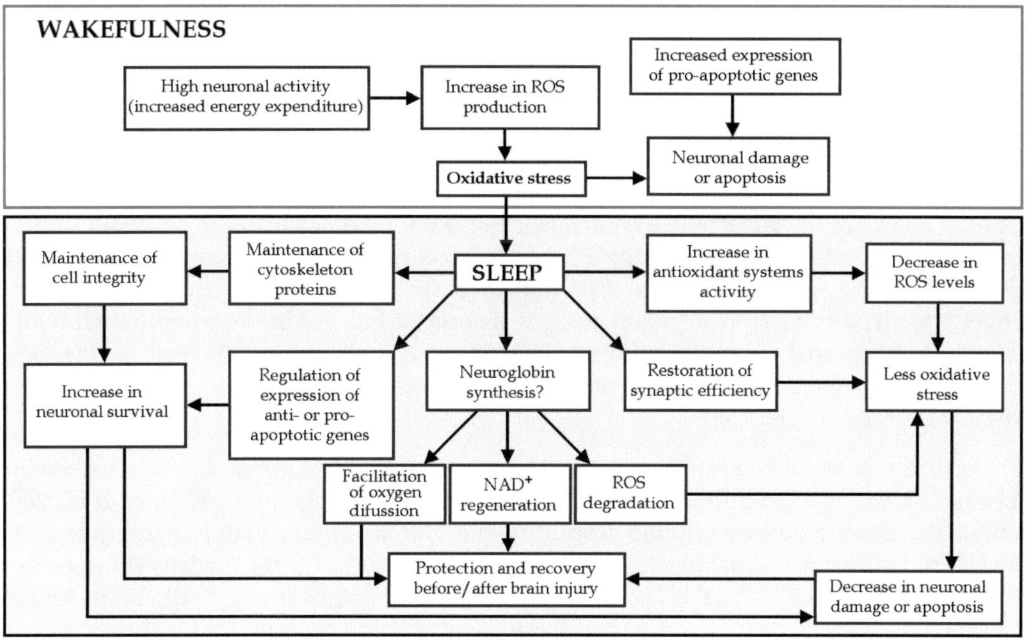

Fig. 3. Possible ways involved in brain restoration during sleep.
High neuronal activity and increased energy expenditure generated during wakefulness (and sleep deprivation, not shown) produce an excess of reactive oxygen species (ROS) becoming oxidative stress, which is able to produce neuronal damage, apoptosis and induce sleep (upper panel); the final aim of this sleep induction (lower panel) could be protect or recover the brain from different kinds of cerebral injuries. This sleep function is probably carried out by increasing antioxidant systems activity and restoration of synaptic efficiency, which decrease oxidative stress and neuronal damage. Another way is probably through maintenance and regulation of cell structure genes and proteins that allow increase neuronal survival. Finally, an extra but unknown (?) way for brain recovery during sleep could be through neuroglobin synthesis; these proteins could help to improve neuronal survival by ROS degradation, oxygen transport facilitation and NAD+ regeneration under hypoxia conditions.

Interestingly, 3 days of sleep recovery after REMSD are sufficient to counteract these cellular changes (Biswas et al., 2006; Majumdar & Mallick, 2005). These results suggest that sleep could prevent neuronal damage through the maintenance of cell integrity and neuronal survival by preservation of cytoskeleton proteins (Biswas et al., 2006), regulation of anti- and pro-apoptotic protein expression (Biswas et al., 2006; Montes-Rodriguez et al., 2009) or through the expression of genes involved in the maintenance of different cellular processes; such as cholesterol and protein synthesis, synaptic vesicle formation, antioxidant enzymes synthesis, etc. (Cirelli et al., 2004; Mackiewicz et al., 2007) (figure 3).

Additionally, it has been proposed that during sleep a synaptic efficiency improvement is necessary in order to prevent the storage of unnecessary information (Tononi & Cirelli, 2003, 2006), which requires high energy expenditure for cells (Attwell & Laughlin, 2001) because, as already mentioned, an overwork of the cell produces an increase in oxidative stress that finally affects the cerebral integrity which is necessary not only for well functioning of cognitive processes, such as memory (Born et al., 2006; Stickgold & Walker, 2007; Tononi & Cirelli, 2001), but also for maintenance of neuronal ways involved in adaptive processes (Shank & Margoliash, 2009). Related to this, in people with acquired brain injury, sleep seems to play a special role in recovery of motor damage, independently of the cerebral region that is affected (Gómez Beldarrain et al., 2008; Siengsukon & Boyd, 2008, 2009a, 2009b) (figure 3). In addition, it is possible to say that neurotrophins (molecules that improve neuronal development and facilitate the synaptic efficiency) are involved in brain restoration occurred during sleep. However, according to its sleep-inducing factor characteristics, i.e. higher level in wakefulness than in sleep, neurotrophins are maybe actively involved in brain restoration along wakefulness but not in sleep and therefore, it is difficult that neuronal restoration during sleep occurs completely by this way. In this sense, an interaction between wakefulness and sleep is necessary to promote cerebral restoration (Montes-Rodriguez et al., 2006).

On the other hand, recent studies have demonstrated that neuronal hypoxia or cerebral ischemia induces an increase in neuroglobin (Ngb) expression (Schmidt-Kastner et al., 2006; Sun et al., 2001); Ngb is a protein belong to the globin family, mainly synthesized and located in neurons from thalamus, hypothalamus, LC and PPT/LDT nucleus (Burmester et al., 2000; Hankeln et al., 2004; Hundahl et al., 2008; Wystub et al., 2003), brain regions involved in sleep generation and regulation. It has been suggested that Ngb plays a neuroprotector role through oxygen transport into neurons, NAD^+ regeneration under anaerobic conditions (to maintain glycolysis) or by ROS degradation (Burmester & Hankeln, 2004; Sun et al., 2003; Wang et al., 2008). The fact that Ngb plays an important role in the recovery of the injured brain, being synthesized in cerebral regions involved in sleep regulation (Hundahl et al., 2008) and, that patients with cerebral damage display a high amount of sleep (Masel et al., 2001; Watson et al., 2007), altogether, let us think that the synthesis of these proteins could be a way by which sleep promotes brain restoration (figure 3); nevertheless, this is a topic that needs to be highly investigated.

5. Conclusion

The biological function of sleep is a topic that has widely been studied; nevertheless, in spite of the great amount of information that already exists, there is not a consensus about why we sleep. At cellular level, little is known about the role that sleep plays in the conservation of cellular integrity in conditions of health and neuronal damage (García-García & Drucker-Colín, 2008). Therefore, it is necessary to continue with the search of detailed mechanisms involved in both physical and brain restoration that occurs total or partially during sleep, which as much as possible increases subjects survival.

6. Acknowledgements

This work was supported by a grant from CONACYT 133178 to FGG.

7. References

Aloe, F., Azevedo, A.P. & Hasan, R. (2005). [Sleep-wake cycle mechanisms]. *Revista Brasileira de Psiquiatria*, Vol. 27 Suppl 1, May 2005, pp. 33-9, ISSN 1516-4446

Aserinsky, E. & Kleitman, N. (2003). Regularly occurring periods of eye motility, and concomitant phenomena, during sleep. 1953. *The Journal of Neuropsychiatry and Clinical Neuroscience*, Vol. 15, No. 4, Novemeber 2003, pp. 454-5, ISSN 0895-0172

Attwell, D. & Laughlin, S.B. (2001). An energy budget for signaling in the grey matter of the brain. *Journal of Cerebral Blood Flow and Metabolism*, Vol. 21, No. 10, October 2001, pp. 1133-45, ISSN 0271-678X

Backhaus, J. & Junghanns, K. (2006). Daytime naps improve procedural motor memory. *Sleep Medicine*, Vol. 7, No. 6, September 2006, pp. 508-12, ISNN 1389-9457

Biswas, S., Mishra, P. & Mallick, B.N. (2006). Increased apoptosis in rat brain after rapid eye movement sleep loss. *Neuroscience*, Vol. 142, No. 2, October 2006, pp. 315-31, ISSN 0306-4522

Born, J., Rasch, B. & Gais, S. (2006). Sleep to remember. *The Neuroscientist*, Vol. 12, No. 5, October 2006, pp. 410-24, ISSN 1073-8584

Burmester, T. & Hankeln, T. (2004). Neuroglobin: a respiratory protein of the nervous system. *News in Physiological Science*, Vol. 19, June 2004, pp. 110-3, ISSN 0886-1714

Burmester, T., Weich, B., Reinhardt, S. & Hankeln, T. (2000). A vertebrate globin expressed in the brain. *Nature*, Vol. 407, No. 6803, September 2000, pp. 520-3, ISSN 0028-0836

Carskadon, M. & Dement, W.C. (2005). Normal human sleep: An overview, In: *Principles and practice of sleep medicine*, M.H. Kryger, T. Roth & W.C. Dement, (Eds.), pp. 13-23, Elsevier-Saunders, ISBN 978-072-160-797-9, Philadelphia

Cirelli, C., Gutierrez, C.M. & Tononi, G. (2004). Extensive and divergent effects of sleep and wakefulness on brain gene expression. *Neuron*, Vol. 41, No. 1, January 2004, pp. 35-43, ISSN 0896-6273

Cirelli, C., Shaw, P.J., Rechtschaffen, A. & Tononi, G. (1999). No evidence of brain cell degeneration after long-term sleep deprivation in rats. *Brain Research*, Vol. 840, No. 1-2, September 1999, pp. 184-93, ISSN 0006-8993

Chase, M.H. & Morales, F.R. (1990). The atonia and myoclonia of active (REM) sleep. *Annual Review of Psychology*, Vol. 41, January 1990, pp. 557-84, ISSN 0066-4308

D'Almeida, V., Lobo, L.L., Hipolide, D.C., de Oliveira, A.C., Nobrega, J.N. & Tufik, S. (1998). Sleep deprivation induces brain region-specific decreases in glutathione levels. *Neuroreport*, Vol. 9, No. 12, August 1998, pp. 2853-6, ISSN 0959-4965

Datta, S. & Siwek, D.F. (2002). Single cell activity patterns of pedunculopontine tegmentum neurons across the sleep-wake cycle in the freely moving rats. *Journal of Neuroscience Research*, Vol. 70, No. 4, November 2002, pp. 611-21, ISSN 0360-4012

Dobato-Ayuso, J.L., Barriga-Hernández, F.J. & Pareja-Grande, J.A. (2002). EEG normal durante el sueño, In: *Manual de electroencefalografía*, A. Gil-Nagel, J. Parra, J. Iriarte & A.M. Kanner, (Eds.), pp. 43-50, McGraw-Hill interamericana, ISBN 978-844-860-420-2, Madrid, España

Drucker-Colín, R. (1995). The function of sleep is to regulate brain excitability in order to satisfy the requirements imposed by waking. *Behavioural Brain Research*, Vol. 69, No. 1-2, July-August 1995, pp. 117-24, ISSN 0166-4328

Drummond, S.P. & Brown, G.G. (2001). The effects of total sleep deprivation on cerebral responses to cognitive performance. *Neuropsychopharmacology*, Vol. 25, No. 5 Suppl, November 2001, pp. S68-73, ISSN 0893-133X

Eiland, M.M., Ramanathan, L., Gulyani, S., Gilliland, M., Bergmann, B.M., Rechtschaffen, A. & Siegel, J.M. (2002). Increases in amino-cupric-silver staining of the supraoptic nucleus after sleep deprivation. *Brain Research*, Vol. 945, No. 1, July 2002, pp. 1-8, ISSN 0006-8993

Everson, C.A., Bergmann, B.M. & Rechtschaffen, A. (1989). Sleep deprivation in the rat: III. Total sleep deprivation. *Sleep*, Vol. 12, No. 1, February 1989, pp. 13-21, ISSN 0161-8105

Finkel, T. & Holbrook, N.J. (2000). Oxidants, oxidative stress and the biology of ageing. *Nature*, Vol. 408, No. 6809, November 2000, pp. 239-47, ISSN 0028-0836

Fischer, S., Hallschmid, M., Elsner, A.L. & Born, J. (2002). Sleep forms memory for finger skills. *Proceedings of the National Academy of Sciences of the United States of America*, Vol. 99, No. 18, September 2002, pp. 11987-91, ISSN 0027-8424

Fuller, P.M., Gooley, J.J. & Saper, C.B. (2006). Neurobiology of the sleep-wake cycle: sleep architecture, circadian regulation, and regulatory feedback. *Journal of Biological Rhythms*, Vol. 21, No. 6, December 2006, pp. 482-93, ISSN 0748-7304

García-García, F., Beltrán-Parrazal, L., Jiménez-Anguiano, A., Vega-González, A. & Drucker-Colín, R. (1998). Manipulations during forced wakefulness have differential impact on sleep architecture, EEG power spectrum, and Fos induction. *Brain Research Bulletin*, Vol. 47, No. 4, November 1998, pp. 317-24, ISSN 0361-9230

García-García, F. & Corona-Morales, A. (2008). Bases biológicas del ciclo vigilia-sueño, In: *Bases celulares y moleculares de los ritmos biológicos*, M. Caba, (Ed.), pp. 127-38, Universidad Veracruzana, ISBN 978-968-834-843-7, Xalapa, México

García-García, F., De la Herrán-Arita, A.K., Juárez-Aguilar, E., Regalado-Santiago, C., Millán-Aldaco, D., Blanco-Centurión, C. & Drucker-Colín, R. (2011). Growth hormone improves hippocampal adult cell survival and counteracts the inhibitory effect of prolonged sleep deprivation on cell proliferation. *Brain Research Bulletin*, Vol. 84, No. 3, February 2011, pp. 252-7, ISSN 1873-2747

García-García, F. & Drucker-Colín, R. (2008). Sleep Factors, In: *Sleep Disorders: Diagnosis and Therapeutics*, S.R. Pandi-Perumal, J.C. Verster, J.M. Monti, M. Lader & S.Z. Langer, (Eds.), pp. 125-32, Informa Healthcare, ISBN 978-041-543-818-6, UK

Gómez Beldarrain, M., Astorgano, A.G., Gonzalez, A.B. & García-Monco, J.C. (2008). Sleep improves sequential motor learning and performance in patients with prefrontal lobe lesions. *Clinical Neurology and Neurosurgery*, Vol. 110, No. 3, March 2008, pp. 245-52, ISSN 0303-8467

Guzmán-Marín, R., Bashir, T., Suntsova, N., Szymusiak, R. & McGinty, D. (2007). Hippocampal neurogenesis is reduced by sleep fragmentation in the adult rat. *Neuroscience*, Vol. 148, No. 1, August 2007, pp. 325-33, ISSN 0306-4522

Guzmán-Marín, R., Suntsova, N., Methippara, M., Greiffenstein, R., Szymusiak, R. & McGinty, D. (2005). Sleep deprivation suppresses neurogenesis in the adult hippocampus of rats. *European Journal of Neuroscience*, Vol. 22, No. 8, October 2005, pp. 2111-6, ISSN 0953-816X

Guzmán-Marín, R., Suntsova, N., Stewart, D.R., Gong, H., Szymusiak, R. & McGinty, D. (2003). Sleep deprivation reduces proliferation of cells in the dentate gyrus of the hippocampus in rats. *Journal of Physiology*, Vol. 549, No. Pt 2, June 2003, pp. 563-71, ISSN 0022-3751

Hankeln, T., Wystub, S., Laufs, T., Schmidt, M., Gerlach, F., Saaler-Reinhardt, S., Reuss, S. & Burmester, T. (2004). The cellular and subcellular localization of neuroglobin and cytoglobin -- a clue to their function? *IUBMB Life*, Vol. 56, No. 11-12, November-December 2004, pp. 671-9, ISSN 1521-6543

Hayashi, M., Watanabe, M. & Hori, T. (1999). The effects of a 20 min nap in the mid-afternoon on mood, performance and EEG activity. *Clinical Neurophysiology*, Vol. 110, No. 2, February 1999, pp. 272-9, ISSN 1388-2457

Hipolide, D.C., D'Almeida, V., Raymond, R., Tufik, S. & Nobrega, J.N. (2002). Sleep deprivation does not affect indices of necrosis or apoptosis in rat brain. *The International Journal of Neuroscience*, Vol. 112, No. 2, February 2002, pp. 155-66, ISSN 0020-7454

Hundahl, C.A., Allen, G.C., Nyengaard, J.R., Dewilde, S., Carter, B.D., Kelsen, J. & Hay-Schmidt, A. (2008). Neuroglobin in the rat brain: localization. *Neuroendocrinology*, Vol. 88, No. 3, October 2008, pp. 173-82, ISSN 1423-0194

Ikeda, M., Ikeda-Sagara, M., Okada, T., Clement, P., Urade, Y., Nagai, T., Sugiyama, T., Yoshioka, T., Honda, K. & Inoue, S. (2005). Brain oxidation is an initial process in sleep induction. *Neuroscience*, Vol. 130, No. 4, n.d., pp. 1029-40, ISSN 0306-4522

Inoué, S., Honda, K. & Komoda, Y. (1995). Sleep as neuronal detoxification and restitution. *Behavioural Brain Research*, Vol. 69, No. 1-2, July-August 1995, pp. 91-6, ISSN 0166-4328

Kannan, K. & Jain, S.K. (2000). Oxidative stress and apoptosis. *Pathophysiology*, Vol. 7, No. 3, September 2000, pp. 153-63, ISSN 0928-4680

Komoda, Y., Honda, K. & Inoue, S. (1990). SPS-B, a physiological sleep regulator, from the brainstems of sleep-deprived rats, identified as oxidized glutathione. *Chemical & Pharmaceutical Bulletin*, Vol. 38, No. 7, July 1990, pp. 2057-9, ISSN 0009-2363

Mackiewicz, M., Shockley, K.R., Romer, M.A., Galante, R.J., Zimmerman, J.E., Naidoo, N., Baldwin, D.A., Jensen, S.T., Churchill, G.A. & Pack, A.I. (2007). Macromolecule biosynthesis: a key function of sleep. *Physiological Genomics*, Vol. 31, No. 3, November 2007, pp. 441-57, ISSN 1531-2267

Majumdar, S. & Mallick, B.N. (2005). Cytomorphometric changes in rat brain neurons after rapid eye movement sleep deprivation. *Neuroscience*, Vol. 135, No. 3, n.d., pp. 679-90, ISSN 0306-4522

Malik, S.W. & Kaplan, J. (2005). Sleep deprivation. *Primary Care*, Vol. 32, No. 2, June 2005, pp. 475-90, ISSN 0095-4543

Mamelak, M. (1997). Neurodegeneration, sleep, and cerebral energy metabolism: a testable hypothesis. *Journal of Geriatric Psychiatry and Neurology*, Vol. 10, No. 1, January 1997, pp. 29-32, ISSN 0891-9887

Markov, D. & Goldman, M. (2006). Normal sleep and circadian rhythms: neurobiologic mechanisms underlying sleep and wakefulness. *The Psychiatric Clinics of North America*, Vol. 29, No. 4, December 2006, pp. 841-53; abstract vii, ISSN 0193-953X

Masel, B.E., Scheibel, R.S., Kimbark, T. & Kuna, S.T. (2001). Excessive daytime sleepiness in adults with brain injuries. *Archives of Physical Medicine and Rehabilitation*, Vol. 82, No. 11, November 2001, pp. 1526-32, ISSN 0003-9993

Montes-Rodriguez, C.J., Alavez, S., Soria-Gomez, E., Rueda-Orozco, P.E., Guzman, K., Moran, J. & Prospero-Garcia, O. (2009). BCL-2 and BAX proteins expression throughout the light-dark cycle and modifications induced by sleep deprivation and rebound in adult rat brain. *Journal of Neuroscience Research*, Vol. 87, No. 7, May 2009, pp. 1602-9, ISSN 1097-4547

Montes-Rodriguez, C.J., Rueda-Orozco, P.E., Urteaga-Urias, E., Aguilar-Roblero, R. & Prospero-Garcia, O. (2006). [From neuronal recovery to the reorganisation of neuronal circuits: a review of the functions of sleep]. *Revista de Neurología*, Vol. 43, No. 7, October 2006, pp. 409-15, ISSN 0210-0010

Nilsson, J.P., Soderstrom, M., Karlsson, A.U., Lekander, M., Akerstedt, T., Lindroth, N.E. & Axelsson, J. (2005). Less effective executive functioning after one night's sleep deprivation. *Journal of Sleep Research*, Vol. 14, No. 1, March 2005, pp. 1-6, ISSN 0962-1105

Ramanathan, L., Gulyani, S., Nienhuis, R. & Siegel, J.M. (2002). Sleep deprivation decreases superoxide dismutase activity in rat hippocampus and brainstem. *Neuroreport*, Vol. 13, No. 11, August 2002, pp. 1387-90, ISSN 0959-4965

Rampin, C., Cespuglio, R., Chastrette, N. & Jouvet, M. (1991). Immobilisation stress induces a paradoxical sleep rebound in rat. *Neuroscience Letters*, Vol. 126, No. 2, May 1991, pp. 113-8, ISSN 0304-3940

Rauchs, G., Bertran, F., Guillery-Girard, B., Desgranges, B., Kerrouche, N., Denise, P., Foret, J. & Eustache, F. (2004). Consolidation of strictly episodic memories mainly requires rapid eye movement sleep. *Sleep*, Vol. 27, No. 3, May 2004, pp. 395-401, ISSN 0161-8105

Reimund, E. (1994). The free radical flux theory of sleep. *Medical Hypotheses*, Vol. 43, No. 4, October 1994, pp. 231-3, ISSN 0306-9877

Roman, V., Van der Borght, K., Leemburg, S.A., Van der Zee, E.A. & Meerlo, P. (2005). Sleep restriction by forced activity reduces hippocampal cell proliferation. *Brain Research*, Vol. 1065, No. 1-2, December 2005, pp. 53-9, ISSN 0006-8993

Sakai, K., Crochet, S. & Onoe, H. (2001). Pontine structures and mechanisms involved in the generation of paradoxical (REM) sleep. *Archives Italiennes de Biologie*, Vol. 139, No. 1-2, February 2001, pp. 93-107, ISSN 0003-9829

Sakai, K. & Koyama, Y. (1996). Are there cholinergic and non-cholinergic paradoxical sleep-on neurones in the pons? *Neuroreport*, Vol. 7, No. 15-17, November 1996, pp. 2449-53, ISSN 0959-4965

Schmidt-Kastner, R., Haberkamp, M., Schmitz, C., Hankeln, T. & Burmester, T. (2006). Neuroglobin mRNA expression after transient global brain ischemia and prolonged hypoxia in cell culture. *Brain Research,* Vol. 1103, No. 1, August 2006, pp. 173-80, ISSN 0006-8993

Shank, S.S. & Margoliash, D. (2009). Sleep and sensorimotor integration during early vocal learning in a songbird. *Nature,* Vol. 458, No. 7234, March 2009, pp. 73-7, ISSN 1476-4687

Siengsukon, C.F. & Boyd, L.A. (2008). Sleep enhances implicit motor skill learning in individuals poststroke. *Topics in Stroke Rehabilitation,* Vol. 15, No. 1, January-February 2008, pp. 1-12, ISSN 1074-9357

Siengsukon, C.F. & Boyd, L.A. (2009a). Sleep enhances off-line spatial and temporal motor learning after stroke. *Neurorehabilitation and Neural Repair,* Vol. 23, No. 4, May 2009, pp. 327-35, ISSN 1545-9683

Siengsukon, C.F. & Boyd, L.A. (2009b). Sleep to learn after stroke: implicit and explicit off-line motor learning. *Neuroscience Letters,* Vol. 451, No. 1, February 2009, pp. 1-5, ISSN 0304-3940

Silber, M.H., Ancoli-Israel, S., Bonnet, M.H., Chokroverty, S., Grigg-Damberger, M.M., Hirshkowitz, M., Kapen, S., Keenan, S.A., Kryger, M.H., Penzel, T., Pressman, M.R. & Iber, C. (2007). The visual scoring of sleep in adults. *Journal of Clinical Sleep Medicine,* Vol. 3, No. 2, March 2007, pp. 121-31, ISSN 1550-9389

Singh, R., Kiloung, J., Singh, S. & Sharma, D. (2008). Effect of paradoxical sleep deprivation on oxidative stress parameters in brain regions of adult and old rats. *Biogerontology,* Vol. 9, No. 3, June 2008, pp. 153-62, ISSN 1389-5729

Smith, M.E., McEvoy, L.K. & Gevins, A. (2002). The impact of moderate sleep loss on neurophysiologic signals during working-memory task performance. *Sleep,* Vol. 25, No. 7, November 2002, pp. 784-94, ISSN 0161-8105

Stenberg, D. (2007). Neuroanatomy and neurochemistry of sleep. *Cellular and Molecular Life Sciences,* Vol. 64, No. 10, May 2007, pp. 1187-204, ISSN 1420-682X

Steriade, M. (2001). Active neocortical processes during quiescent sleep. *Archives Italiennes de Biologie,* Vol. 139, No. 1-2, February 2001, pp. 37-51, ISSN 0003-9829

Stickgold, R. & Walker, M.P. (2007). Sleep-dependent memory consolidation and reconsolidation. *Sleep Medicine,* Vol. 8, No. 4, June 2007, pp. 331-43, ISSN 1389-9457

Stickgold, R., Whidbee, D., Schirmer, B., Patel, V. & Hobson, J.A. (2000). Visual discrimination task improvement: A multi-step process occurring during sleep. *Journal of Cognitive Neuroscience,* Vol. 12, No. 2, March 2000, pp. 246-54, ISSN 0898-929X

Sun, Y., Jin, K., Mao, X.O., Zhu, Y. & Greenberg, D.A. (2001). Neuroglobin is up-regulated by and protects neurons from hypoxic-ischemic injury. *Proceedings of the National Academy of Sciences of the United States of America,* Vol. 98, No. 26, December 2001, pp. 15306-11, ISSN 0027-8424

Sun, Y., Jin, K., Peel, A., Mao, X.O., Xie, L. & Greenberg, D.A. (2003). Neuroglobin protects the brain from experimental stroke in vivo. *Proceedings of the National Academy of Sciences of the United States of America,* Vol. 100, No. 6, March 2003, pp. 3497-500, ISSN 0027-8424

Tononi, G. & Cirelli, C. (2001). Some considerations on sleep and neural plasticity. *Archives Italiennes de Biologie,* Vol. 139, No. 3, April 2001, pp. 221-41, ISSN 0003-9829

Tononi, G. & Cirelli, C. (2003). Sleep and synaptic homeostasis: a hypothesis. *Brain Research Bulletin,* Vol. 62, No. 2, December 2003, pp. 143-50, ISSN 0361-9230

Tononi, G. & Cirelli, C. (2006). Sleep function and synaptic homeostasis. *Sleep Medicine Reviews*, Vol. 10, No. 1, February 2006, pp. 49-62, ISSN 1087-0792

Wang, X., Liu, J., Zhu, H., Tejima, E., Tsuji, K., Murata, Y., Atochin, D.N., Huang, P.L., Zhang, C. & Lo, E.H. (2008). Effects of neuroglobin overexpression on acute brain injury and long-term outcomes after focal cerebral ischemia. *Stroke*, Vol. 39, No. 6, June 2008, pp. 1869-74, ISSN 1524-4628

Watson, N.F., Dikmen, S., Machamer, J., Doherty, M. & Temkin, N. (2007). Hypersomnia following traumatic brain injury. *Journal of Clinical Sleep Medicine*, Vol. 3, No. 4, June 2007, pp. 363-8, ISSN 1550-9389

Wystub, S., Laufs, T., Schmidt, M., Burmester, T., Maas, U., Saaler-Reinhardt, S., Hankeln, T. & Reuss, S. (2003). Localization of neuroglobin protein in the mouse brain. *Neuroscience Letters*, Vol. 346, No. 1-2, July 2003, pp. 114-6, ISSN 0304-3940

Young, I.S. & Woodside, J.V. (2001). Antioxidants in health and disease. *Journal of Clinical Pathology*, Vol. 54, No. 3, March 2001, pp. 176-86, ISSN 0021-9746

11

Dynamic Brain Function Monitoring a New Concept in Neuro-Intensive Care

E. Bosco and P. Zanatta
Department of Anesthesia and Intensive Care, Treviso Hospital
Italy

1. Introduction

Multimodality neuromonitoring has became increasingly complex, and although advances in neuromonitoring have provided insight into pathophysiology and physiological response to therapy, beneficial effects on patient outcomes have not been definitively established. The attitude towards the benefits of monitoring equipment has often been guided by wishful thinking. Rosner and colleague (Rosner MJ,1986) popularized the notion that cerebral perfusion pressure (CPP) should be aggressively managed at levels above 70-90 mmHg, if necessary by using vasopressors. At the same time, however, the "Lund concept" urged for a reduction of microvascular hydrostatic pressures to minimize oedema formation, accepting CPP as low as 50 mmHg in adults (Grände PO,2002). Following an update of the Brain Trauma Foundation guidelines in 2003, the consensus target value for CPP has been set at 60 mmHg. Even so, the controversy described above exemplifies the frustrating lack of good evidence that is available to make rational treatment decisions in the setting of intracranial pressure (ICP)-guide care. It is important to consider that there is large heterogeneity within the head trauma population, the intracerebral hemorrhage, the subarachnoid hemorrhage and the physiopathology between them. Therefore it is possible that many commonly used interventions that are aimed to reduce intracranial hypertension are ineffective, unnecessary or even harmful for some patient at certain times, at certain values. There is an increasing awareness that an aggressive ICP and CPP targeted approach may result in cardiorespiratory complications. A key limitation in the demonstration of efficacy of monitoring in neurocritical care is the complexity of care generated by multimodality monitoring. If one considers continuously monitoring 10-20 interrelated physiological parameters in a modern neurocritical care unit and each parameter has 10 possible interventions, the enormous potential number of co-interventions represents a formidable challenge in clinical trial design. The application of continuous neurophysiological monitoring with somatosensory evoked potential (SEP) and electroencephalography (EEG) have an intuitive appeal, since these techniques yeald a direct measure of brain function in patients whose neurological status might otherwise be difficult to evaluate. The early components of SEP are used in the acute phase of cerebral damage when the patient, as result of sedatives, neuromuscular blockade or the severity of coma, is difficult to assess on a clinical level. Short latency SEP are largely resistant to analgo-sedation and have a waveform, which is easily interpretable and comparable in subsequent recordings. They have peripheral, spinal, brainstem and intracortical components, which are identifiable in all subject exploring an extended Cerebral Nervous

System (CNS) pathway. In the absence of a relevant lesion along afferent sensory pathways, a "global" index of brain function (reflected of brainstem, thalamo-cortical and intracortical transmission in both emispheres) can be extrapolated from them. The concept of secondary insults occurring after the primary neurologic injury was put forth by Jennet and colleagues (Rose et al., 1977), Andrew et al. (1990) and later by Miller et al. (1994), who reported that the majority of patients (91%) suffered secondary insults. The secondary insults that occurred most frequently were raised intracranial pressure, hypotension, and pyrexia. Moreover, several investigator have reported ongoing transient and dynamic changes in brain metabolism and neurochemistry (Bullock et al., 1995; Vespa et al., 2003) after brain injury. Continuous EEG monitoring is a valuable clinical instrument "to detect and protect"; to detect seizures and protect the brain from seizures-related injury in critically ill patients, whose brain are often in a particular vulnerable state.

2. The Importance of the aetiology of coma

2.1 Anoxic coma

The prognostic value of SEP patterns in anoxia is complex

Preserved short or middle-latency SEP do not prognosticate awakening with sufficient certainty,but absent cortical SEP are among the most powerful predictors of non-awakening from anoxic coma.

The bilateral absence of N20 in anoxic coma (and only in anoxic coma) is a very reliable indicator of poor prognosis,since none of the patients reported in literature did better than PVS. Therefore ,this pattern provides strong information for decision making in intensive care .

2.2 Head trauma

Can be associated with both "primary" and "secondary" dysfunction.

Primary dysfunction can be a consequence of mechanical lesions,which are usually irreversible,of associated brain oedema,which may be reversible. Mechanical lesions can consist either of brain contusion or diffuse axonal lesions (white matter of the cerebral hemispheree, corpus callosum,midbrain).

Secondary dysfunction may be ischemic (systemic hypoperfusion),epileptic, or due to intracranial hypertension and its complications (transtenorial herniation,brain death).

Short latency SEP are normal in about 50% of cases. Moreover, in contrast with brain anoxia, in which it has no prognostic meaning,the observation of bilaterally normal short-latency SEP constitutes a favourable sign in head trauma (predictive positive value of awaikening of about 90% and 75% to 80% probability of good outcome). Level 1a abnormalities (Table I) are still a relatively good sign too (69% of good outcome). These situations with preserved short latency SEP include brain oedema and/or diffuse axonal lesion without brainstem involvement. By contrast, level 2 or 3 abnormalities have been associated with death or vegetative states in more than 90% of cases, and with severe disability in almost 100%. Therefore, normal or absent cortical SEP are the strongest prognostic indicators, with an occurrence of about 70% in severly injured patients;

Level	Description	Remarks
0	Normal	
1a	Inter Peak Latency (IPL) increas without peak distorsion	Drugs,metabolic disturbances,hypothermia,usually reversible
1b	Distorsion or disappearance,without proof of the integrity of the sensory receptors or proximal afferent pathways	Uncertain pattern
2	Distorsion without disappearance, with proof of the integrity of the sensory system	
3	Disappearance,with proof of the integrity of the sensory system	

Table 1. Classification of short-latency EP abnormalities

3. The EEG

The electroencephalogram (EEG) provides a non invasive way to dynamically assess brain function. Recent advances in computer technology, networking, and data storage have made continuous EEG (cEEG) monitoring practical, and its use is common in many Neuro Intensive Care Unit (NICU). Methods for analyzing and compressing the vast amounts of data generated by cEEG have allowed neurophysiologists to more efficiently review recordings from many patients monitored simultaneously and provide timely information for guiding treatment. There are still many hurdles in making monitoring of brain function truly real time, reliable, practical, and widely available, but the technology is progressing rapidly. The most common reason for performing cEEG is to detect nonconvulsive seizures (NCSzs) or non convulsive status epilepticus (NCSE). Although previously thought to be uncommon NCSzs and NCSE are being recognized more frequently. The current indications and potential uses for cEEG in the critically ill are summarized in Table II

1.Detection of nonconvulsive seizures
2.Detection of convulsive status epilepticus
3.Stereotyped activity such as paroxysmal movements, nystagmus, twitching, jerking, hippus, autonomic variability
4. Monitoring of ongoing therapy:
a)Induced coma for elevated intracranial pressure or refractory status epilepticus
b) Assessing level of sedation
5. Ischemia detection:
a)Vasospasm in subarachnoid hemorrhage
b)Cerebral ischemia in other patients at high risk for stroke
6. Prognosis:
a)Following cardiac arrest
b)Following acute brain injury

Table 2. Indications for Continuous Electroencephalogram (cEEG) Monitoring (Friedman D et al.2009)

NCSzs and NCSE are increasingly recognized as common occurrences in the ICU, where 8%–48% of comatose patients may have NCSzs, depending on which patients are studied. NCSzs are electrographic seizures with little or no clinical manifestations, so EEG is necessary for detection. NCSE occurs when NCSzs are prolonged; a common definition is continuous or near-continuous electrographic seizures of at least 30 min duration. The most common manifestation is a depressed level of consciousness.Most patients with NCSzs have purely electrographic seizures, but other subtle signs can be associated with NCSzs, such as face and limb myoclonus, nystagmus, eye deviation, pupillary abnormalities (including hippus), and autonomic instability.None of these signs are highly specific for NCSz, and they are often seen under other circumstances in the critically ill patient; thus, cEEG is usually necessary to diagnose NCSzs. The etiologies for NCSzs and NCSE in ICU patients are similar to the causes of convulsive seizures in these patients. These include acute structural lesions, infections, metabolic derangements, toxins, withdrawal and epilepsy, all common diagnoses in the critically ill patient (Table III). However, NCSzs are the more common ictal manifestation in ICU patients and should be considered when evaluating the cause of or contributors to altered mental status, especially in high-risk populations.

a)Primary criteria
Any pattern lasting at least 10 s satisfying any one of the following three primary criteria:
-Repetitive generalized or focal spikes, sharp-waves, spike-and-wave complexes at 3/s
-Repetitive generalized or focal spikes, sharp-waves, spike-and-wave or sharp-and-slow wave complexes at 3/s and the secondary criterion
-Sequential rhythmic, periodic, or quasi-periodic waves at _1/s and unequivocal evolution in frequency (gradually increasing or decreasing by at least 1/s, e.g. 2-3/s), morphology, or location (gradual spread into or out of a region involving at least two electrodes).
-Evolution in amplitude alone is not sufficient. Change in sharpness without other change in morphology is not enough to satisfy evolution in morphology
b)Secondary criterion
Significant improvement in clinical state or appearance of previously absent normal electroencephalogram (EEG)-patterns (such as posterior-dominant "alpha" rhythm) temporally coupled to acute administration of a rapidly acting antiepileptic drug.
Resolution of the "epileptiform" discharges leaving diffuse slowing without clinical improvement and without appearance of previously absent normal EEG patterns would not satisfy the secondary criterion.
Adapted from Chong DJ, Hirsch LJ, J Clin Neurophysiol, 2005, 22, 79–91, who modified the criteria of Young et al.13

Table 3. Criteria for Nonconvulsive Seizure (Chong DJ et al.,2005)

4. Which patients are most likely to have nonconvulsive seizures?

In our experience subarachnoid haemorrhage with severe vasospasm shows a higher incidence of epileptiform discharge 24-48 hours before detection of vasospasm Table IV

Study	**Study population**	**EEG type**	**Design**	**N**	**Percentage of patients with any seizures (%)**
Jordan	Neuro ICU patients	cEEG	Retrospective	124	35
De Lorenzo et al.	prior convulsive SE	cEEG	Prospective	164	48
Vespa et al.	moderate to severe traumatic brain injury	cEEG	Prospective	94	22
Vespa et al.	stroke or intracerebral hemorrhage.	cEEG	Retrospective	109	19
Claassen et al.	decreased level of consciousness or suspected subclinical seizures.	cEEG	Retrospective	570	19
Pandian et al.	Neuro ICU patients	cEEG	Retrospective	105	68
Jette	Patients _18 yr old with suspected subclinical seizures.	cEEG	Retrospective	117	44
Claassen et al.	Patients with intracerebral hemorrhage	cEEG	Retrospective	102	31
Oddo et al.	suspected subclinical seizures	cEEG	Retrospective	201	27
Bosco et al.	Subarachnoid hemorrhage with severe vasospasm	cEEG	Retrospective	68	35

Table 4. Studies Using Continuous Electroencephalogram (EEG) Monitoring in Critically Ill Patients for Detection of Nonconvulsive Seizures

5. Cost-effectiveness

Little information is available regarding the cost-effectiveness of cEEG monitoring. In part, this is due to the early stage of development of this technique. This also is related to rapid changes in the technology used to perform cEEG monitoring. Each year provides new capabilities, often at decreased overall cost, making timely assessment of cost-effectiveness difficult. Vespa PM et al.assessed available data from their monitoring experience at UCLA, and concluded that cEEG accounted for only 1% of hospital costs and, during its use, significantly affected critical decision making in >90% of 300 patients who underwent monitoring.They concluded, "cEEG is cost-effective and appears to offer additional quality to intensive care." Claassen et al evaluating their experience in 15 patients undergo cEEG for evaluation of status epilepticus or nonconvulsive seizures associated with altered consciousness,determined that cEEG monitoring influenced clinical management—usually decisively—in 50 of 109 monitoring days. Assessing the cost-effectiveness of cEEG will, however, remain a difficult task. This is because the technology and capabilities continue to evolve rapidly, and because, given the clear diagnostic and therapy-guiding benefits evident to many patients undergoing monitoring, randomization of comatose and obtunded patients to receive or forego such monitoring may not be ethical.

6. Methods (from a personal experience of continuous EEG-SEP monitoring in Neurosurgical Intensive Care of Treviso Hospital Italy 2007-2009)

Quantitative brain function monitor consisted of an EEG-SEP recording system located far from the patient bedside connected by a serial interface to a small amplification head box with 28 channels and a multimodal stimulator (NEMUS-EB Neuro, Italy) FIG 1. The acquired data were transmitted to the PC by means of optical fiber. This software allows the setting of cycles of SEP for each channel obtained to electrical stimulation of the right and left median nerve at the wrist. We used straight stainless steel needle electrodes. Stimulus intensity was set above motor threshold (15-20 mAmp), pulse duration was 0,2 ms; stimulus rate 3Hz. Electrodes were placed at Erb's point (referred to posterior muscle), spinous process Cv7 (referred to anterior neck), P3 and P4 (referred both to Fz). Time base was 100 ms; bandwidth 5 Hz-3KHz. An average of 200 responses were repeated and superimposed. The length of the SEP session was set through a user-defined macro. We used a recording macro of 12 minutes of EP every 50 minutes. EEG was recorded continuously. We recorded a first trace of EP as the template, to which the following traces were compared. We manually located the markers of the principal waves (N20 latency and N20-P25 amplitude), than we started the session. The software automatically recognize N20 and P25 peaks and puts the marker on the maximum negative and positive deflection within a narrow window of ±1msec. Traces are displayed in cascades on one side of the screen, while the trends of SEP latencies and amplitude are displayed on the other side. A horizontal baseline represents latency and amplitude of the template; latency and/or amplitude modifications cause the lines diverge from baseline. Digital EEG is acquired through eight electrodes at the location F3,C3,T3,P3,F4,C4,T4,P4 of the International 10-20 System. These are referred to a reference electrode at midpoint between Fz and Cz. The needles were covered with a plastic transparent dressing. According to Amantini et al SEP of each side were graded on a 3-point scale as normal (N) if cortical complex N20/P25 amplitude and central conduction time (CCT) were normal (1,2 mcV=5° percentile); pathological (P) if CCT was prolonged and /or N20/P25 amplitude was<1,2mcV or the left-right amplitude asymmetry was greater than 50%; absent (A) if cortical responses were absent with preserved N13. Taking into account responses in both hemispheres, 6 patterns were defined: NN, NP, PP, AN, AP and AA. We used an electroencephalographic classification for coma based on Synek modificated system (Synek VM ,1988). According to this, all the recordings were reviewed and classified, by a single expert EEGer in:

IA-Delta/theta>50% reactivity,
IB-Delta/theta>50% without reactivity,
II-Triphasic waves,
IIIA-Burst suppression with epileptiform activity,
IIIB-Burst suppression without epileptiform activity,
IV-Alpha/theta/spindle coma unreactive,
VA-Epileptiform activity Generalized,
VB-Epileptiform activity focal or multifocal,
VIASuppression<20 mcV,but>10mcV,
VIBsuppression< 10mcV.

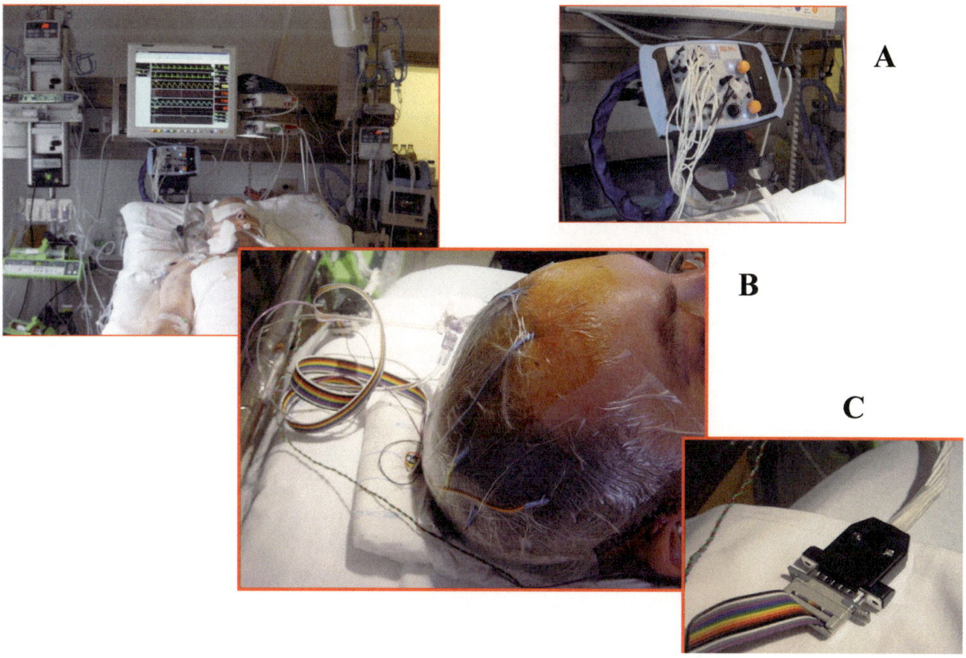

Fig. 1. Example of continuous EEG–SEP monitoring setting in ICU
A-Small amplification head-box with 28 channels and a multimodal stimulator (NEMUS-EB Neuro, Italy)The acquired data are transmitted to the PC by means of an optical fiber.
B-We use straight stainless steel needle electrodes these are gathered in plaits of colored strings.The needles were covered with a plastic transparent dressing
C-Plug-in to deconect the patient

EEG traces were displayed on one side of the screen, and quantitative elettroencephalographic (QEEG) on the other side. QEEG consists of both frequency Color Spectral Density Array (CDSA) and amplitude (percentage of burst-suppression) analysis. The ICP was monitored with a an intraventricular catheter. ICP, CPP, Mean artery pressure (MAP) were stored in a database file. From these informations, the peak ICP level and the time of its occurrence were established for each patient during the monitoring period. In the SAH, Transcranial Doppler (TCD) was used for detecting vasospasm and guiding therapy. TCD monitoring by using bilateral 2 MHz Probes with probe holder were lasted at least 30 minutes per day through temporal windows and eye windows to explore the cerebral arteries flow. Vasospasm was diagnosed in the presence of TCD mean velocities above 120 cm/s (or a daily change in mean transcranial Doppler velocities of >50 cm/s) or angiographic arterial narrowing. Patients were treated with a standard protocol including intravenous muscle relaxants, mechanical ventilation, osmotic diuresis and cerebrospinal fluid (CSF) drainage for elevations in ICP>20-25 mmHg. The respective lengths of EEG and SEP sessions were decided on the basis of clinical features. Monitoring went on until the monitorated parameters were stable and the patient was no more considered at risk of developing brain complications. Acquired data were saved on the recording remote PC used as a server. A follow up telephone interview was conducted at least 3 month after discharge from the hospital. The outcome was assessed using the 5 point Glasgow Outcome Scale (GOS,Jennet and Bond,1975).

7. Statistical analysis

Our interest focused on assessing the degree to which level of SEP and EEG monitoring predicts GOS levels, in particular considering evolutions in time, independently from other concomitant variables. Hence, we fitted a model in which the ratio between probability that GOS shows a certain level and the probability to observe a lower level depends on levels and changes in SEP and EEG by taking into account the joint effect of other related variables. A proportional odds model (e.g. Agresti, 2002) has been fitted to data, by assuming, as reasonable first approximation, that the effect of each variable does not vary with the CGS score at admittance. We also fit a binary logistic model (e.g. Agresti, 2002) to estimate the effect of monitors on the probability of dying (GOS equal to 1). Both families of models, logistic and proportional odds, have been fitted by Maximum Likelihood and the partial effect of each variable has been tested by Likelihood Ratio test.

8. Results

A total of 68 patients (34 males and 34 females, mean age 53.19±14.44 years, range 18-83 years) were monitored with continuous EEG-SEP for an average of 10±4 days and were included in the study. We observed that in all the patients who were clinically stable SEP never showed modification in latency or amplitude. On the contrary, whenever a neurological deterioration occurred with GCS decrease (in 20 patients, 29,4%) SEP always showed significant increase in latency and decrease in amplitude. In these 20 patients the EEG-SEP worsening was not correlated with an immediate increased ICP. In 16 out of 20 patients EEG-SEP worsening appeared 24-48 hours before ICP rising. These patients had developed angiographic vasospasm with ischemic lesion at CT Scan. Moreover, EEG-SEP worsening appeared after ICP increase in 4 patients with brain swelling documented at a serial CT scan. In the first 16 patients, analysis of EEG showed nonconvulsive seizures with periodic discharges and rhythmic delta activity in a range of 48 hours before a documented TCD and angiographyc vasospasm. After EEG epileptiform discharge, SEP showed an instability of amplitude with increments and decrements upper 50% of baseline with a final reduction or dissapereance of cortical SEP (Fig II and Fig III). These patients documented cortical ischemia at a serial CT scan (TableV).

	No of patients	SEP Stable	Decrease SEP BEFORE ICP increase	Decrease SEP AFTER ICP increase	No of Vasospasm	Epileptiform discharge(periodic discharges,rhythmic delta activity,spike-wave or sharp-Wave)	Increase ICP>25mmHg	CTscan Secondary damage
SAH	51 (75%)	35 (68,6%)	16 (31,4%)	0	16 (31,4%)	18 (35,2%)	27 (52,9%)	18 ischemic lesion
ICH	17 (25%)	13 (76,5%)	0	4 (23,5%)	0	6 (40%)	12 (70,5%)	12 mass effect
tot	68 (100%)	48 (70,5%)	16 (23,5%)	4 (5,8%)	18 (26,4%)	24 (35,2%)	39 (57,3%)	30 (48,5%)

Table 5. Temporal analysis of ICP and EEG worsening related to ICP increase, vasospasm and CT scan ischemic evidence.

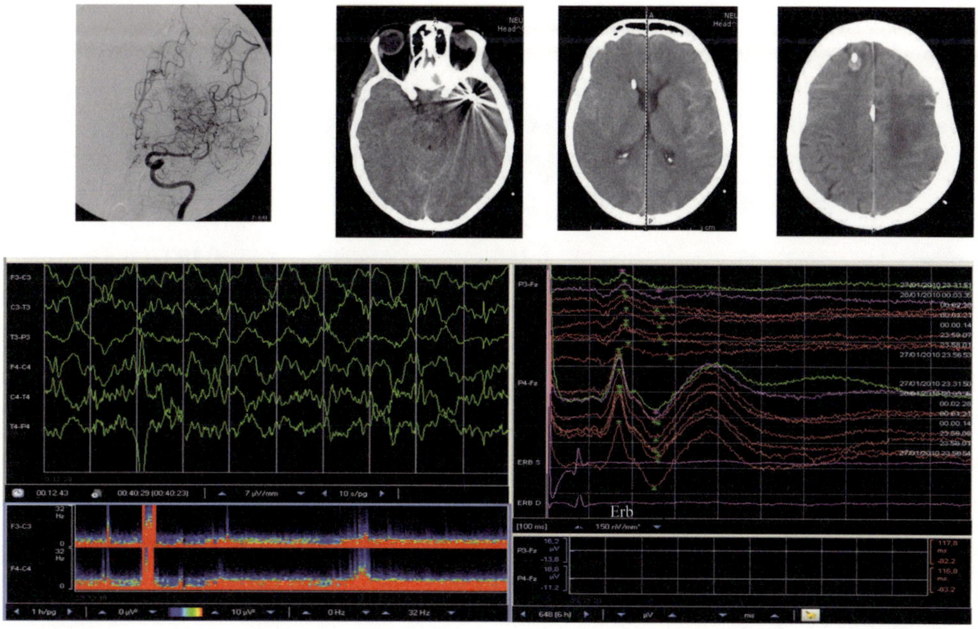

Fig. 2. Multimodality monitoring for vasospasm after subarachnoid hemorrhage (SAH): SEP traces and trend, on right and with raw EEG and CDSA, on left. Angiographic vasospasm with ischemic lesion at CT Scan upper screen

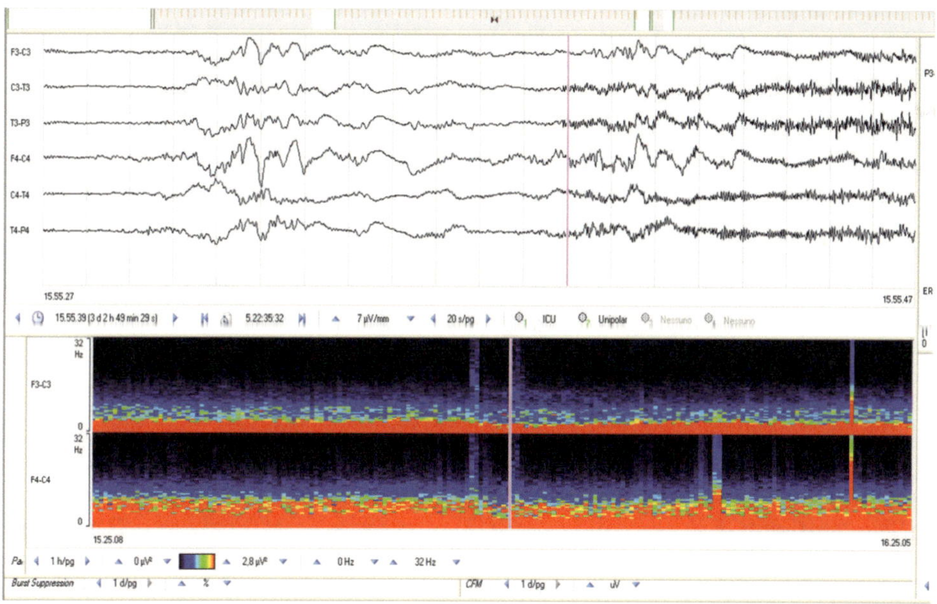

Fig. 3. The EEG segment documents a nonconvulsive seizure discovered during an EEG performed to evaluate a 62-year-old women with subarhanoic hemorrhage Clinical seizure activity was not evident despite the repetitive occurrence of electrographic seizures. Continuous EEG monitoring was initiated to evaluate the effects of therapy.

In the table VI we show the p-values obtained by univariate association tests.

Variable	Association with GOS	Association with mortality
Age	0.637	0.363
Duration	0.253	0.037
Gender	0.488	0.183
CGS-M	< 0.001	< 0.001
EEG initial	0.717	0.205
EEG second	0.747	0.214
EEG final	0.136	0.002
SEP initial	0.001	0.514
SEP second	0.002	0.152
SEP final	< 0.001	< 0.001
EEG from first to second time interval (worsened)	0.766	0.349
EEG from second to third time interval (worsened)	0.012	0.001
EEG from first to third time interval (worsened)	0.005	0.001
SEP from first to second time interval (worsened)	0.227	0.221
SEP from second to third time interval (worsened)	< 0.001	< 0.001
SEP from first to third time interval (worsened)	0.001	< 0.001
Embolization	0.275	0.734
Craniotomy	0.252	1
Cr. Dec	0.407	0.215
ICP	0.007	< 0.001

Table 6. Univariate association measures: p-values

We included in the logistic model all the available variables: age, sex, initial observed EEG and SEP levels, each of the dichotomised decrease of EEG and SEP level, ICP, available treatment and clinical variables during hospitalization, and extent of the observation time (table VII). Regarding ICP in particular, we divided patients accordingly to ICP major values during the monitoring time, and in particular accordingly to ICP values<20mmHg, 20<ICP<40mmHg, and ICP>40mmHg. We selected the variables with a forward stepwise procedure by using the AIC criterion (Claeskens G et al). Note that differences between ICP< 20mmHg and 20<ICP<40mmHg were not significant (p>0,05), so the two classes were collapsed. The overall fit of this model is quite good, since goodness-of-fit of Chi Square statistics is 47.87 on 62 degrees of freedom, giving a p-value of 0.9.

Variable	Coefficient estimate	p-value	Odds
Intercept	-6.1706	0.034	0.002
Age	0.0914	0.040	1.096
ICP >40 mmHg	6.5074	0.006	670.1
Duration (days)	-0.5866	0.020	0.556
EEG, from first to third time observation (worsened)	3.1839	0.028	24.14
SEP, from first to third time observation (worsened)	3.4769	0.005	32.36

Table 7. Summary of the final logistic model for the probability of GOS 1

Considering the obtained estimates, when the EEG gets worse during the time of observation, the odds for dying increase of about 24% with respect to similar patients that did not get worse. SEP decrease is also significant: patients with worsening SEP show an odds-of-dying increase of about 32%. Moreover, the longer the duration of hospitalization, the lower the risk of dying. Each day of hospitalization decreases the odds of dying of about 50%.

To assess whether the inclusion of EEG and SEP variations in the model improves prediction, we compared ROC curves of four models: the final model including both EEG and SEP variations, the two models obtained by removing either EEG or SEP variations, respectively, and the model fitted removing both EEG and SEP variations.

The joint contribution of both variables was significant (p-value for comparisons between ROC curves is 0.046) even if each variable alone does not seem to be significant (p-value=0.21 for eliminating from the final model EEG variation and p-value=0.15for eliminating SEP variation).

Table VIII illustrates the coefficients and the p-values for the proportional odds model. As for the logistic model, we selected the most significant variables via a forward stepwise procedure considering the AIC index. Since very few patients showed GOS levels 2 and 5, we aggregated them to levels 3 and 4 respectively. Therefore, we obtained a three-level GOS.

Variable	Coefficient estimated	p-value	exp(coefficient)
Intercept 1|2	-1.799	<0.001	0.16
Intercept 2|3	2.156	0.015	8.63
CGS-M - worsened	-4.453	<0.001	0.01
CGS-M - improved	2.660	0.004	14.29
SEP, from first to second time observation (worsened)	-2.807	0.002	0.06

Table 8. Summary of the proportional odds model.

Also this model has a good fit to data: Chi-square goodness-of-fit statistic is 85.86 on 131 degrees of freedom, giving a p-value of almost 1. Here, only modifications of GCS-M and SEP during hospitalization are significant to predict the GOS level. Patients showing worsening SEP during the last time interval are less likely (1/20) to have a high GOS level than patients with stable SEP. Patients with a GCS-M getting worse during the entire observational period have a probability of a high GOS level of 1%, if compared to patients with stable GCS-M. Moreover, an improved GCS-M increases the probability of a high GOS level of about 14 times (Table VII).

We also tested a model excluding the GCS-M modifications in time. However, it did not fit as well, showing the importance of GCS-M changes during hospitalization. It is interesting to observe that the initial SEP level and its changes during hospitalization, the changes of EEG in the last period of observation, and the presence of ICP higher than 40 mmHg are significant variables when GCS-M is not considered, similarly to what we obtain with the logistic model.

It is worth noting that demographic variables, like age and sex, are not significant in any of the models used to predict the GOS level. They were not significant even when considered alone (Table V). The treatments effect is not significant neither in association with the other variables, nor when considered alone (Table V).

9. Discussion

Continuous EEG-SEP is a relatively new, non-invasive, bedside monitoring tool that allows a functional measurement of neurological impairment. There are two main advantages of clinical neurophysiology with respect to clinical examination:it can be employed in sedated and/or curarized patients, and it provides quantitative data for comparison with follow up studies. Compressed presentations like cerebral function monitor (CFM) or CDSA may help visualize these long term changes that are due to variations in the level of sedation. These tools, should be carefully used with the collaboration of a competent neurophysiologist. It should be kept in mind that,like any other clinical or technical examination,clinical neurophysiology only evaluates the current functional brain status, so that any prognostic information needs to be updated in case of eventual complication. Moreover, SEP trend is based on two simple parameters, amplitude and latency. Amplitude decrease and latency increase are dependent on the physiopathology of brain damage. Amplitude is related to the number of fibers carrying the signal to the primary somatosensory cortex. In the central nervous system, latency is mainly associated to white matter swelling. In the peripheral nervous system, it is related to temperature and focal myelin dysfunctions. There is good evidence that serial evoked potential studies provide useful information about the functional recovery of impaired areas [Amantini A et al.2008, Moulton RJ et al. 1998]. This is particularly true during the early post-injury stage, as SEP are a sensitive measure of secondary damage. Our results clearly show that SEP frequently change over time. The SEP-EEG deterioration is probably related to many different pathogenetic mechanisms: In the case of ischemia following vasospasm, SEP modifications precede 24-48 hours ICP increasing (18 patients), in the case of brain oedema without hypoxic damage SEP modifications cames later (2 patients) The most likely explanation for this temporal sequence of events is that uncontrollable ICP may simply be a sign of large volumes of non-viable brain in fatally injured patients [Moulton RJ et al 1998]. A continuous SEP monitoring has a strong prognostic power, because amplitude modifications usually precede clinical manifestation of functional integrity. As continuous SEP monitoring reveal the potential for recovery, it can sometimes direct the physician towards a more aggressive clinical management. SEP provide important information about patients who are pharmacologically paralyzed and sedated to help ventilation and ICP management. In this setting, we have frequently relied on SEP measurement to direct the therapy. We discourage aggressive treatment (barbiturate coma, decompressive craniectomy) to control refractory ICP in patients who lost cortical SEP activity. Other investigators have also observed the absence of correlation between increased ICP and SEP deterioration. Focal injury results in primary damage to neurons and to the surrounding cerebral vessels. The secondary damage is due to ischemia and the cytotoxic cascade. Cytotoxic and vasogenic oedema in neurons leads to excitotoxic swelling. The SEP deterioration can have different timing, and it can occur before or after an ICP increase. Trends for ICP did not demonstrate a clear seizure-related effect on ICP or CPP in the hours directly before or during a seizure. The ICP always increased after vasospasm. Vasospasm is a primary source of neurologic co-morbidity after SAH. Trans-cranial Doppler ultrasounds (TCD) and cerebral angiography cannot be continuously performed; in contrast, EEG can constantly monitor the cerebral activity. In our series, the most sensitive QEEG monitoring parameter to detect seizures was CDSA. Seizures are often associated with transient increases in EEG power, although they have to be confirmed with the review of the raw EEG. Similarly, QEEG should never be interpreted without reviewing portions of the original waveforms. Most epileptiform activity occurred in the form of repetitive sharp waves. This activity shows a clear related predictive effect on vasospasm 24-48 hours in advance. QEEG data can be displayed with many methods [Jordan KG et al.1995, Rennie CJ et al 2002, Vespa PM et al. 1999]. CDSA depicts ictal and interictal data after a quantitative transformation of raw EEG data (Figure IV).

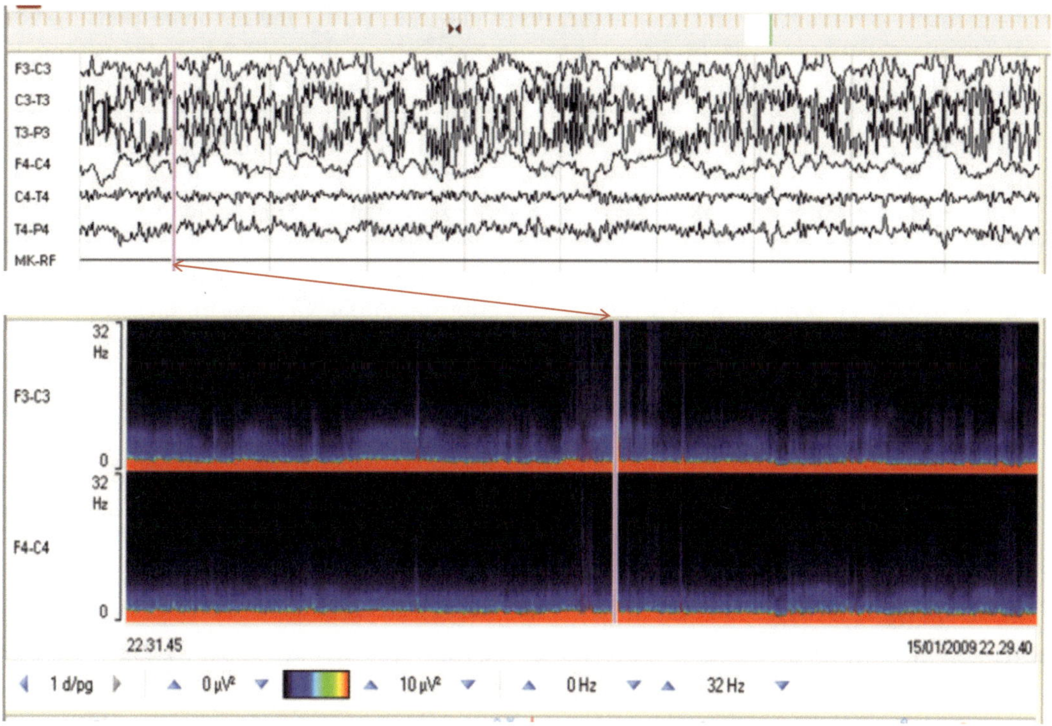

Fig. 4. The spectrogram shows high frequency activity : non convulsive status epilepticus

Time is displayed on the x-axis. The upper graph is a colour spectrogram showing averaged root EEG power from 0 to 32 Hz (y-axis), created from consecutive 10-second EEG epochs (each composed of five 2-second windows) obtained from F3-C3, F4-C4. The patient's repetitive seizures are now clear in the spectrogram as vertical bands of increased power. These graphs usually express power amplitude as a colour scale. Amplitude-integrated EEG graph can also provide a reasonable indication of the presence of suppression-burst activity. The somatosensory evoked potentials have not only a strong predictive power on outcome. They provide a feedback tool to modify and correct the treatment, according to the correlated neurological instability. If SEP are stable, the patient is neurologically stable even though ICP and CPP values are not in the normal range. Moreover, SEP can be pathological despite normal ICP and CPP values: in this case it is necessary to find the best ICP and CPP settings to re-establish "normal" evoked potentials values.

10. Conclusions

Our approach is based on the choice of an integrated EEG-SEP continuous monitoring,the respective parts of each test are individually evaluated,according to which one is likely to be more informative in these patients. SEP were always monitorable despite the frequent use of high level of neurosedation. As SEP monitoring shows high correlation with patient's outcome, it defines a measurable level of initial damage basing on the template SEP baseline, and on measurable parameters like amplitude and latency. The temporal variation of these two parameters, evaluated with the continuous monitoring, can confirm whether the treatment is tailored to the neurological changes induced by the lesion responsible for the secondary damage. The findings from our experience show that SEP worsening is independently associated with a poor outcome in patients with coma after intracranial hemorrhage. It is measured by specific parameters that quantify the damage and it replaces the clinical data that are often not quantifiable due both to the patient sedation and to the subjective evaluation performed by the physician. The precocious SEP deterioration can detect neurological impairment earlier than other hemodynamic variables like ICP and CPP, allowing the improving of the treatment. However it is not always possible to block the pathophysiological process, despite its early identification. In patients with SAH, the early changes in SEP amplitude allow a timely detection of initial vasospasm. QEEG changes preceded clinical evidence of vasospasm. cEEG use has documented a surprisingly high incidence of nonconvulsive seizures and nonconvulsive status epilepticus in patients with acute cerebral ischemia and intracranial hemorrhages. The combined use of SEP and continuous EEG monitoring is a unique example of dynamic-brain-monitoring.

11. References

Agresti A: *Categorical Data Analysis*, 2nd Edition. Wiley; 2002.

Amantini A, Amadori A, Fossi S: Evoked potentials in the ICU. *Eur J Anaesthesiol Suppl* 2008, 42:196-202.

Amantini A, Grippo A, Fossi S, Cesaretti C, Piccioli A, Peris A, Ragazzoni A, Pinto F: Prediction of "awakening" and outcome in prolonged acute coma from severe traumatic brain injury: evidence for validity of short latency SEP. Clin Neurophysiol 2005, 116:229-235.

Bosco E, Marton E, Feletti A, Scarpa B, Longatti P, Zanatta P, Giorgi E, Sorbara C. Dynamic monitors of brain function: a new target in neurointensive care unit.Crit Care. 2011 Jul 15;15(4):R170.

Bullock R, Zauner A, Myseros JS, Marmarou A, Woodward JJ, Young HF: Evidence for prolonged release of excitatory amino acids in severe human head trauma. Relationship to clinical events. Ann N Y Acad Sci 1995, 765:290-297.

Chong DJ, Hirsch LJ. Which EEG patterns warrant treatment in the critically ill? Reviewing the evidence for treatment of periodic epileptiform discharges and related patterns. J Clin Neurophysiol 2005;22:79–91

Claassen J, Jette N, Chum F, Green R, Schmidt M, Choi H,Jirsch J, Frontera JA, Connolly ES, Emerson RG, Mayer SA,Hirsch LJ. Electrographic seizures and periodic discharges after intracerebral hemorrhage. Neurology 2007;69:1356–65.

Claassen J, Mayer SA, Kowalski RG, Emerson RG, Hirsch LJ.Detection of electrographic seizures with continuous EEG monitoring in critically ill patients. Neurology 2004;62:1743–8

Claeskens G, Hjort NL: *Model selection and model averaging.* Cambridge University Press; 2008.

DeLong, Elizabeth R., DeLong, David M., Clarke-Pearson Daniel L. (1988) Comparing the Areas under Two or More Correlated Receiver Operating Characteristic Curves: A Nonparametric Approach. Biometrics, Vol. 44, pp.837-845

DeLorenzo RJ, Waterhouse EJ, Towne AR, Boggs JG, Ko D,DeLorenzo GA, Brown A, Garnett L. Persistent nonconvulsive status epilepticus after the control of convulsive status epilepticus. Epilepsia 1998;39:833–40

Friedman D, ClassenJ, Hirsh LJ. Continuous electroencephalogram monitoring in the intensive care unit. Anesth Analg 2009;109:506-523

Grände PO, Asgeirsson B, Nordström CH. Volume-targeted therapy of increased intracranial pressure: the Lund concept unifies surgical and non-surgical treatments.Acta Anaesthesiol Scand. 2002 Sep;46(8):929-41. Review

Greenberg RP, Mayer DJ, Becker DP, Miller JD: Evaluation of brain function in severe human head trauma with multimodality evoked potentials, methods and analysis. *J Neurosurg* 1977, 47:150-162.

Jennett B, Bond M: Assessment of outcome after severe brain damage. *Lancet* 1975, 7905:480-484.

Jette N, Claassen J, Emerson RG, Hirsch LJ. Frequency and predictors of nonconvulsive seizures during continuous electroencephalographic monitoring in critically ill children. Arch Neurol 2006;63:1750–5

Jordan KG: Neurophysiologic monitoring in the neuroscience intensive care unit. *Neurol Clin* 1995, 13:579-626.

Miller JD, Piper IR, Jones PA: Integrated multimodality monitoring in the neurosurgical intensive care unit. Neurosurg Clin N Am 1994, 5:661-670.

Moulton RJ, Brown JI, Konasiewicz SJ: Monitoring severe head injury: a comparison of EEG and somatosensory evoked potentials. *Can J Neurol Sci* 1998, 25:S7-S11.

Oddo M, Carrera E, Classen J, Mayer SA, Hirsch LJ. Continuous electroencephalography in the medical intensive care unit. Crit Care Med 2009;37:2051-2056

Pandian JD, Cascino GD, So EL, Manno E, Fulgham JR. Digital videoelectroencephalographic monitoring in the neurologicalneurosurgical intensive care unit: clinical features and outcome. Arch Neurol 2004;61:1090–4

Rennie CJ, Robinson PA, Wright JJ: Unified neurophysical model of EEG spectra and evoked potentials. *Biol Cybern* 2002, 86:457-471.

Rose J, Valtonen S, Jennett B: Avoidable factors contributing to death after head injury. Br Med J 1977, 2:615-618.

Rosner MJ, Coley IB. J Cerebral perfusion pressure, intracranial pressure, and head elevation Neurosurg. 1986 Nov;65(5):636-41.

Synek VM: Prognostically important EEG coma pattern in diffuse anoxic and traumatic encephalopathies in adults. J Clin Neurophysiol 1988, 5:161-174.

Vespa PM, McArthur D, O'Phelan K, Glenn T, Etchepare M, Kelly D, Bergsneider M, Martin NA, Hovda DA: Persistently low extracellular glucose correlates with poor outcome 6 months after human traumatic brain injury despite a lack of increased lactate: a microdialysis study. J Cereb Blood Flow Metab 2003, 23:865-877.

Vespa PM, Nenov V, Nuwer MR: Continuous EEG monitoring in the intensive care unit: early findings and clinical efficacy. *J Clin Neurophysiol* 1999, 16:1-13.

Young GB, Lachlan MC, Kreeft JH and Demelo JD.An Electroencephalographic Classification for Coma. Can.J.Neurol.Sci.1997;24:320-32

12

Carotid Endarterectomy

Mustafa Karaçelik
Izmir Tepecik Research and Training Hospital, Turkey

1. Introduction

Carotid endarterctomy (CEA) is still remain a good therapeutic modality for carotid artery disase in some medical centers if these centers do not have any endovascular surgical options. CEA may reduce the risk of possible neurological deficits, but has some surgical complications. Benefit in patients with stroke and to decline progressively in patients with cerebral TIA and retinal events in both the 50% to 69% and 70% to 99% stenosis groups, and also showed a trend towards greater benefit in patients with irregular plaque than a smooth plaque in both stenosis groups.This chapter summarises the CEA as a surgical therapy and its components.

2. Indications

In patients with 70% to 90% diameter reduction of an ipsilateral internal carotid artery measured on a conventional biplane angiogram, ipsilateral to either focal hemispheric symptoms (transient ischemic attack [TIA] or small stroke) or amaurosis fugax, surgically treated by CEA(1)

There have been five randomised controlled trials of endarterectomy in patients with a recent symptomatic carotid stenosis. CEA is of some benefit for 50% to 69% symptomatic stenosis and highly beneficial for 70% to 99% stenosis without near occlusion.(**Fig.1**) Benefit from endarterectomy depends not only on the degree of carotid stenosis, but also on several other factors, including the delay to surgery after the presenting event(2). For 70% stenosis (excluding near occlusion) absolute risk reduction (ARR) of 16% over 5 years (number needed to treat 6.3); 50% to 69% stenosis ARR of 4.6% over 5 years (number needed to treat_22); near occlusion, ARR of 5.6% over 2 years (p= 0.19) but 1.7% over 5 years (p=0.9); and CEA is not appropriate for symptomatic patients with 49% stenosis(13).

3. Diagnosis

Carotid angiogram is still "gold standard" for measuring the degree of carotid stenosis. Nowadays, *computed tomography angiography* (CTA) is more common used to visualize carotid arteries. Doppler ultrasonography is a helpful another noninvasive method, but it is not enough for desicion making of operation.

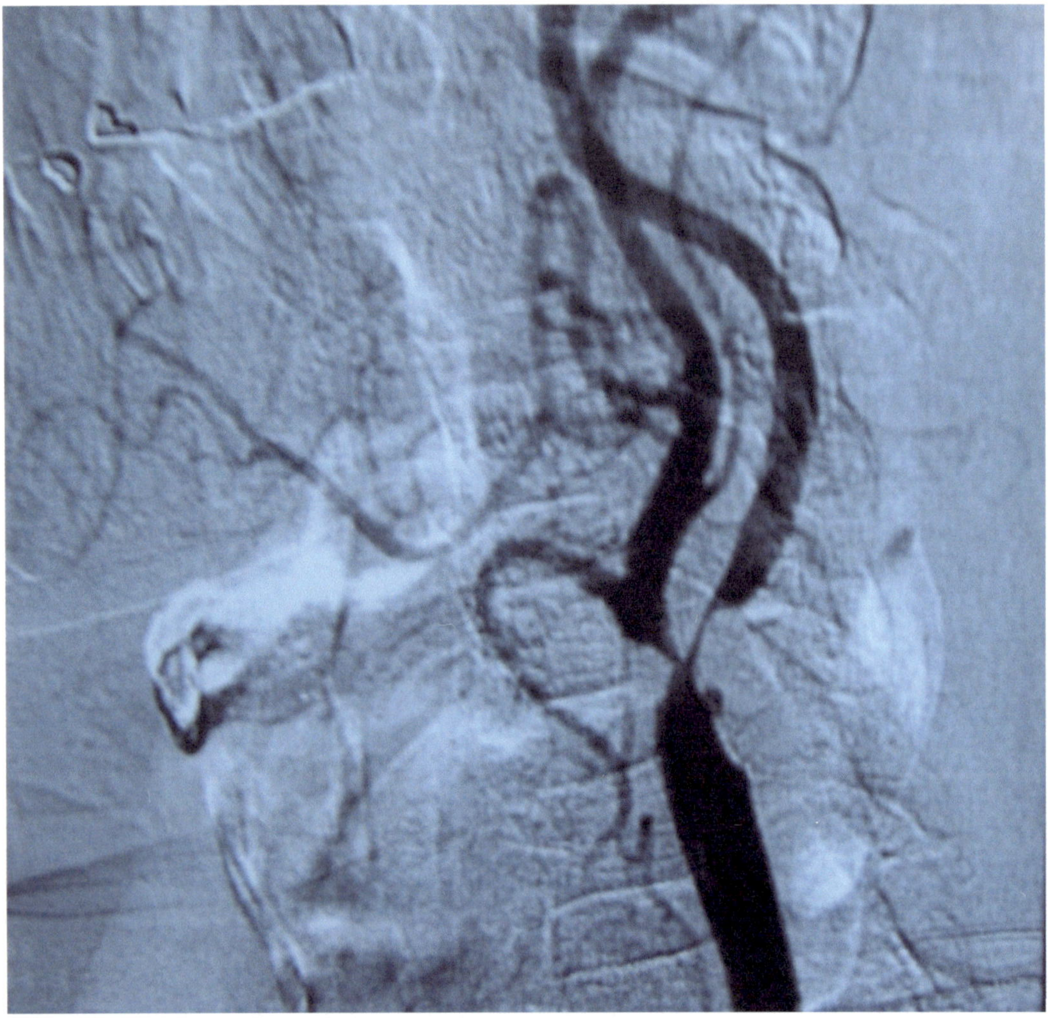

Fig. 1. Digital substraction Angiography of the carotid arteries

4. Techniques for Carotid Endarterectomy

4.1 The choice of anaesthetic

CEA may be performed under local or general anaesthesia. Meta-analysis of the randomised studies showed that there was no evidence of a reduction in the odds of operative stroke or death (odds ratio (OR) 0.85, 95% confidence interval (CI) 0.63 to 1.16). Patients and surgeons can choose either anaesthetic technique, depending on the clinical situation and their own preferences. Local anaesthesia reduces need for intraoperative shunting and as a result a reduction in hospital stay occurs(3)(**Fig.2**).

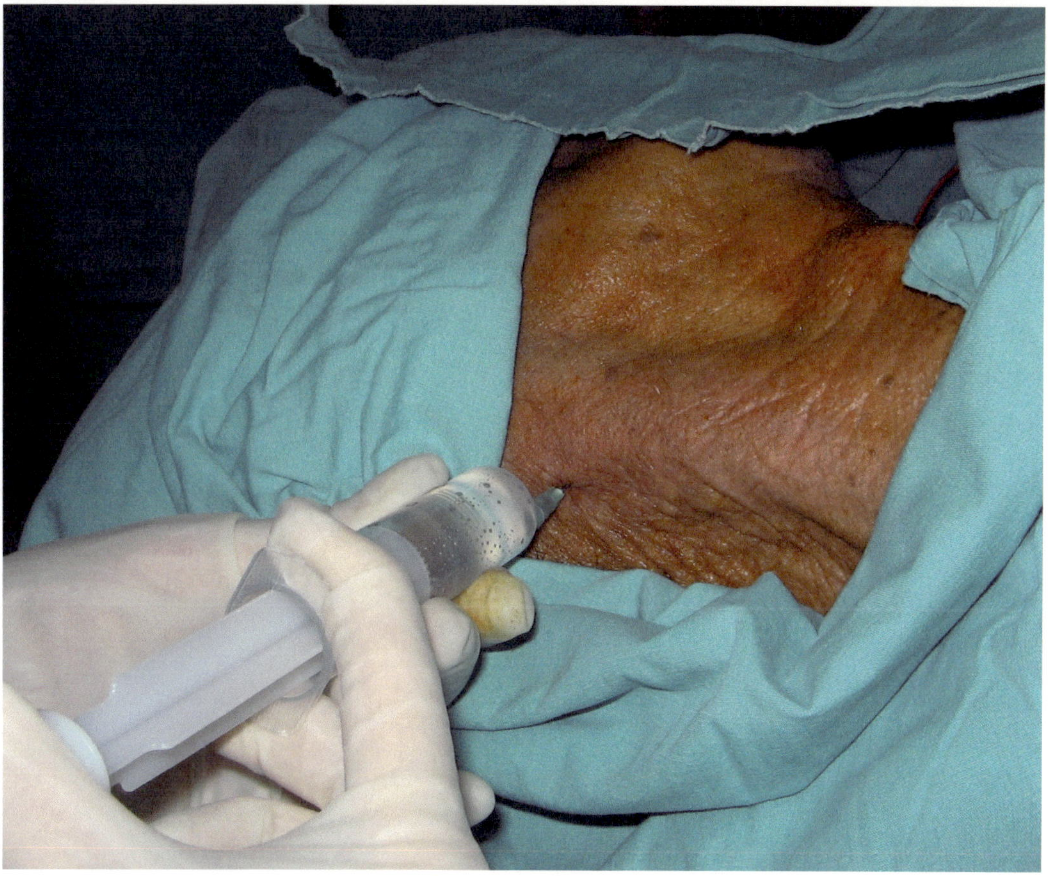

Fig. 2. Local anaesthesia application

4.2 Patch or no patch?

Choosing the method of closure of arteriotomy depends on diameter of the internal carotid artery(ICA). Small diameter (less than 5mm) of ICA should be closed by a native or nonnative tissue patch. The main issue regarding patch angioplasty is patching increases clamp time and infection risk. **Rerkasem** mentioned that a significant reduction in perioperative and long-term risks of ipsilateral stroke and of perioperative carotid occlusion and later restenosis associated with the use of patching. A policy of selective patching of only those arteries thought to require a patch at the time of operation compared with no patching has not been tested in randomized, controlled trials. These reseachers support a policy of routine patching, but most included trials were small and some had methodological shortcomings(4).There is no evidence that patch type influences stroke rate, mortality or arterial restenosis in any way at all(5).There is some evidence that other synthetic (e.g. PTFE) patches may be superior to collagen impregnated Dacron grafts in terms of perioperative stroke rates and restenosis. Pseudoaneurysm formation may be more common after use of a vein patch compared with a synthetic patch(6).

4.3 Shunt desicion

The main aim of shunting is to reduce the risk of perioperative stroke but it could possibly be associated with an increased risk of restenosis and late recurrent stroke.The data on the use of routine shunting from randomised controlled trials were limited. There were promising but non-significant trends favouring a reduction in both deaths and strokes within 30 days of surgery with routine shunting. The data available were too limited to either support or refute the use of routine or selective shunting in carotid endarterectomy. It was suggested that large scale randomised trials between routine shunting versus selective shunting were required. No one method of monitoring in selective shunting has been shown to produce better outcomes(7).The most recent trial used stump pressure measurement and patients with stump pressure < 50 mmHg required shunting(8).

4.4 Surgical technique

Following intravenous heparinisation (5000units), vascular clamps are applied to the ICA, CCA and ECA respectively. A longitudinal arteriotomy is made from the CCA across the plaque and into the ICA beyond the stenosis. A shunt can be deployed at this stage if it is necessary.**(Fig.3)**

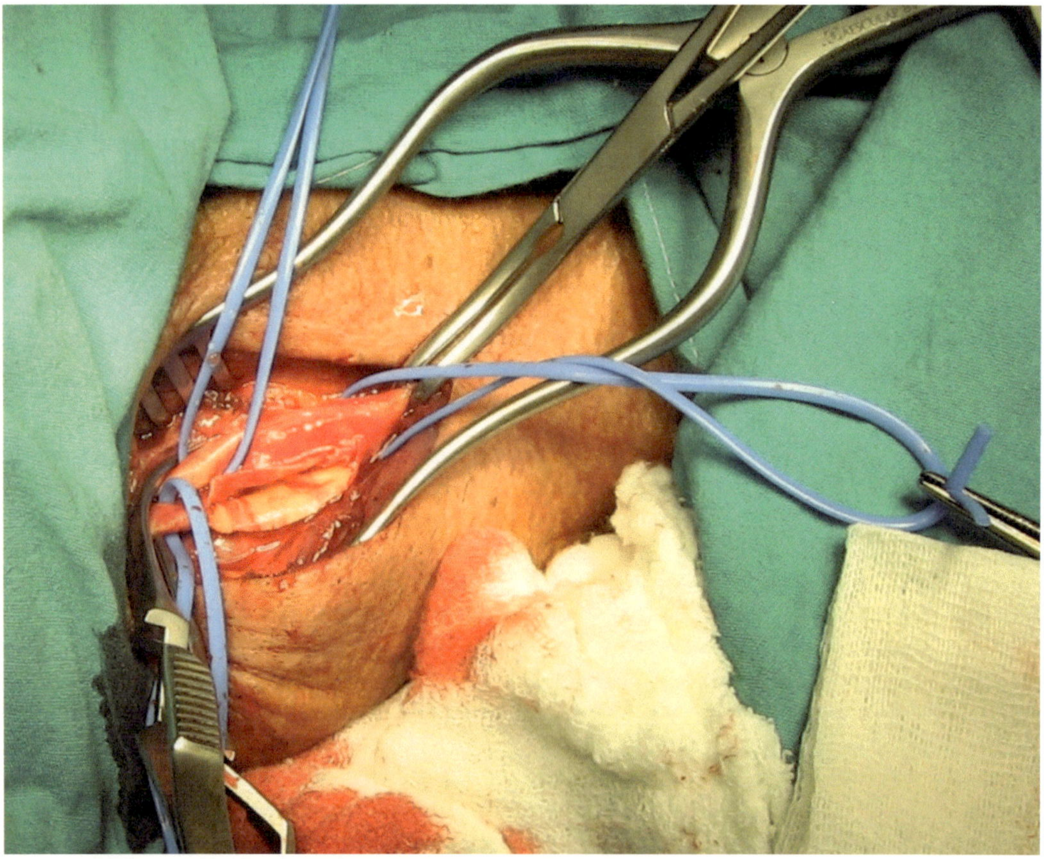

Fig. 3. Carotid endarterectomy

The endarterectomy plane is entered using a dissector or clamp and it is conventional to divide the plaque first at the CCA aspect and then carefully mobilise it free up into the ICA where it is cut transversly using micro scissors to avoid leaving a flap. Sometimes an additional 7,0 prolene sutures could be needed to restore without a flap in the vessel wall(5). The "eversion" endarterectomy is an alternative technique. The origin of the ICA is transected and re-implanted after eversion endarterectomy of the ICA and conventional endarterectomy of the CCA and ECA(8).In ACST-1 3000 patients were randomised between medical treatment only or medical treatment and immediate surgery. CEA involved a small (~3%) but definite peri-procedural risk of stroke or death, a substantial (~3%vs ~12%) reduction in the subsequent stroke rate over the next 5 years and hence a net reduction (~6% vs~12%) in the overall 5-year risk of stroke or peri-procedural death. The 5-year findings of ACST-1 are already changing surgical practice, and long-term follow-up of stroke rates continues(9,10). Avoidance of patch-closure techniques particularly in thin arteries is an important advantage of carotid endarterectomy with anterior transverse arteriotomy(11).

4.5 Difficult anatomy, make a desicion for CEA or CAS?

Schneider and **Kasirajan** mentioned that anatomy influences decision-making in carotid disease management(12). Patients who have comorbidities, but complicated arterial anatomy, are best candidates for CEA.(**Fig.4**) Patients with a hostile neck are best suited to CAS. Patients with neck immobility, skin cancer at incision site, previous radical neck dissection, or a tracheostomy, can be treated with CAS. **Arya** et al. emphasized that CAS 30 day stroke and death/stroke rates are statistically significantly higher compared to CEA; however this superiority did not reach statistical significance when RPCTs were analyzed alone and those results did not justify the widespread use of CAS for treatment of suitable carotid bifurcation disease(13).

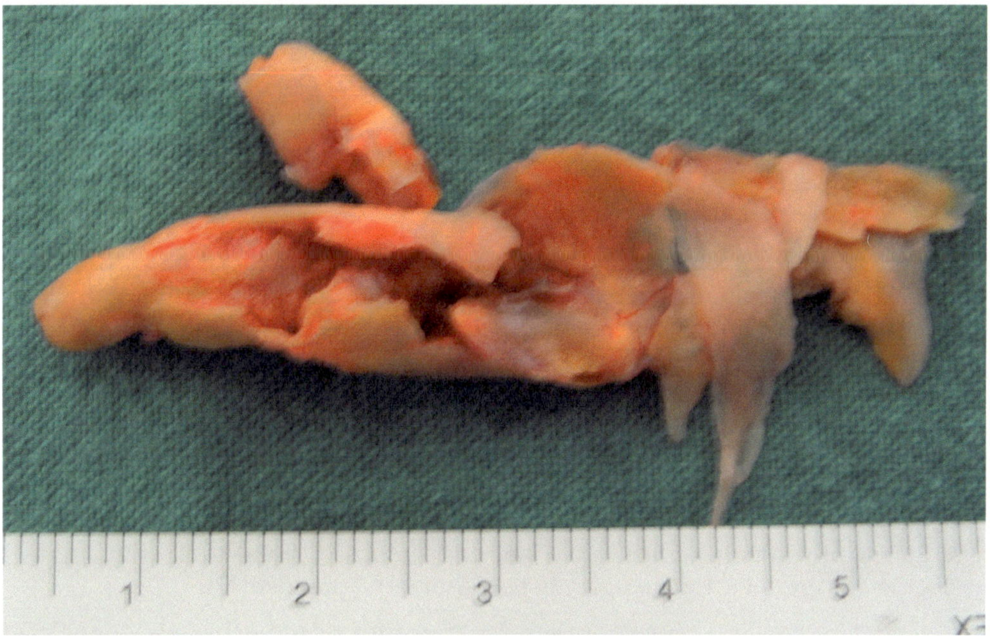

Fig. 4. An atherom plaque excised from carotid artery bifurcation

5. General complications of Carotid Endarterctomy

As with all CEA's, acute coronary syndrome(ACS) is the main problem during and after CEA. In addition, even clinically "silent" myocardial injury detected by enzyme (troponin) leak has a negative effect on both perioperative and long-term survival. Postoperative hypertension is an another major matter after CEA and affects 66% of patients. This phenomenon triggers the ACS easily and resolve spontaously 48-72 hours postoperatively. The annual risk of MI or nonstroke vascular death after an ischemic stroke or TIA is 2%. A prospective study by **Kawahito** et al using Holter monitoring to detect myocardial ischemia identified a history of angina (p= 0.001) and hypertension (p=0.020) as being independently associated with perioperative myocardial ischemia in patients having CEA(14).

5.1 Neurological complications of Carotid Endarterctomy

Neurological complications may be aline as follows; mild deficits: visual disturbances, dysphagia, monoparesis, moderate deficits: severe deficits: hemiplegia. High-risk group for neurological complications are diffuse atherosclerotic disease and by the presense of a previous neurologic deficit. However, reoperation carries higher perioperative stroke and cranial nevre injury rates than primary CEA. Major causes of postoperative ischemia are perioperative thrombosis and embolism, and most strokes were within 24 hours of the procedure, whereas 3% after 24 hours of the operation. Manupulation of the carotid arteries causing stroke by embolization is avoided by prior mobilization of its branches. The risk of postoperative stroke can be determined by postoperative Transcranial Doppler measurement. In a study of Abbott et al., the risk of postoperative neurological deficit was 15 times higher in patients with clinically significant microembolism detected by TCD recording(15).

Other cause of postoperative ischemia is intracerebral hemorrhagic stroke which is resulted from a hyperperfusion syndrome is a rare complication after CEA with range of 0.2–0.75% and it is a fatal outcome. A strategy to prevent intracerebral hemorrhagic stroke consists in close blood pressure monitoring and control and reasonable handling of anticoagulant and antiplatelet agents. For example; Dextran 70 and 40 have been used to prevent thrombosis by decreasing platelet adhesiveness. If there is a large amount of using this product this may cause bleeding from operation side(16).

Postoperative evaluation of neuroligical outcome may be explained in a study Nouraei et al. following CEA, the distribution of saccades initiated by the cerebral hemisphere distal to the operated artery significantly changed in 25 patients. By contrast, there were 14 significant contralateral-hemisphere saccadic changes ($P<.001$) significantly greater postoperative reduction was detected in early saccades generated by the ipsilateral hemisphere than by the contralateral hemisphere ($P<.02$) CEA leads to significant hemisphere-specific subclinical changes in saccadic performance and, in particular, differentially affects the proportion of early saccades, a measure of the ability of the frontal cortex to successfully inhibit lower centers, generated by the 2 hemispheres. Saccadometry, a bedside test, provides data that can be statistically compared for individual and groups of patients. It could allow the neurological outcome of carotid surgery to be objectively quantified(17).

Navin et al. 12 randomized controlled trials (RCT) enrolling 6,973 patients were included in a meta-analysis. Carotid artery stenting was associated with a significantly greater odds of periprocedural stroke (OR 1.72, 95% CI 1.20 to 2.47) and a significantly lower odds of periprocedural myocardial infarction (OR 0.47, 95% CI 0.29 to 0.78) and cranial neuropathy (OR 0.08, 95% CI, 0.04 to 0.16). The odds of periprocedural death (OR 1.11, 95% CI 0.56 to 2.18), target vessel restenosis (OR 1.95, 95% CI 0.63 to 6.06), and access-related hematoma were similar following either intervention (OR 0.60, 95% CI 0.30 to 1.21). In comparison with CEA, CAS was associated with a greater odds of stroke and a lower odds of myocardial infarction. While the results in this meta-analysis support the continued use of CEA as the standard of care in the treatment of carotid artery stenosis, CAS is a viable alternative in patients at elevated risk of cardiac complications(18).

Chronic tissue damage may occur in a subset of individuals with 70% ICA stenosis, globally exhibiting more extensive WMH. Overall, the median volumetric magnetic resonance (WMH) volume was greater in the hemisphere ipsilateral to the stenotic ICA (1.13±2.65 vs. 0.77±2.26 cm^3; p=0.005), but there were no differences in hemispheric brain volumes between the stenotic and nonstenotic sides. In the subgroup of patients with moderate and severe WMH (n=41), the hemispheric volume ipsilateral to the stenotic ICA was significantly smaller (543.46±22.17 vs. 548.66±26.7 cm^3; p=0.03). Multivariate linear regression analysis revealed an independent effect of WMH grade on interhemispheric volume differences relative to the side of stenosis. (19).

Goldberg et al. evaluated the mechanisms of neurologic injury, the measurement of neurobehavioral outcomes, and use of neuroimaging to evaluate carotid revascularization outcomes. They found that neurologic injury after carotid revascularization results from three broad etiologies: atheroembolic, thrombotic, and hypo/hyperperfusion. Of the 47 studies examining the effect of carotid endarterectomy on neurobehavioral functioning, 25 found that some aspect of cognition improved, 12 revealed no change in cognition, and 10 revealed declines in some aspect of cognition. There is a wide variation in the measurement of neurologic outcomes in clinical registries and trials. Future efforts to correlate neuroimaging with cognitive outcomes may offer insight into methods to decrease neurologic injury after carotid revascularization. (20)

Chronic progressive tissue damage as another possible consequence of high-grade ICA stenosis, which can be detected using MRI volumetric methods for assessing volumetric magnetic resonance (WMH) lesion load and hemispheric brain volume differences to clarify if the morphologic changes observed are associated with neuropsychological deficits, and to investigate their relationship with regional cerebral perfusion measurements preferentially in a longitudinal manner(21)

Cerebral hyperperfusion after carotid endarterectomy (CEA) impairs cognitive function and is often detected on cerebral blood flow (CBF) imaging. In this study 158 patients with ipsilateral internal carotid artery stenosis (> or = 70%) underwent CEA. Neuropsychological testing was performed preoperatively and at the 1st postoperative month. Cerebral blood flow was measured using single-photon emission computed tomography before, immediately after, and 3 days after surgery. Magnetic resonance imaging was performed before and 1 day after surgery. The incidence of postoperative cognitive impairment was significantly higher in patients with post-CEA hyperperfusion on CBF imaging (12 [75%] of 16 patients) than in those without (6 [4%] of 142 patients; p<0.0001). Postoperative cognitive impairment developed in all 5 patients with cerebral hyperperfusion syndrome regardless of the presence or absence of new lesions on MR images. Although cerebral hyperperfusion syndrome after CEA sometimes results in reversible brain edema visible on MR imaging, postoperative cerebral hyperperfusion often results in impaired cognitive function without structural brain damage on MR imaging(22).

Two groups (A and B) of 15 patients each, with internal carotid backpressure >30 mmHg were operated and they did not use a shunt in Group A during CEA and group B was operated upon with a shunt. They measured gradual increase of levels of IL-1b and TXB2 during cross-clamping and during reperfusion in group A ($P<0.05$). The levels of TNFa increased only during reperfusion ($P<0.05$). The concentration of IL-1b and TNFa remained almost stable in group B, whereas the concentration of TXB2 reduced but not significantly ($P>0.05$). The levels of PGE2 remained stable in both groups. The increase of proinflammatory mediators during carotid cross-clamping when no shunt is used. The critical concentration of these mediators that threaten the brain's vitality is not yet detected. However, the clinical significance of this is unclear, since there were no perioperative strokes(23).

Reperfusion injury is a dangerous cituation in the critical care unit and free radicals and lytics toxicity may play a role as well. Patients with critical stenosis with maximally dilated blood vessels at baseline (optimized cerebrovascular reserve) are also at risk for hyperperfusion injury. Presentation may include headache, seizure, status epilepticus, cerebral edema, ICH, or subarachnoid hemorrhage. There was no benefit from surgery in the near-occlusion group in ECST where the rate of endarterectomy in the medical group was lower than in NASCET. Prevention with tight blood pressure control during the periprocedural period is as critical as management of the injury itself (24).

A case series of Pappada et al. of 413 CEAs in 390 patients who suffered from the new onset of an ischaemic hemispheric deficit or the worsening of a pre-existing deficit within 72 h after surgery were included in this study. A major stroke after CEA is caused, in most of cases, by the acute ICA occlusion with or without intracerebral embolic occlusion. Reopening of the occluded ICA gives good results when intracerebral vessels are patent and when the occluded ICA is satisfactorily reopened(25).

Diffusion-weighted imaging (DWI) has indicated that CAS is associated with a significantly higher burden of microemboli. This prospective study analyzed the neuropsychologic outcomes after revascularization in 24 CAS and 31 CEA patients with severe carotid stenosis compared with a control group of 27 healthy individuals. The cognitive performance was similar between CEA and CAS patients at all points. The new brain lesions, as detected with DWI after CAS or CEA, do not affect cognitive performance in a manner that is long-lasting or clinically relevant. Despite the higher embolic load detected by DWI, CAS is not associated with a greater cognitive decline than CEA(26).

The North American Symptomatic Carotid Endarterectomy trial(NASCET), enrolled 2885 symptomatic patients had carotid stenosis were categorized as follows: 1) low, moderate stenosis (<50%), 2) moderate stenosis (50-69%), and 3) severe stenosis (70-99%). Patients were assigned to either CEA and best medical management or best medical management alone. Primary stenting for the treatment of post-CEA stroke is encouraging clinical result may be also explained by the fact that the interval between onset of neurological symptoms and stent implantation(27).

6. References

[1] Haimovici H. (1996)Haimovici's Vascular Surgery Principles and Techniques, Blackwell Science, USA
[2] Rerkasem K, Rothwell PM. Carotid endarterectomy for symptomatic carotid stenosis. *Cochrane Database of Systematic Reviews* 2011, Issue 4.
[3] Rerkasem K, Rothwell PM. Local versus general anaesthesia for carotid endarterectomy. *Cochrane Database of SystematicReviews* 2008, Issue 4.
[4] Rerkasem K, Rothwell P.M. Systematic Review of Randomized Controlled Trials of Patch Angioplasty Versus Primary Closure During Carotid Endarterectomy *Stroke* 2010;41;e55-e56
[5] Beard J.D, Gaines P.A.(1998) Vascular and Endovascular Surgery, W.B. Saunders Company Ltd, UK
[6] Rerkasem K, Rothwell PM. Patches of different types for carotid patch angioplasty. *Cochrane Database of Systematic Reviews* 2010, Issue 3.
[7] Rerkasem K, Rothwell PM. Routine or selective carotid artery shunting for carotid endarterectomy (and different methods of monitoring in selective shunting). *Cochrane Database of Systematic Reviews* 2009, Issue 4.
[8] Palombo D, Lucertini G, Mambrini S, Zettin M. Subtle cerebral damage after shunting vs non shunting during carotid endarterectomy. *European Journal of Vascular and Endovascular Surgery* 2007;34:546–51.
[9] Kasprzak P, Raithel D. Eversion carotid endarterectomy: technique and early results. J Cardiovasc Surg 1989, 30: 49.
[10] Halliday A. The Asymptomatic Carotid Surgery Trial has changed clinical practice. Pages 56-60 in: Vascular and Endovascular Controversies. Biba Publishing, 2006.
[11] Çinar B, Göksel O, Aydogan H, Filizcan U, Çetemen S, Eren E. Early and mid-term results of carotid endarterectomy with anterior transverse arteriotomy. Türk Gögüs Kalp Damar Cer Derg 2005;13(3):255-259
[12] Schneider PA, Kasirajan K. Difficult Anatomy: What Characteristics Are Critical to Good Outcomes of Either CEA or CAS? Semin Vasc Surg 2007, 20:216-225
[13] Arya S, Garg N, Johanning JM, Longo GM, Lynch TG, Pipinos II. Carotid Endarterectomy and Stentıng: A Meta-analysis of Current Literature.j.jss.2007,12, 610
[14] Ritesh Maharaj. A Review of Recent Developments in the Management of Carotid Artery Stenosis. Journal of Cardiothoracic and Vascular Anesthesia, Vol 22, No 2 (April), 2008: pp 277-289
[15] Abbott AL, Levi CR, Stork JL, Donnan GA, Chambers BR Timing of clinically significant microembolism after carotid endarterectomy. Cerebrovasc Dis 2007; 23: 362–367.
[16] Wilson PV, Ammar AD: The incidence of ischemic stroke versus intracerebral hemorrhage after carotid endarterectomy: a review of 2,452 cases. Ann Vasc Surg 2005; 19: 1–4.
[17] Nouraei SA, Roos, J; Walsh SR, Ober, JK, Gaunt, ME; Carpenter, RH. Objective Assessment of the Hemisphere-Specific Neurological Outcome of Carotid Endarterectomy: A Quantitative Saccadometric Analysis. Neurosurgery 2010: 67;6, 1534-1541

[18] Yavin D, Roberts DJ, Tso M, Sutherland GR, Eliasziw M, Wong JH. Carotid Endarterectomy Versus Stenting: A Meta-Analysis of Randomized Trials. The Canadian Journal of Neurological Sciences 2011; 38, 2; 230 - 235
[19] Enzinger C, Ropele S, Gattringer T, Langkammer C, Schmidt R, Fazekas F. High-grade internal carotid artery stenosis and chronic brain damage: a volumetric magnetic resonance imaging study. Cerebrovasc Dis. 2010;30(6):540-6.
[20] Goldberg JB, Goodney PP, Kumbhani SR, Roth SM, Powell RJ, Likosky DS. Brain Injury After Carotid Revascularization: Outcomes, Mechanisms, and Opportunities for Improvement. Annals of Vascular Surgery Volume 2011, 25, 2, 270-286
[21] Enzinger C, Ropele S, Gattringer T. High-Grade Internal Carotid Artery Stenosis and Chronic Brain Damage: A Volumetric Magnetic Resonance Imaging Study. Cerebrovasc 544 is 2010;30:540–546
[22] Hirooka R, Ogasawara K, Sasaki M, Yamadate K, Kobayashi M, Suga Y, Yoshida K, Otawara Y, Inoue T, Ogawa A. Magnetic resonance imaging in patients with cerebral hyperperfusion and cognitive impairment after carotid endarterectomy. J Neurosurg. 2008 Jun;108(6):1178-83.
[23] Tachtsi M, Pitoulias G, Kostoglou C, Papadimitriou D. The proinflammatory mediator's production from ischemic brain during carotid endarterectomy. Int Angiol. 2011 Oct;30(5):429-33.
[24] Badruddin A, Taqi MA, Abraham MG, Dani D, Zaidat OO. Neurocritical Care of a Reperfused Brain. Curr Neurol Neurosci Rep (2011) 11:104–110
[25] Pappadà G, Vergani F, Parolin M, Cesana C, Pirillo D, Pirovano M, Santoro P, Landi A, Ferrarese C.Early acute hemispheric stroke after carotid endarterectomy. Pathogenesis and management. Acta Neurochir (Wien). 2010;152(4):579-87.
[26] Wasser K, Pilgram-Pastor SM, Schnaudigel S, Stojanovic T, Schmidt H, Knauf J, Gröschel K, Knauth M, Hildebrandt H, Kastrup A. New brain lesions after carotid revascularization are not associated with cognitive performance. Journal of Vascular Surgery 2011, 53, 1, 61-70.
[27] Anzuini A, Briguori C,Roubin GS, Rosanio S, Airoldi F, Carlino M, Pagnotta P,Mario CD, Sheiban I, Magnani G, Jannello A, Melissano G, Chiesa R, Colombo A. Emergency Stenting to Treat Neurological Complications Occurring After Carotid Endarterectomy. J Am Coll Cardiol 2001;37:2074 –9